Manipal
Textbook of
Biochemistry
for Dental Students

Second Edition

Manipal

Textbook of Biochemistry
for Dental Students

Second Edition

CBS Publishers

Manipal
Textbook of
Biochemistry
for Dental Students

Second Edition

Shivananda Nayak B MSc, PhD, FAGE, NRCC-CC (USA), FACB (USA), FABM

Visiting Professor of Biochemistry
Subbaiah Institute of Medical Sciences,
Shimoga, India

Professor of Biochemistry
Department of Preclinical Sciences
Faculty of Medical Sciences
The University of the West Indies
Trinidad and Tobago, West Indies

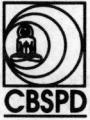

CBS Publishers & Distributors Pvt Ltd

New Delhi • Bengaluru • Chennai • Kochi • Kolkata • Lucknow • Mumbai
Hyderabad • Jharkhand • Nagpur • Patna • Pune • Uttarakhand

Manipal
**Textbook of
Biochemistry**
for Dental Students

ISBN: 978-81-239-2504-2

Second Edition: 2015
Reprint: 2016, 2024
First Edition: 2007

Published by **Satish Kumar Jain** and produced by **Varun Jain** for

CBS Publishers & Distributors Pvt Ltd
4819/XI Prahlad Street, 24 Ansari Road, Daryaganj, New Delhi 110 002, India.
Ph: 011-23289259, 23266861   Website: www.cbspd.com
                                    e-mail: delhi@cbspd.com

Corporate Office: 204 FIE, Industrial Area, Patparganj, Delhi 110 092
Ph: 011-4934 4934   Fax: 011-4934 4935 e-mail: publishing@cbspd.com;
                                               publicity@cbspd.com

Branches

- **Bengaluru:** Seema House 2975, 17th Cross, K.R. Road, Banasankari 2nd Stage, Bengaluru 560 070, Karnataka, India
  Ph: +91-80-26771678/79   Fax: +91-80-26771680   e-mail: bangalore@cbspd.com
- **Chennai:** 7, Subbaraya Street, Shenoy Nagar, Chennai 600 030, Tamil Nadu, India
  Ph: +91-44-26680620, 26681266   Fax: +91-44-42032115   e-mail: chennai@cbspd.com
- **Kochi:** 42/1325, 1326, Power House Road, Opp KSEB, Ernakulam 682 018, Kochi, Kerala, India
  Ph: +91-484-4059061-67   Fax: +91-484-4059065   e-mail: kochi@cbspd.com
- **Kolkata:** 147, Hind Ceramics Compound, 1st Floor, Nilgunj Road, Belghoria, Kolkata 700 056, West Bengal, India
  Ph: +91-33-25633055/56   e-mail: kolkata@cbspd.com
- **Lucknow:** Basement, Khushnuma Complex, 7-Meerabai Marg (Behind Jawahar Bhawan), Lucknow 226 001, UP, India
  Ph: +0552-4000032   e-mail:tiwari.lucknowi@cbspd.com
- **Mumbai:** PWD Shed. Gala no. 25/26, Ramchandra Bhatt Marg, Next to JJ Hospital Gate no. 2, Opp. Union Bank of India, Noorbaug, Mumbai 400 009, Maharashtra, India
  Ph: 022-66661880/89   e-mail: mumbai@cbspd.com

Representatives

• **Hyderabad**	0-9885175004	• **Jharkhand**	0-9811541605	• **Nagpur**	0-8692091830
• **Patna**	0-9334159340	• **Pune**	0-9664372571	• **Uttarakhand**	0-9716462459

Printed at: Glorious Printers, Dilshad Garden, Delhi

to
my parents
and
family

Foreword to the Second Edition

I am extremely happy to write a Foreword to the second edition of *Manipal Textbook of Biochemistry for Dental Students* authored by Professor Shivananda Nayak. In my Foreword to the first edition, I had emphasized the need for a concise book of biochemistry for dental students. Professor Shivananda Nayak fulfilled this need very convincingly in the first edition. The first edition has been received extremely well by students and the faculty members, as a result of which the book is seeing its second edition. I congratulate Professor Shivananda Nayak for his dedication and commitment in addressing the educational needs of dental students. With his extensive experience in teaching in India and the West Indies, Professor Shivananda is fully aware of the demands of dental students studying biochemistry. He has revised this book thoroughly and produced a student-friendly edition. I am certain that the students of dentistry and other health professions will find this book highly useful.

S R Prabhu BDS, MDS, FDS RCS (Edin), FFD RCSI (Oral Med), FDSRCPS (Glasg), FDS RCS (Eng), MO Med RCS (Ed), MFGDP RCS (UK), FICD
School of Dentistry, Charles Sturt University School of Dentistry and Health Sciences, Orange NSW, Australia and Visiting Adjunct Professor, Manipal University, Manipal, India

Foreword to the First Edition

Dental students are expected to have a basic understanding of the range of chemical changes that occur in the human body. This knowledge is of paramount importance in understanding the status of health and disease of those who come in contact during their training and later in their professional practice.

It is a well-known fact that the available books on Biochemistry are too exhaustive. Generally, with a heavy workload, students of dental sciences often find it difficult to cope with the information provided in these voluminous books. A need for a book that provides relevant information in a concise manner, therefore, becomes real. *Manipal Textbook of Biochemistry for Dental Students* written by Dr. Shivananda Nayak is a timely addition to the dental and literature.

Topics discussed in this book are highly relevant to the dental professions. These conform to the curricular requirements of the Dental Council of India and other dental institutions in India. Chapters are concise, well written, and the contents are easy to understand. Information provided is also examination-oriented, hence students of dentistry would find the book very useful to prepare for their examinations. Although this book is targeted primarily at the undergraduate dental students, medical students and those pursuing postgraduate courses in dentistry would also find the contents useful for quick revision.

Dr. Shivananda Nayak, with his extensive teaching and research experience is to be congratulated for his excellent authoring task. I am absolutely sure that the students of dentistry would find this book highly useful.

S R Prabhu BDS, MDS, FDS RCS (Edin), FFD RCSI (Oral Med), FDSRCPS (Glasg), FDS RCS (Eng), MO Med RCS (Ed), MFGDP RCS (UK), FICD

School of Dentistry, Charles Sturt University School of Dentistry and Health Sciences, Orange NSW, Australia and Visiting Adjunct Professor, Manipal University, Manipal, India

Message

The publication of this textbook is a welcome addition to the corpus of knowledge available to undergraduates in dentistry for the study of Biochemistry. Since an understanding of the principles of Biochemistry is basic to the syllabus for medical sciences and allied health sciences, it is a most timely teaching and learning tool that undoubtedly meets an important need.

It is generally agreed that successful undergraduate teaching and learning depend upon a considerable extent of well-written and straightforward texts. This is particularly important in dentistry disciplines that are the critical component in the comprehensive approach to healthcare, since the graduates of those disciplines are tasked with an important responsibility in providing healthcare across all levels of society.

Dr. Nayak's work, as a member of the teaching staff of the Faculty of Medical Sciences, The University of the West Indies, is well known, particularly his ability to impart to his students on the most relevant and significant knowledge in the field of Biochemistry. He is following in the tradition set by his peers by being cognizant of the importance of disseminating his knowledge and research to the wider public and taking concrete steps to do so. Such dissemination is enriched by the lessons obtained from the teaching and learning processes, and from the constant and lively debates that take place between students and lecturers, leading to a product that meets the needs of students as well as lay people who are seeking information.

It is a great pleasure for me to congratulate Dr. Nayak for recognizing the need to produce a student-friendly textbook that addresses the requirements of undergraduates for knowledge in these fields that are an integral component of the curriculum of the Faculty of Medical Sciences.

Bhoendradatt Tewarie
Minister of Planning and Sustainable
Development, Republic of Trinidad and Tobago

Preface to the Second Edition

I have great pleasure in presenting this second edition of the *Manipal Textbook of Biochemistry for Dental Students*. The previous edition of this title has been popular among the dental and other students and it has been recommended by various dental colleges as a reference book. The overwhelming response from the student community and support from the teachers of various institutions has encouraged me to bring out this second edition. The simple, concise, diagram-based explanation and self-assessment question formats have been maintained in this revised edition. The suggestions and criticisms of teachers and the students to my first edition have been used as a basis of revision. I tried best to incorporate new contents which are essential for both dental and allied health students. We attempted to incorporate diagram-based explanation, self-assessment questions and additional multiple choice questions in each chapter.

The salient features of the revised edition are as follows:
- Content of the handbook is divided into 20 chapters
- Two new chapters have been included on:
  - Organ function tests
  - Practical experiments
- A number of new illustrations and figures have been included to facilitate understanding of the contents easily.

I take this opportunity to thank all those who warmly received my first edition of *Manipal Handbook of Biochemistry*. I am always grateful to Professor Samuel Ramsewak (Dean, Faculty of Medical Sciences, The University of the West Indies), it is my pleasure to thank Prof S R Prabhu (Deputy Dean, School of Dentistry). I would like to thank Dr Geetha Bhaktha for contributing practical experiments and helped during editing process of this title. Last but not the least, I thank each and everyone who encouraged me to bring this title in a right time.

A textbook will be improved only by successive revisions. I will try to revise this book in every two years. The comments, suggestions and constructive criticisms from the faculty, students and other readers are always welcome. Please feel free to communicate at my e-mail address as: shiv25@gmail.com, if you have any suggestions. The success of the book was due to the active participation of the publishers. This is to record my appreciation for the support extended by V K Jain, Chairman, Mr Y N Arjuna and his associates of CBS Publishers & Distributors, New Delhi, India for readily conceding my request to publish this second edition in two colors and taking all pains to bring this edition to my utmost satisfaction.

Shivananda Nayak B

Preface to the First Edition

I am glad to present the *Manipal Textbook of Biochemistry for Dental Students*. There are ample of textbooks, which deal with the theoretical aspects of Biochemistry in a simple way. My experience of more than 15 years in teaching Biochemistry to dental and medical students in India as well as abroad enabled me to write this title in a simple way that can be easily understood by the students. I tried my level best to incorporate diagram-based explanation wherever necessary, that may help the readers. Also, I made an attempt to present SELF TEST at the end of each chapter. The suggestions and support from both the teacher and student community inspired me to bring this title with interesting diagrams.

I take this opportunity to thank all those who warmly received my other title *Manipal Manual of Clinical Biochemistry*. I am always grateful to Dr Sudhakar Nayak (Head, Department of Biochemistry) and Dr Shivaraj (Professor of Biochemistry) for their excellent support throughout my service. I am indebted to Dr Bhoendradatt Tewarie (Principal and Pro-Vice-Chancellor, The University of the West Indies) for writing message to this title. It is my pleasure to thank Prof Prabhu for support. Last but not the least, I thank each and everyone who encouraged me to bring this title in the right time.

A textbook will be improved only by successive revisions. I will try to revise this book in every two years. The comments, suggestions and constructive criticism from the faculty, students and other readers are always welcome. Please feel free to communicate at my e-mail address as: shiv25@gmail.com, if you have any suggestions. The success of the book was due to the active participation of the publishers. This is to record my appreciation for the support extended by Mr YN Arjuna, Publishing Director, and his associates of CBS Publishers & Distributors, New Delhi, India, for readily conceding my request to publish this book in color and taking all pains to bring this title to my utmost satisfaction.

Shivananda Nayak B

Contents

8. Lipid Chemistry   98

9. Metabolism of Lipids   111

10. Integration of Metabolism   128

11. Hemoglobin Synthesis   133

1

The Cell

Cells are the structural and functional units of all living organisms. Man is a multicellular organism, contains at least 10^{14} cells. These cells differ considerably in shape, structure and function as a result of specialization. An aggregation of cells those are similar in origin, structure and function forms tissue. Most of the metabolic activities occur at cellular level. Hence, it is essential, first to understand the basic organization of cell and functions of its components.

A typical cell, as seen by the light microscope is illustrated in Figure 1.1. It contains two compartments, inner nucleus and outer cytoplasm. Nucleus contains nucleoplasm suspended with genetic material. Nuclear envelope separates nucleus from cytoplasm. Cytoplasm composed of aqueous cytosol, suspended with particles and membrane bound organelles. Externally cytoplasm is limited by plasma membrane.

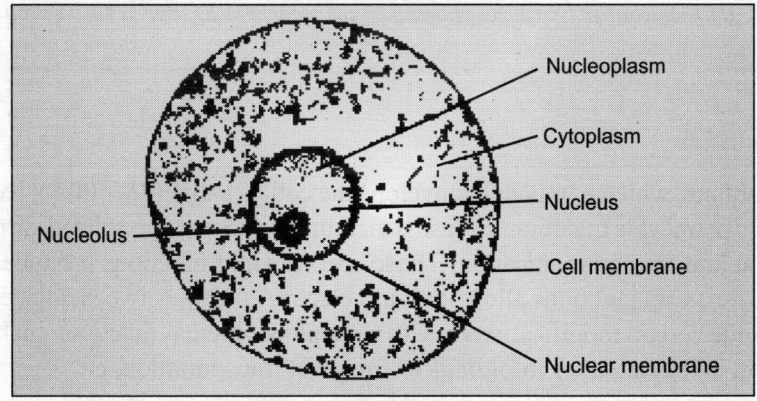

Figure 1.1: *Structure of the cell as seen with light microscope*

Ultra structure

Normal cell ranges between 10 and 30 μm in diameter. Figure 1.2 shows the ultra structure or finer details of typical cell, which has been revealed by the electron microscope.

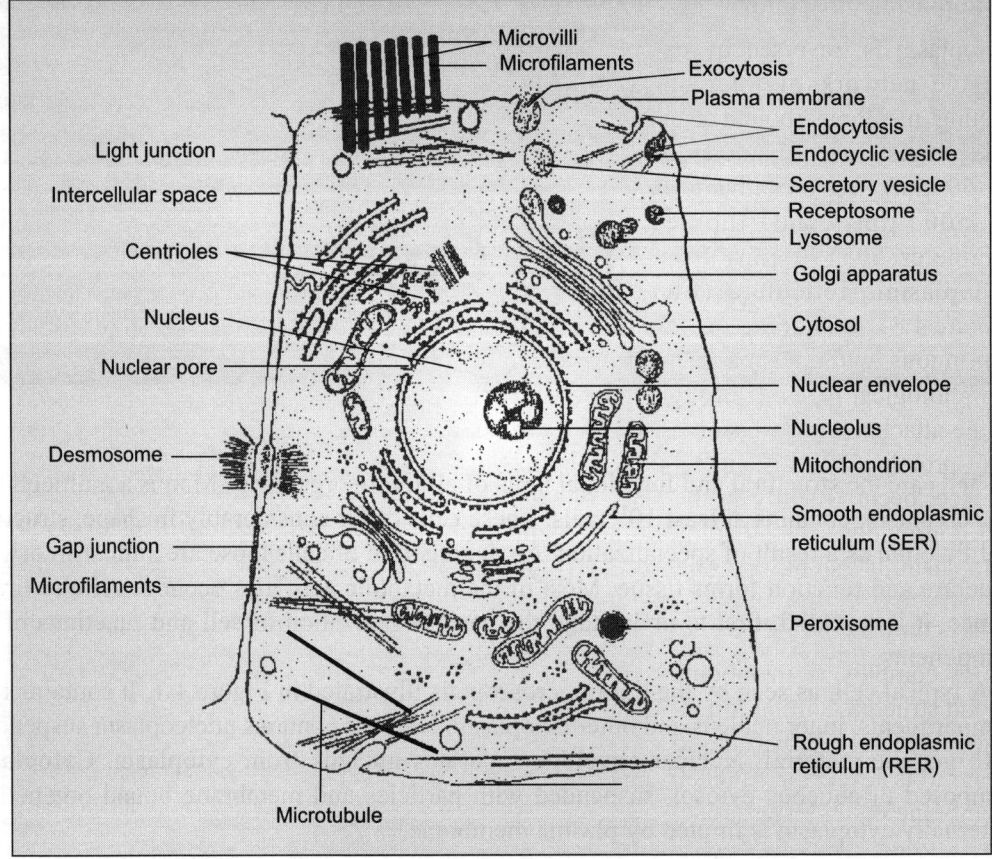

Figure 1.2: *Ultra structure of typical cell showing all cell organelles as seen in the electron microscope*

Plasma membrane

The cell membrane, which completely envelops the cell, is a thin (75–100Å), living, dynamic and selectively permeable membrane. Plasma membrane consists specialized surface structures for attachment and for communication. Those are: (i) Tight junctions produce seal between adjacent cells. (ii) Gap junctions allow ions and electric current between adjacent cells. They may also include certain modifications to carry out physiological functions such as microvilli for absorption, invagination or infoldings to carry out transportation, etc.

All biological membranes including the plasma membrane and internal membranes which form the sub-cellular structures such as endoplasmic reticulum, mitochondria, lysosomes, nuclear envelope, peroxisomes, Golgi complex, etc. are similar in structure, lipoprotein in nature, consists lipids (60–40%), proteins (40–60%) and carbohydrates (1–10%). The membranes separate the cell from external environment and separates different parts of the cell from one another so that cellular activities are compartmentalized.

Endoplasmic reticulum

Cytoplasm is traversed by extensive network of interconnecting membrane-bound channels or cisternae (diameter of 40–50 μm), vesicles (diameter 25–500 μm) and tubules (diameter 50–190 μm) form endoplasmic reticulum (ER) (Figure 1.3). Membranes of ER

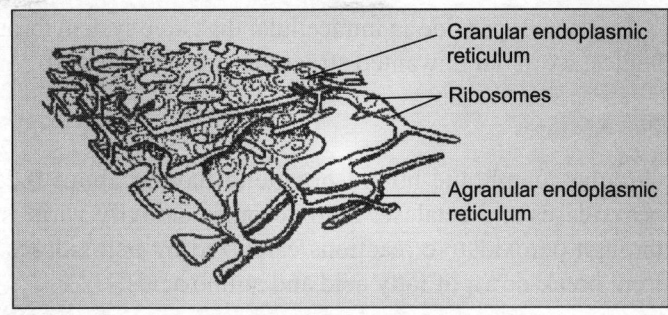

Figure 1.3: *Endoplasmic reticulum*

continuous with plasma membrane and outer nuclear envelope. There are two basic morphological types: (i) Rough endoplasmic reticulum (RER) possesses rough surface due to the attachment of ribosomes. RER occurs mainly in the form of cisternae and concerned with protein synthesis. (ii) Smooth endoplasmic reticulum (SER) lacks ribosomes on their surface, occurs mainly in the form of tubules. SER is concerned with lipid synthesis.

ER provides skeletal framework to cells and gives mechanical support to the colloidal cytoplasm. It also plays a role in detoxifying the xenobiotics.

Golgi complex

Golgi complex is membrane bound structure similar to ER, discovered in 1873 by Camillo Golgi. It is a stack of flattened membrane vesicles (cisternae) surrounded by networking of tubules of 300–500Å diameter. Cisternae gently curved, convex part *cis* side faces ER and concave part *trans* side locates near plasma membrane (Figure 1.4).

Golgi complex functions in association with ER, is a center

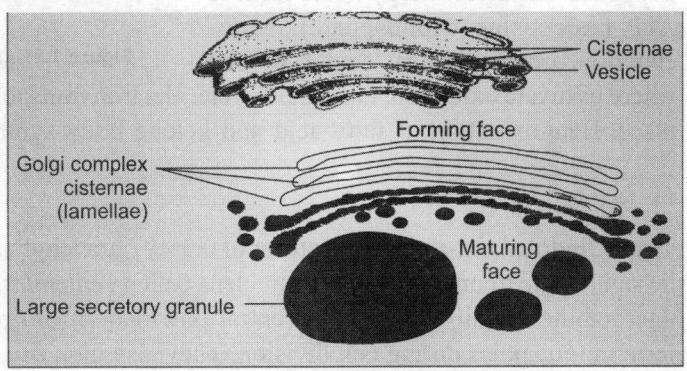

Figure 1.4: *Golgi apparatus*

of reception, finishing, packaging and transportation of variety of materials. Proteins synthesized in ER added with sulfate, carbohydrates, lipid moieties, etc. and dispatched in the form of secretory vesicles. Golgi complex also gives rise to lipoprotein of plasma membrane and lysosomes.

Lysosomes

Lysosomes are packets of hydrolases. These are spherical with 1 μm in diameter surrounded by tough carbohydrate-rich lipoprotein membrane enclosing about 50 types hydrolases such as proteases, lipases, carbohydrases, nucleases, transferases, sulfatases, etc.

Lysosomes provide an intracellular digestive system through which macromolecules, foreign bodies, worn out unwanted structures are got digested.

Peroxisomes

Circular membrane-bound organelle having about 0.25 µm diameter contain enzymes peroxidases and catalase. Peroxiosomes detoxify various toxic substances and metabolites through peroxidative reactions catalyzed by peroxidases. Catalase degrades H_2O_2 resulted from break-down of fatty acid and amino acids.

Mitochondria

They are spherical, oval or rod like bodies, about 0.5–1 µm in diameter and up to 7 µm in length. DNA (Deoxyribonucleic acid) molecules, which encode information for certain mitochondrial proteins (Figure 1.5).

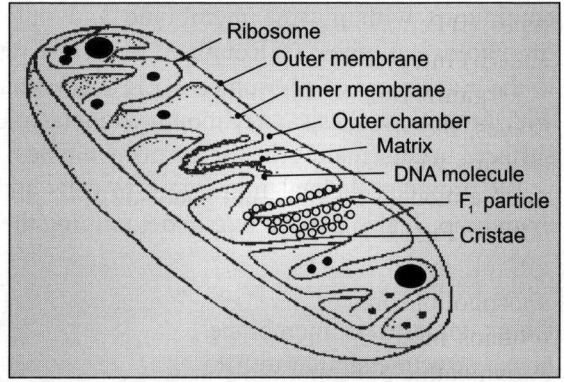

Figure 1.5: *Longitudinal section of mitochondrion*

Mitochondria are considered to be the powerhouse of the cell, where energy released from oxidation of foodstuffs is trapped as chemical energy in the form of ATP (Adenosine triphosphate). Mitochondria are respiratory center of cell where pyruvate oxidation, citric acid cycle, electron transport chain and ATP generation takes place. Beta-oxidation of fatty acid and ketone body synthesis also taking place.

Centrioles

Two cylindrical rod-shaped structures of 0.3–0.7 µm length and 0.1–0.25 µm diameter, which lie right angle to one another near nucleus called *centrioles*. Centriole is an array of 9-triplet microtubules equally spaced from central axis, made up of structural protein tubulin. Centrioles form mitotic poles during cell division. They also give rise to cilia and tail of sperm.

Nucleus

Cell center, prominent spherical structure where genetic material is confined. All cells in the human body contain nucleus, except matured RBCs and upper dead skin cells. Generally, nucleus is spherical or oval in shape and of 3–25 µm in diameter. But squamous epithelial cells contain discoidal and multilobed in polymorphonuclear leucocytes. Nuclear envelope, which encircles the nucleus, consists of outer and inner nuclear membranes, typical lipoprotein membranes. Outer nuclear membranes continuous with membranes of ER and found attached with ribosomes on its outer surface. Nuclear envelope contains numerous nuclear pores of 100–1000Å diameter, which regulate nucleocytoplasmic trafficking of ions, nucleotides, proteins, mRNA, tRNA and ribosomal subunits.

Nucleoplasm consists of genetic material (chromosomes), and nucleolus. Nucleolus is ribonucleoprotein structure is the site of formation of ribosomal subunits. Nucleoplasm composed of mainly the nucleoproteins, proteins, enzymes, minerals, organic and inorganic substances.

TRANSPORT ACROSS MEMBRANE

Biological membranes are lipoprotein viscous barriers exist around all living cell and also form structural and functional components of all cell organelle. Membranes contain mainly lipids, proteins and very little amount carbohydrates. The contents of these vary according to the nature of the membrane. Lipids are mainly amphipathic phospholipids, glycolipids and cholesterol. Proteins are of two types: (i) Peripheral or extrinsic proteins and (ii) Integral or intrinsic proteins.

Organization of biological membranes, the arrangement of lipids and proteins were best explained in fluid mosaic model of Singer and Nicolson (1972) (Figure 1.6). According to this model, membrane is viscous fluid phospholipid bilayer, in which globular proteins inserted in a mosaic pattern. Amphipathic phospholipid consists of polar phosphate head, glycerol neck and nonpolar two fatty acid tails. Hydrophobic tails or fatty acids form the middle core of lipid bilayer. Hydrophilic heads line both sides. Both phospholipids and proteins are amphipathic, form permeability barrier. Degree of saturation and unsaturation of fatty acids, presence of cholesterol and carbohydrates regulate the fluidity and

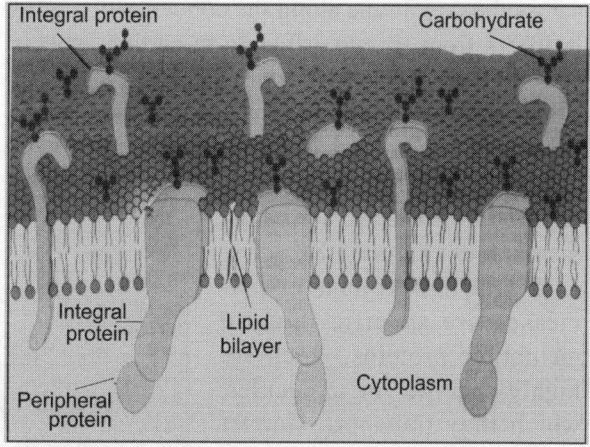

Figure 1.6: *Fluid mosaic model of plasma membrane*

movement of molecules. Hydrophilic heads of inner and outer surfaces keep constant circulation of water. But hydrophobic fatty acid core acts as selective permeable barrier saves the cells and cell organelles from osmotic shocks.

Important function of the membrane is to withhold unwanted molecules but permit entry of molecules necessary for cellular metabolism. Transport across the membrane occurs in following ways: (i) Passive transport, (ii) Active transport (Figure 1.7), (iii) Exocytosis, (iv) Endocytosis.

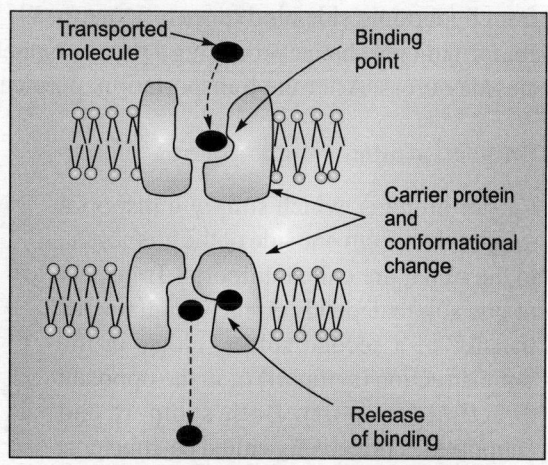

Figure 1.7: *Mechanism of facilitated diffusion*

Passive transport

Passive transport of molecules across the membrane is along the concentration gradient without using energy. Movement of molecules from higher concentration to lower concentration takes place without using energy. Solutes and gases enter into the cells passively. They are driven by the concentration gradient. The rate of transport is directly proportional to the concentration gradient of that solute across the membrane. Passive transport of molecules across the biomembranes is in two ways: (i) Simple diffusion, (ii) Facilitated diffusion.

1. Simple diffusion: Small uncharged molecules such as H_2O, O_2, CO_2, CH_4, other gases, urea ethanol, etc. cross lipid bilayer by simple diffusion.

2. Facilitated diffusion or carrier mediated passive transport: Diffusion of molecules across the membrane along the concentration gradient through carrier proteins or permeases. It differs from simple diffusion in certain aspects. Firstly, the process is stereospecific, i.e. only one of the two possible isomers, L and D, is transported. Secondly, it shows saturation kinetics. Thirdly, a carrier is required for transport across the membranes (Figure 1.8).

The carrier proteins or permeases are specific integral membrane proteins which are highly specific for molecules, which they transport. Carrier proteins specific for individual sugars, amino acids, phosphate, etc. Whenever there is concentration gradient of a solute across the membrane, solute molecules

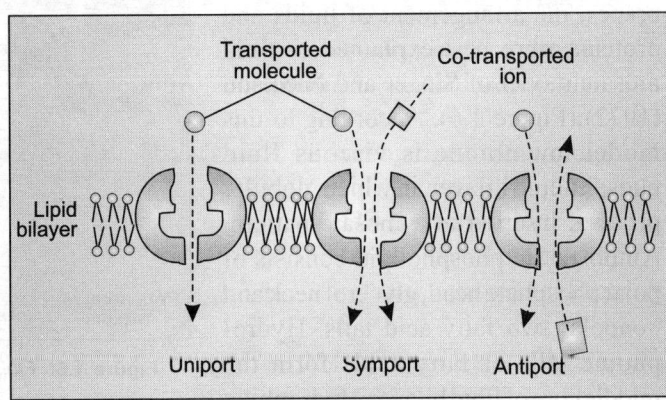

Figure 1.8: *Carrier proteins of membrane functioning as uniports, symports and antiports*

from hypertonic side bind to specific permease of the membrane. This binding triggers some conformational change producing a pore or tunnel in carrier protein through which ions, glucose, etc. may cross. After the transportation, permease regains its original structure.

Uniport, symport and antiport

Carrier proteins, which simply transport a single solute from one side of the membrane to the other, are called uniports. Transport of one solute depends on the simultaneous transfer of a second solute, either in the same direction (symport) or in the opposite direction (antiport). Both symport and antiport are collectively called co-transport (Figure 1.9).

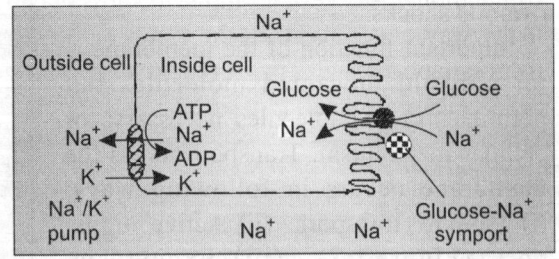

Figure 1.9

Symport: For example: Glucose-Na$^+$ symport protein in intestinal epithelial cell.

Antiport: For example: Na$^+$/K$^+$-ATPase pump, Cl$^-$ HCO$_3^-$ anion exchange permease in erythrocytes.

Active transport

Active transport of molecules across the membrane against the concentration gradient using energy. Molecules are transported from lower concentration (hypotonic) to higher concentration (hypertonic) with the use of energy. In all cells, a significant portion of energy goes in maintaining concentration gradient of ions across plasma membrane and intracellular membranes. In human RBC 50% of (cellular metabolism) energy is used for the above purpose. Active transport is mainly of two types:

1. ATP-driven active transport or primary active transport

Transmembrane proteins or carrier proteins form channels to bring the transport of molecules and ions across biological membranes using energy from ATP. The most important active transport in cells is Na$^+$/K$^+$-ATPase pump. All cells maintain high internal concentration of K$^+$ and low concentration of Na$^+$. This Na$^+$/K$^+$ gradient across the membrane is maintained using energy from hydrolysis of ATP. ATPase (Adenosine triphosphatase) is a large carrier protein, hydrolysis of ATP brings the binding of 3Na$^+$ to ATPase, which brings some conformational changes in ATPase so that 3Na$^+$ pumped outside and in exchange of 2K$^+$ pumped in opposite direction.

2. Ion-driven active transport or secondary active transport

Secondary active transport takes place in the presence of ionic gradient maintained across the membrane by primary active transport. Example: Glucose absorption in intestinal epithelial cells. Concentration gradient maintained by Na$^+$/K$^+$-ATPase pump across the cell brings the symport of Na$^+$ and glucose molecules into the cell.

Exocytosis

Secretions of cell such as proteins, lipids and carbohydrates are released out of the cell through exocytosis. These secretions are packed in the form of secretary vesicles. As per necessary stimulation, these vesicles move towards plasma membrane and fuse with plasma membrane. In this way, materials inside the vesicles are externalized. For example: Release of acetylcholine from synaptic vesicles in presynaptic cholinergic nerves; release of trypsinogen by pancreatic cells; release of insulin by β cells of Langerhans, etc.

Endocytosis

Endocytosis is the mechanism by which cells uptake macromolecules in the form of endocytic vesicles. Plasma membrane invaginates and encloses the materials which results into vesicles. These are two types (Figure 1.10).

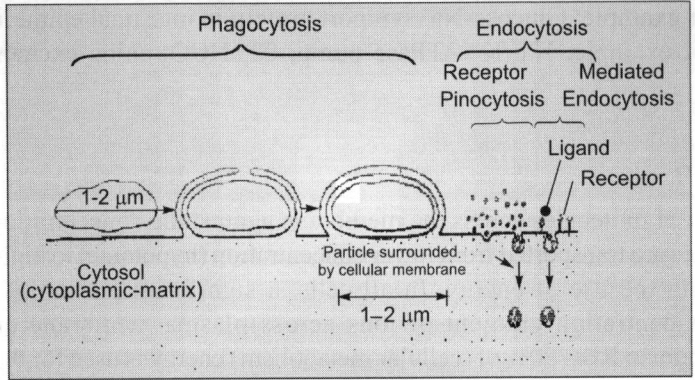

Figure 1.10: *The process of phagocytosis and endocytosis*

1. Phagocytosis: Ingestion of large particles such as bacteria, cell debris, etc. and plasma membrane invaginates in the form of pseudopodia and encloses particles in the form of phagosome. Materials of phagosomes will be digested by lysosomes. For example: Engulfment of bacteria by macrophages and granulocytes.

2. Pinocytosis: Uptake of nonspecific or specific extracellular molecules in the form of endocytic vesicles. Later is termed receptor mediated endocytosis. Plasma membranes internalize these receptor-attached molecules in the form of vesicles. For example: Uptake of chylomicrons by liver cells; internalization of LDL (Low-density lipoproteins) through LDL receptors of plasma membrane.

Self Test

1. Briefly discuss the ultra structure of a typical cell.

2. Add a note on the structural aspects of mitochondria and mention the metabolism which takes place in mitochondria.

3. Explain the fluid mosaic model of plasma membrane.

4. Write the features and importance of active transport mechanism.

5. How do you explain the ATP-driven active transport and ion-driven active transport?

6. Mention a few significances of endocytosis and exocytosis.

2

Enzymes

Enzymes are **biological catalysts** produced by the living cells and they catalyze several reactions in the body.

- They are **proteins** in nature.
- They are **specific in action**, i.e. each enzyme can catalyze only one type of reaction.
- They are required in very small quantities.
- The loss of catalytic activity was observed when they are subjected to heat or strong acids or bases or organic solvents.
- The enzymes mainly catalyze the **metabolic pathways** in the human body.
- The **deficiency** of the enzyme leads **to inborn errors of metabolism**.
- Most of the enzymes are produced by the cells of a particular tissue and function within that cell. Such enzymes are called **intracellular enzymes.**

  For example: Enzymes of glycolysis, TCA cycle and fatty acid synthesis.
- On the other hand, there are certain enzymes, which are produced by the cells of a particular tissue from where these are liberated for use in the other tissues. Such enzymes are called as **extracellular enzymes.**

  For example: Various proteolytic enzymes of gastrointestinal tract (Trypsin, chymotrypsin).

  The enzyme binds with its specific substrate and forms an enzyme-substrate complex. At the end of the reaction the substrate is converted into the product and the enzyme remains unchanged.

$$E + S \longrightarrow ES \longrightarrow E + Product.$$

Chemical nature of enzymes

- All most all enzymes are protein in nature.
- Enzymes with two or more subunits (polypeptides) are called oligomeric enzymes.
- Several enzymes occur in the form of multienzyme complex. In this case, several enzymes occur in a single complex form.

  For example, pyruvate dehydrogenase, Fatty acid synthase complex.

- Some enzymes require the presence of certain additional organic or inorganic substances and are conjugated proteins. Such enzymes are called as **holoenzymes.** The protein part of the conjugated protein is called as apoenzymes. The nonprotein part is called as prosthetic group.

  Apoenzyme + Prosthetic group [coenzyme] → Holoenzyme

- **Coenzymes** are dialyzable, thermostable, low molecular weight organic substances, which may be regarded as a co-substrate or second substrate, e.g. Thiamine pyrophosphate (vitamin B_6) derivative is required for the action of pyruvate dehydrogenase enzyme.

  NAD^+ is required for the activity of lactate dehydrogenase.

- Several apoenzymes require the presence of metal ions such as Mg^{2+} (for Hexokinase), Zn^{2+} (for the activity of carboxypeptidase). Such inorganic ions are called as **cofactors.** If the metal ion is the integral part of the enzyme, such enzymes are called as metalloenzymes.

Factors affecting the enzyme activity

1. pH
2. Temperature
3. Concentration of substrate
4. Concentration of enzyme

Effect of pH

Each enzyme has an optimum pH at which the activity of the enzyme is maximum (Figure 2.1). Either decreased or increased pH causes a decrease in enzyme activity. For example,

1. Pepsin has an optimum pH at 1–2 (its activity is maximum at this pH).
2. Optimum pH for amylase is 6.8.
3. Optimum pH for ALP is 9.0.
4. Optimum pH for ACP is 5.0.

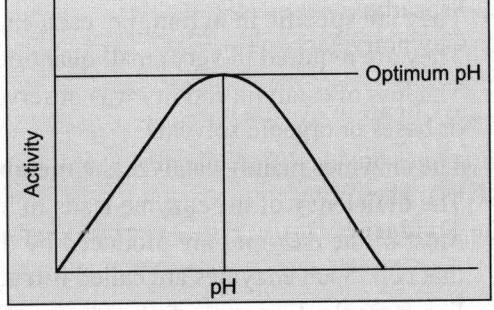

Figure 2.1: *Effect of pH*

Effect of Temperature

The temperature at which the enzyme activity is more is called optimum temperature (Figure 2.2). Any strong change in the optimum temperature results in the loss of enzyme activity. Optimum temperature of enzymes in the human body is 37°C.

Effect of substrate concentration

At low substrate concentration, enzyme molecules are free initially and the ES complex (ES = enzyme-substrate) formation is proportional

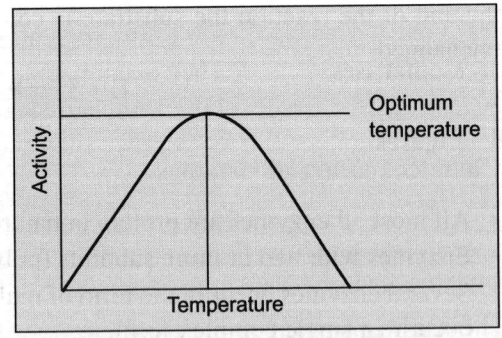

Figure 2.2: *Effect of temperature*

to the substrate concentration. At higher concentration, all the enzyme molecules are saturated
with substrate. There will be no change in the
activity further (Figure 2.3). Hence, in an enzyme
reaction system more substrate is taken than the
requirement.

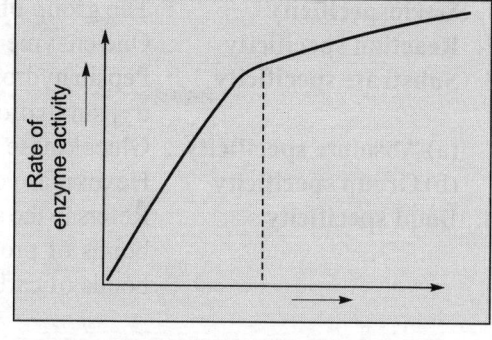

Figure 2.3: *Effect of substrate concentration*

Effect of enzyme concentration

The velocity of the enzyme reaction is directly
proportional to the enzyme concentration.

Zymogens or proenzymes: The protein
digesting enzymes (proteolytic enzymes) of gastrointestinal tract are produced in the form of
precursor. This is to prevent unwanted degradation of body self-protein. These precursor forms
of enzymes (zymogen) are converted into active form by HCl and trypsin.

For example, Pepsinogen → pepsin (HCl activates the pepsinogen)

Trypsinogen → trypsin (trypsin and enteropeptidase activates the enzymes)

Procarboxypeptidase

Chymotrypsinogen

Classification of enzymes

Enzymes are classified into six groups according to the International Union of Biochemistry
(IUB). They are:

1. **Oxidoreductases** : Enzymes involved in oxidation-reduction reactions.
   For example, lactate dehydrogenase, Glyceraldehyde-3-phosphate
   dehydrogenase.
2. **Transferases** : Enzymes transfer a particular group from one substrate to another.
   For example, alanine transaminase, hexokinase.
3. **Hydrolases** : Hydrolyse the substrate with the addition of water molecule.
   For example, glucose-6-phosphatase amylase, pepsin.
4. **Lyases** : Catalyze the removal of a small molecule from a large substrate
   without the addition of water.
   For example, fumarase and enolase.
5. **Isomerases** : They isomerise substrates.
   For example, racemases, isomerase, etc.
6. **Ligases** : Synthesize substance by joining two substrates with the utilisation
   of energy.
   For example, glutamine synthetase.

Enzyme specificity

The most important property of enzyme is its specificity. They exhibit several types of
specificities.

1. **Steriospecificity**   : The group of enzymes catalyzes either L or D isomer.
2. **Reaction specificity**   : One enzyme catalyzes only one type of reaction.
3. **Substrate specificity**   : Pepsin hydrolyzes residues of only aromatic amino acids while trypsin hydrolyzes residues of the basic amino acids only.
   (a) **Absolute specificity** : Glucokinase acts on glucose only.
   (b) **Group specificity**   : Hexokinase catalyzes hexoses.
4. **Bond specificity**   : Refers to the action of proteolytic enzymes, which act on peptide bonds of proteins. Glycosidase and lipase acts on glycosidic bonds of carbohydrates and ester bonds of lipids respectively.

Michaelis-Menten Equation

Introduction

Study of the impact made on the rate of an enzyme-catalyzed reaction by changes in experimental conditions is known as **enzyme kinetics**.

Knowledge of kinetics can be a very useful tool in understanding the mechanism by which an enzyme carries out its catalytic activity.

The effect of substrate concentration on the initial rate of an enzyme-catalyzed reaction is a main concept in enzyme kinetics. When data are generated from experiments of this type and the results plotted as a graph of initial rate (**v, y-axis**) against substrate concentration (**[S], x-axis**), many enzymes exhibit a rectangular hyperbolic curve like the one shown in Figure 2.4.

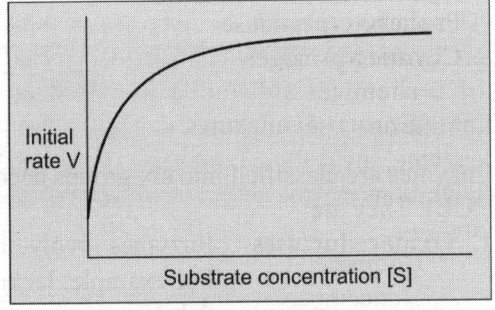

Figure 2.4

Observations of this type set Leonor Michaelis and Maud Menten thinking about the underlying reasons why a curve should follow this shape and led them to derive an algebraic equation that now bears their names. There are several modern ways to explain the way in which the Michaelis-Menten equation is derived, and one is mentioned below.

For most enzymes, if increased the **substrate concentration [S]** and hold **enzyme concentration [E]** constant, the resulting **initial velocities**, or **reaction rates of the reaction** (*v*) produce a hyperbolic curve. In other words, *v* increases rapidly at first as we increase substrate concentration [S]. Then, the rate of increase in *v* decreases, and *v* approaches a **limit of the reaction rate**, called v_{max}. No further increases in [S] will increase velocity. With some assumptions, the **Michaelis-Menten equation** describes this relationship between [S] and *v*, as follows:

$$v = \frac{v_{max}[S]}{K_m + [S]}$$

K_m is **Michaelis-Menten constant** and is equal to the [S], where $v = v_{max}/2$. K_m is also an indicator of the enzyme's affinity for the substrate. The lower the K_m value, the higher the affinity, so it takes less substrate to reach half of v_{max} and the enzyme is a better catalyst for the reaction.

Lineweaver-Burke Plot

$$v = VA/(K + A)$$

Invert: $1/v = K/V \; 1/A + 1/V$

Plot $1/v$ against $1/A$: y-intercept = $1/V$, slope = K/V, x-intercept = $-1/K$

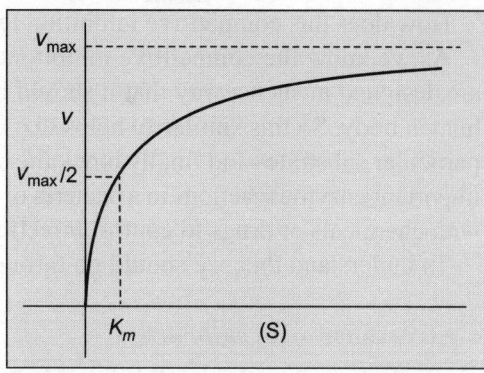

Figure 2.5: *Initial reaction velocity versus substrate concentration for Michaelis-Menten equation*

Enzyme inhibitor

The phenomenon of the decrease in the rate of enzymatic reaction brought about by the addition of a chemical substance is called enzyme inhibition. The substances, which inhibit the enzyme, are called inhibitors. Three types of inhibitions may be observed with enzymes. They are:

1. Competitive inhibition
2. Noncompetitive inhibition
3. Feedback inhibition

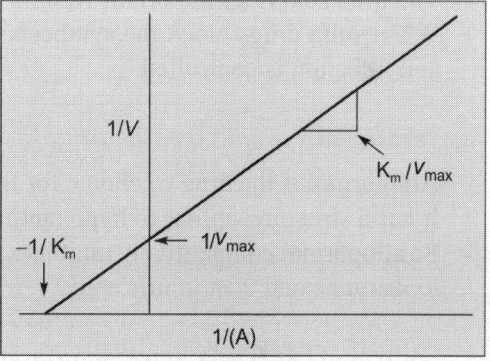

Figure 2.6

1. Competitive inhibition: The competitive inhibitor closely resembles with that of substrate. Hence, the inhibitor competes with the substrate for substrate binding sites on the enzymes. By increasing the concentration of the substrate, enzyme inhibition can be relieved.

A competitive inhibitor does not alter v_{max}, but it increases K_m value.

For example, inhibition of succinate dehydrogenase by malonate.

Succinate dehydrogenase is the enzyme, catalyzing the conversion of succinate to fumarate.

The malonate has the close structural resemblance to succinate.

That is why, the malonate tries to occupy the active site of the enzyme.

Some of the competitive inhibitors are made use in the treatment of disorders are as follows:

Enzyme	Substrate	Inhibitor	Therapeutic use
Dihydrofolate reductase	FH_2	Methotrexate	Treatment of cancer
Xanthine oxidase	Hypoxanthine	Allopurinol	Treatment of gout
Carbonic anhydrase	H_2CO_3	Acetazolamide	To treat hypertension

How does this competitive inhibition technique can apply in drug therapy?

As we know the competitive inhibitors available are mostly synthetic compounds which are designed in such a way that it should have similarities with the substances present in the human body. So this similarity helps that compound to inhibit the enzymes which act on the particular substrates and finally block the reaction. Such type of inhibitors or drugs inhibit the important enzyme reactions in a bacteria or virus to control the infection. This type of treatment with chemicals or drugs to control infection is called **chemotherapy**.

To understand this, we should go through some of the examples.

a. Treatment with *sulfa drugs*

➤ Bacteria can synthesize folic acid from para amino benzoic acid (PABA).
➤ Sulfa drugs like sulfanilamide have a structure similar to PABA.
➤ When a person treated with sulfa drugs, it inhibits the synthesis of folic acid in bacteria.
➤ The folic acid is an important vitamin required for bacterial multiplication.
➤ When sulfa drugs block the synthesis of folic acid, the bacterial multiplication inhibited and infection is controlled.

b. Treatment for gout by *allopurinol*

➤ Allopurinol is the drug of choice for the treatment of gout.
➤ It has a structure similar to hypoxanthine.
➤ So allopurinol competitively inhibits xanthine oxidase, the enzyme converts hypoxanthine to xanthine and then to uric acid.

c. Control of cancer by *amethopterin* and *aminopterin*

➤ Amethopterin and aminopterin are antifolic compounds having structure similar to folic acid.
➤ Coenzyme (tetrahydrofolic acid) of this folic acid helps in the transfer of one carbon unit in the reactions like the synthesis of purines and pyrimidines.
➤ Purines and pyrimidines are required for the synthesis of nucleic acids for growth and cell multiplication.
➤ Aminopterin or amethopterin competitively inhibits folate reductase and interferes with the synthesis of tetrahydrofolate.
➤ These compounds are used in the treatment of blood cancer where there is excessive production of WBC.
➤ Because of the coenzyme deficiency the multiplication of WBC inhibited.

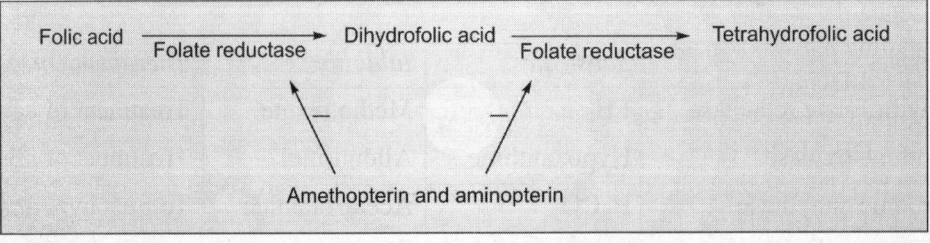

d. *Dicumarol* to thromboembolic condition

➤ Vitamin K is involved in the γ-carboxylation (see details in Vitamin K) of glutamic acid residues of the clotting factors like **Prothrombin, Proconvertin factor, Christmas factor and Stuart-Prower factor.**
➤ There are various anticoagulants to treat the thromboembolic conditions.
➤ Clinically coumarins and heparins are important and useful. Dicumarol and warfarin are the coumarins to treat the thromboembolic condition.
➤ When the patient treated with dicumarol, it competes with vitamin K and decreases the formation of prothrombin by liver.

e. Isonicotinic acid hydrazide (INH) treatment for tuberculosis

➤ The INH drug has structural similarity with pyridoxine.
➤ This drug may be interfering with the formation of PLP, a coenzyme of pyridoxine in TB bacillus.
➤ That is the reason, patients with treated with INH always supplemented with vitamin B_6.

2. **Noncompetitive inhibition:** In this type, the inhibitor does not resemble the substrate and do not bind to the substrate binding site of the enzyme. It binds to the enzyme other than the active site.

For example, inhibition of enzymes by heavy metals like Hg^{2+}, iodoacetate, etc.

A noncompetitive inhibitor lowers the v_{max} with no change in the K_m value.

3. **Feedback inhibition:** Feedback inhibition refers to the inhibition of the enzyme by the end product of the reaction.

For example, inhibition of hexokinase by glucose-6-phosphate, inhibition of HMG CoA reductase by cholesterol.

4. **Allosteric enzymes:** These enzymes have more than one subunit and have a catalytic site and a regulatory site. Allosteric activator or inhibitor binds to the regulatory site and regulate the activity of the enzyme.

For example, HMG CoA reductase enzyme is a regulatory enzyme of cholesterol biosynthesis.

ADP and glucose-6-phosphate are the allosteric activator and inhibitor of hexokinase respectively.

Isoenzymes

Defined as the different forms of a single enzyme and exist in the same species, which have same catalytic activity but differ structurally, physically, electrophoretically and chemically.

For example,

Lactate dehydrogenase—LDH (Has 5 different forms),

Creatine phosphokinase—CK (Has 3 different forms).

LDH: LDH has 5 different forms each consists of four subunits (polypeptide chains). It is made up of two types of subunits (H and M) and contains 4 of them in different proportions as LDH_1, LDH_2, LDH_3, LDH_4 and LDH_5.

CK: It is dimeric enzymes having two types of subunits (B and M). There are three isoenzyme forms of CK (CK_1 [BB], CK_2 [MB], CK_3 [MM]).

Diagnostic enzymes

The cells produce enzymes and they remain within the cells. Very small amount of enzymes are released into the blood stream, due to the normal breakdown of the cells. Hence, the enzymes are present even in the blood in very small amounts under normal conditions. The levels of these enzymes are greatly increased in blood under certain diseased conditions, which leads to breakdown of cells. Estimation of these enzyme levels in blood or plasma is useful in the diagnosis of various diseases. These enzymes indicate from which organ they are released and on this it is easy to find out which organ is affected.

The diagnostic enzymes are grouped according to the organ they belong. Important groups are as follows:

1. Liver enzymes   (AST, ALT, ALP and GGT)
2. Cardiac enzymes   (LDH, LD_1, CK, CKMB, AST)
3. Muscle enzymes   (CK, LDH, AST)
4. Pancreatic enzymes   (Amylase, lipase)
5. Bone enzymes   (ALP and ACP)

Table 2.1 gives the diagnostic significance of certain serum enzymes.

Lactate Dehydrogenase (LDH)

The LDH is present in almost all the tissues of the body. There are different forms of LDH and they are known as isoenzymes, it is one of the best examples of isoenzymes.

Isoenzyme	Subunits	Source
LD_1	HHHH	Heart, RBC
LD_2	HHHM	RBC, Heart
LD_3	HHMM	Liver, lung and spleen
LD_4	HMMM	Liver, lung and spleen
LD_5	MMMM	Skeletal muscle

Since LDH is present in almost all the tissues, its increase in the serum is nonspecific. LDH level mainly increases in the following condition.

➤ Myocardial infarction (LD_1 and LD_2 increased)
➤ Skeletal muscle diseases (LD_5 increased)
➤ Liver diseases (LD_3 and LD_4 increased)
➤ Cancer of lung, liver and many other organ diseases (LD_3 and LD_4 increased)

Note: The hemolysed serum samples are not used because the LDH will be high, due to the release of LD_1 and LD_2 from the RBC.

Table 2.1

Serum enzymes	Diagnostic significance
1. Acid phosphatase	Increases in carcinoma of prostate
2. Alkaline phosphatase	Increases in obstructive jaundice and bone disorders like ricket, Paget's disease, hyperthyroidism
3. Amylase	Increases in acute pancreatitis, intestinal obstruction, decreases in acute liver disease
4. Creatine phosphokinase CPK 1 (BB) CPK 2 (MB) CPK 2 (MB)	Brain disorder Myocardial infarction (within 4 hours of onset) Muscular dystrophy
5. Ceruloplasmin	Increases in liver cirrhosis, decreases in Wilson's disease
6. Cholinesterase	Increases in nephrotic syndrome and decreases in acute liver disease and organophosphorous poisoning
7. Glutamate oxaloacetate transaminase (GOT) or aspartate transaminase (AST)	Increases in myocardial infarction, toxic liver cell necrosis and acute liver diseases
8. Glutamate pyruvate transaminase (GPT) or Alanine transaminase (ALT)	Increases in viral hepatitis and other liver diseases
9. Lactate dehydrogenase LDH_1, LDH_2 LDH_4, LDH_5	Myocardial infarction Acute viral hepatitis
10. Lipase	Increases in acute pancreatitis
11. 5′ nucleotidase	Increases in liver disease, obstructive jaundice
12. γ-glutamyl transpeptidase	Alcoholic liver disease

Normal range

Alkaline phosphatase	:	40–200 U/L (35–140 U/L)
GGT	:	5–40 U/L
Amylase	:	80–240 U/L
Lipase	:	40–200 U/L

Self Test

1. What are enzymes?
2. What are extracellular and intracellular enzymes? Explain with examples.
3. Briefly discuss the factors affecting enzyme activity.
4. Classify enzymes with an example for each class.
5. What is inhibitor? Give three examples.
6. What are the antimetabolites? Mention any two importances of it.
7. Is competitive inhibition can be reversed by increasing substrate concentration?
8. How do you explain the competitive type of inhibition? Mention some of the uses of competitive inhibitors in drug therapy.
9. How the noncompetitive inhibition differs from competitive type of inhibition?
10. What are proenzymes? Give an example.
11. How trypsinogen converted to trypsin?
12. Briefly discuss the isoenzymes with some examples.
13. Mention the clinical importance of diagnostic enzymes.
14. Add a note on the specificity of enzymes.
15. Give the formula for Michaelis-Menten Constant.
16. Give the normal serum value for LDH and alkaline phosphatase.
17. Mention the importance of G-6-P dehydrogenase and which pathway needs this enzyme?
18. How many isoenzyme forms of lactate dehydrogenase are possible?
19. Mention the five organs which releases alkaline phosphatase.
20. Derive the Michaelis-Menten equation.
21. Give the clinical significance of GGT estimation.
22. Write the different forms of CK.
23. Which form of LDH increases in MI?
24. Which form of LDH moves fast on electrophoresis?
25. Give the cardiac enzyme panel.

3

Chemistry of Amino Acids and Proteins

Proteins are the group of organic compounds of carbon, hydrogen, oxygen and nitrogen (sulfur and phosphorus may also present). They are of prime importance to the living systems. All the biologically active proteins comprise the nearly 22 different amino acids (α-L-amino acids), which are called building blocks of proteins.

Definition of an α-amino acid

Amino acids are organic compounds, which contain two functional groups. They are basic $-NH_2$ group (amino group) and the $-COOH$ group (carboxyl group).

$$NH_2 - \underset{\alpha}{\overset{\overset{\displaystyle COOH}{|}}{C}} - H$$
$$|$$
$$R$$

L-amino acid

The carbon atom attached to $-NH_2$ group and $-COOH$ group is α-carbon. Where R- is the side chain of amino acid and can be hydrogen or an aliphatic group, aromatic or heterocyclic group.

Following are the 20 different amino acids, which occur in nature.

Name	Abbr.	Structural formula
Alanine	ala	$CH_3-CH(NH_2)-COOH$

Name	Abbr.	Structural formula
Arginine	arg	$HN=C(NH_2)-NH-(CH_2)_3-CH(NH_2)-COOH$
Asparagine	asn	$H_2N-CO-CH_2-CH\,(NH_2)-COOH$
Aspartic acid	asp	$HOOC-CH_2-CH\,(NH_2)-COOH$
Cysteine	cys	$HS-CH_2-CH\,(NH_2)-COOH$
Glutamine	gln	$H_2N-CO-(CH_2)_2-CH\,(NH_2)-COOH$
Glutamic acid	glu	$HOOC-(CH_2)_2-CH\,(NH_2)-COOH$
Glycine	gly	NH_2-CH_2-COOH

Name	Abbr.	Structural formula
Histidine	his	$NH–CH=N–CH=C–CH_2–CH\,(NH_2)–COOH$ (ring closure between NH and C)
Isoleucine	ile	$CH_3–CH_2–CH\,(CH_3)–CH\,(NH_2)–COOH$
Leucine	leu	$(CH_3)_2–CH–CH_2–CH\,(NH_2)–COOH$
Lysine	lys	$H_2N–(CH_2)_4–CH\,(NH_2)–COOH$
Methionine	met	$CH_3–S–(CH_2)_2–CH\,(NH_2)–COOH$
Phenylalanine	phe	$Ph–CH_2–CH\,(NH_2)–COOH$
Proline	pro	$NH–(CH_2)_3–CH–COOH$ (ring closure between NH and CH)

Name	Abbr.	Structural formula
Serine	ser	$HO–CH_2–CH\,(NH_2)–COOH$
Threonine	thr	$CH_3–CH\,(OH)–CH\,(NH_2)–COOH$
Tryptophan	trp	$Ph–NH–CH{=}C–CH_2–CH\,(NH_2)–COOH$
Tyrosine	tyr	$HO–p–Ph–CH_2–CH\,(NH_2)–COOH$
Valine	val	$(CH_3)_2–CH–CH\,(NH_2)–COOH$

Classification of amino acids

Amino acids are classified mainly into three groups depending on their reaction in solution as **neutral, acidic** and **basic** amino acids.

They are also classified on the basis of charge they carry, as well as on their essentiality in the diet. Those which carry a net negative charge at pH 6.0 are called acidic amino acids and those which carry a net positive charge are called basic amino acids. Neutral amino acids carry no net charge at pH 6.0.

I. Neutral amino acids

Glycine, alanine

Serine and threonine (–OH group containing amino acids) $\Longrightarrow$ Aliphatic amino acids

Valine, leucine and isoleucine (branched chain amino acids)

Phenylalanine, tyrosine and tryptophan (heterocyclic) $\Longrightarrow$ Aromatic amino acids

II. Acidic amino acids

Aspartic acid, asparagine, glutamic acid and glutamine $\Longrightarrow$ Aliphatic amino acids

III. Basic amino acids

Lysine and arginine $\Longrightarrow$ Aliphatic amino acids

Histidine $\Longrightarrow$ Heterocyclic amino acids

*IMINO ACID: For example, **proline** (Heterocyclic amino acid)

❖ According to their chemical structure they are also classified as aliphatic, aromatic and heterocyclic amino acids.

Essential and nonessential amino acids

Nutritionally, amino acids are classified as **essential** and **nonessential** amino acids. Of the 20 amino acids, our body has the ability to synthesize 10. Even if they are absent in our dietary proteins, our body can synthesize them. Hence, they are known as **nonessential amino acids**. On the other hand, our body cannot synthesize the remaining 10 amino acids, should be supplied through diet. Hence, they are called as **essential amino acids**.

Essential amino acids

*M*ethionine	*V*aline	*P*henylalanine
*A*rginine	*I*soleucine	*H*istidine
*T*hreonine	*L*eucine	*L*ysine
*T*ryptophan		

The code word to remember them is ***MATTVILPHLy***.

Glucogenic and ketogenic amino acids

• After the removal of amino group of amino acid, if the carbon skeleton of amino acid can be converted into glucose in the body, such amino acids are called **glucogenic amino acids**.

• Similarly, if the carbon skeleton of amino acid is converted into ketone body (acetoacetic acid), such amino acids are called **ketogenic amino acids**.

• If one part of the carbon skeleton is converted into glucose and the other part is converted into ketone body, such amino acids are termed both **glucogenic and ketogenic amino acids.**

Glucogenic AA		Ketogenic AA	Glucogenic and ketogenic AA	
Glycine	Methionine	Leucine	Lysine	Phenylalanine
Alanine	Aspartic acid		Isoleucine	Tyrosine
Serine	Glutamic acid			Tryptophan
Threonine	Asparagine			
Valine	Glutamine			
Cysteine	Histidine			
Proline	Arginine			

Peptides and peptide bond

The amino acids are joined by **peptide bonds** in proteins.

$$H_2N\text{–}R_1\text{–}COOH + H_2N\text{–}R_2\text{–}COOH \longrightarrow H_2N\text{–}R_1\text{–}CO\text{–}HN\text{–}R_2\text{–}COOH$$

Amino acid 1   Amino acid 2 H_2O Dipeptide

Peptide bond

The dipeptide formation from two amino acids occurs by a loss of a molecule of water.

If amino acid **1** is glycine and **2** is alanine then the dipeptide formed is glycylalanine. If the amino acids are interchanged then the resulting peptide is alanylglycine. Always the amino group of the first amino acid in the peptide is free and the carboxyl group of the last amino acid is also free. The amino terminal of the peptide is always written on the left side and carboxyl terminal will be on the right side.

Naturally occurring peptides

1. Dipeptide: It is made up of two amino acids.

For example,   (a) Carnosine

(b) Anserine.

The two amino acids are β-alanine and histidine. Anserine is the derivative of carnosine. Both these peptides are found in muscle.

2. Tripeptide: Made up of three amino acids.

For example, a. Glutathione. [Abbreviated as GSH]

The three amino acids present are glutamic acid, cysteine and glycine.

Contains –SH group [sulfydryl group] from amino acid cysteine as active group. The oxidized form of glutathione is represented as GS-SG.

Glutathione present in RBC in large amount.

Plays a major role in oxidation-reduction reaction.

It protects the –SH group of various other proteins.

It decomposes H_2O_2, and maintains the integrity of cells and keeps hemoglobin in reduced state (Fe^{2+} form) when it is oxidized to Fe^{3+} form.

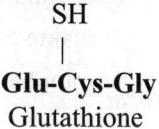

Glu-Cys-Gly
Glutathione

b. TRH (also called thyrotropin-releasing hormone): This hormone is secreted from hypothalamus.

3. Pentapeptide: Made up of five amino acids, e.g. Enkephalins. They influence transmission in some parts of the brain.

4. Nanopeptide: Made up of 9 amino acids.

Oxytocin and vasopressin (ADH—antidiuretic hormone) secreted by posterior pituitary gland are the best examples for nanopeptides.

5. Polypeptide: They are made up of large number of amino acids.

Hemoglobin, myoglobin and insulin are the examples.

Hemoglobin (made up of four polypeptide chains): Each polypeptide chain contains several amino acids.

The insulin is the hormone secreted from β cells of pancreas. It is made up of 51 amino acids. Insulin contains two polypeptide chains joined by disulfide bridge.

Charge properties of amino acids and proteins

- Each amino acid has at least two ionizable groups.

  i. The $-NH_2$ group

  ii. The $-COOH$ group (in addition, charged groups present in the side group of amino acid if present)

- In acidic medium, the $-NH_2$ group behaves as a base and accepts a proton and becomes positively charged (cationic form).

- In basic medium, the $-COOH$ group acts as a proton donor and the amino acid becomes negatively charged (anionic form).

- This property in which amino acids act as acid or both is known as amphoteric nature of amino acids.

- At specific pH, the amino acids carry both the charges in equal number and thus exist as dipolar ion or zwitterions. At this point, the net charge on the amino acid is zero. The number of positive charges is equal to number of negative charges at this condition.

- The pH at which the amino acid or protein exists in zwitterionic form is called isoelectric pH or pI.

$$
\begin{array}{ccc}
\text{COOH} & \text{COO}^- & \text{COO}^- \\
| & | & | \\
{}^+\text{H}_3\text{N}-\text{C}-\text{H} & {}^+\text{H}_3\text{N}-\text{C}-\text{H} & \text{H}_2\text{N}-\text{C}-\text{H} \\
| & | & | \\
\text{R} & \text{R} & \text{R}
\end{array}
$$

1. Cation form	**2. Zwitterion form**	**3. Anionic form**
at (1) acidic pH	at (2) isoelectric pH	at (3) basic pH

- Proteins are made up of amino acids and hence, they also exhibit charged properties similar to amino acids.

For example, isoelectric pH of:

  i. albumin is 4.7.

  ii. hemoglobin is 6.7.

  iii. casein is 4.6.

- Proteins do not move under electrical field at their isoelectric pH (pI). Hence, for the electrophoretic separation, selection of pH of the medium should be different from the pI.

- Proteins tend to aggregate and precipitate at their isoelectric pH. As a result, they exhibit least solubility.

CLASSIFICATION OF PROTEINS

There are several classifications of proteins.

I. Based on solubility: Different proteins of different soluble properties.

Class	Soluble in	Example
Albumins	Water	Serum albumin, egg albumin
Globulins	Dilute salt solutions	Serum globulins
Histones (Basic proteins)	Dilute acids	Nucleoproteins, histones
Scleroproteins	Insoluble in H_2O	Collagen, elastin

II. Based on composition: They are classified into simple, conjugated and derived proteins.

1. Simple proteins: Proteins made up of only amino acids are simple proteins.

For example, serum albumin, keratin, lactalbumin.

2. Conjugated proteins: Proteins containing amino acid and an additional nonprotein part are called conjugated proteins. Nonprotein part is called prosthetic part. Table below gives the examples of conjugated proteins and their composition.

Example for conjugated proteins	Nonprotein part present + protein
1. Hemoglobin (Hb)	Heme + globin
2. Nucleoprotein	DNA + histone
3. Lipoprotein	Lipids + apolipoprotein
4. Phosphoprotein (Casein)	Phosphate + protein
5. Glycoprotein (egg albumin)	Carbohydrate + protein
6. Rhodopsin	11-*cis* retinal + opsin (protein)
7. Ferritin	Iron + apoferritin

3. Derived proteins: Are those which are formed on partial hydrolysis of high molecular weight proteins. Peptone and gelatin are the examples.

Gelatin is formed from native protein collagen.

III. Based on the shape (conformation)

a. **Globular proteins**

These are spherical in shape.

For example, hemoglobin and albumin.

b. **Fibrous proteins**

They are long and fiber like.

For example, keratin, myosin, collagen.

Biological role of proteins

General functions of proteins

1. Proteins play a central role in **cell functions** and **cell structure**. It constitutes 17% of body weight.
2. Proteins form an essential part of the particular **structure** in the body. Membrane, muscle, connective tissues and organs are the examples.
3. Various proteins are **enzymes** in nature and catalyze biological reactions.
4. Several proteins act as **hormones** and thus regulate various metabolic processes of the body.
5. A number of proteins serve as carrier for the **transport** of various substances.
6. Some proteins act as **receptor** molecule for the transport of the compounds, across the cell membrane, such as hormone receptor.
7. Various proteins bind to certain substances and store them in different tissues, acting as **storage** proteins.
8. Some proteins like γ-globulins act as antibodies and provide **immunity**.
9. Proteins function as buffers to maintain pH of the cell.

Biological importance of proteins

The following table gives biological role of proteins and functions with examples.

Biologic role	Proteins	Function
1. Structural proteins	Collagen, keratins	Bone and hair respectively
2. Enzymes	Pepsin, amylase	Help in digestion of food
3. Hormones	Insulin, prolactin	Regulate the metabolism
4. Transport proteins	Hemoglobin (Hb)	Transport of oxygen
5. Protein receptor	Hormone receptor	Insulin receptor on liver cell
6. Storage proteins	Ferritin	Storage form of iron in liver
7. Immune proteins	γ-globulins	Act against antigens
8. Contractile proteins	Actin, myosin	Muscle contraction
9. Buffering proteins	Plasma protein and Hb	Maintain the pH of blood

STRUCTURE OF PROTEINS

Proteins are made up of one or more polypeptide chains. Four levels of structural organization can be recognized in proteins.

They are called:
a. Primary structure
b. Secondary structure
c. Tertiary structure
d. Quaternary structure.

(a) **Primary structure:** Primary structure of proteins refers to the order and sequence of α-L-amino acids in a polypeptide chain in which these different amino acids are linked through the peptide linkage. It has an N-terminus (amino terminus) and a C-terminus (carboxyl terminal).

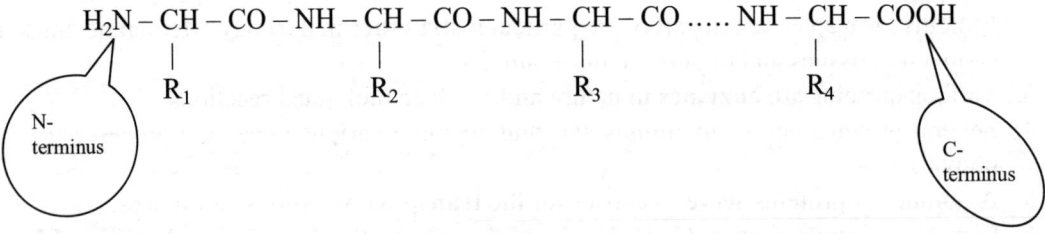

$$H_2N - CH - CO - NH - CH - CO - NH - CH - CO ..... NH - CH - COOH$$

Peptide structure: R_1, R_2, R_3 and R_4 are the side groups of the amino acids.

(b) **Secondary structure:** Folding or twisting the large polypeptide molecule possessing primary structure obtains secondary level of structure.

For the secondary level of protein structure hydrogen bonds and disulfide linkages are involved.

Hydrogen bonds: They are weak, low energy noncovalent bond sharing single H between two electronegative atoms such as O and N. These are occurred between polar side chains of amino acids.

Disulfide linkages: It occurs between two cysteine residues. These are strong, high-energy covalent bonds. Cystine contains the disulfide (–S–S–) bridge formed by the oxidation of two cysteine molecules.

These forces cause indefinite number of configurations in protein structure. Hydrogen bond in secondary structure may form one or all of the following structure.

1. α-Helix (This is coiling up like a slinky or spring.)
2. β-Pleated sheets (This is a fan-shaped bending.)
3. Random coils (This is when we cannot describe any real pattern to the folding.)

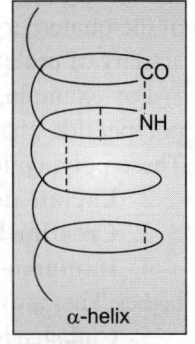

α-Helix: Hydrogen bonds may be formed between –CO and –NH groups within the same polypeptide chain (intrachain peptide linkage) resulting in its folding and forming a coil or helix (Figure 3.1).

The right-handed folding of protein chain results in the formation of α-helix. For example, α-helix of many globular proteins like myoglobin and hemoglobin.

Figure 3.1: *Secondary structure of protein*

β-Pleated sheets: β-pleated sheets are formed by the formation of H bonds between –CO and –NH groups of different polypeptides (interchain peptide linkage) (Figure 3.2).

Stretching the helices of the polypeptide chains, results in β-pleated sheets.

For example, β-pleated sheets of ribonuclease and fibroin protein of silk.

(c) Tertiary structure: Refolding of the polypeptide chain possessing secondary level of structure like: (1) α-helix, (2) β-pleated sheets and (3) Random coils lead to the formation of tertiary structure.

The forces responsible for the interaction between different groups of amino acids are—hydrogen bonds, hydrophobic interactions, ionic interactions and Van der Waal forces (Figure 3.3).

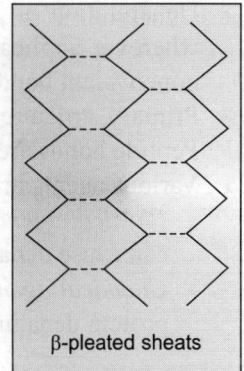

β-pleated sheats

Figure 3.2: *Secondary structure of protein*

Hydrogen bonds: It is formed between –CO and –NH groups of two different peptide bonds. It is also formed between –OH group of serine and –COOH group of acidic amino acids.

Hydrophobic interactions: Hydrophobic interactions occur between nonpolar side chains of amino acids like alanine, phenylalanine, etc.

Ionic interactions: Ionic or electrostatic interactions occur between oppositely charged polar side groups of amino acids. They are lysine, arginine, histidine and acidic amino acids.

Van der Waal forces: These forces occur between nonpolar side chains of amino acids.

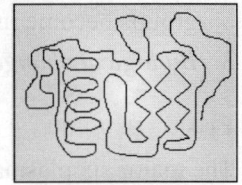

Figure 3.3: *Tertiary structure of protein*

(d) Quaternary structure: Some proteins contain more than one polypeptide chain. They are known as oligomeric (multisubunit) proteins. Each subunit possesses primary, secondary and tertiary level of structures as explained above. When these subunits are held together by non-covalent interactions, or by covalent cross-links (–S–S– bridge), it is referred to as quaternary structure. Same weak bonds involved in the secondary and tertiary structures are also involved here. Disintegration of the quaternary structure leads to the loss of biological activity of proteins.

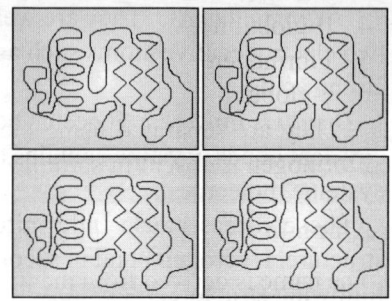

Figure 3.4: *Hemoglobin*

For example, 1. **Hemoglobin**. A tetramer having 4 polypeptide chains held together by noncovlent bonds. These polypeptide chains are called α_1, α_2, β_1 and β_2 chains (Figure 3.4).

2. **Lactate dehydrogenase (LDH)**. Have 4 polypeptide chains.

3. **Creatine kinase** (CK) has 2 polypeptide chains.

4. **Immunoglobulin (Ig)**: They are also called anti-bodies. They are made up of two heavy and two light chains.

5. **Collagen** is a fibrous protein containing three helical polypeptide chains wound together. Glycine, proline and lysine are the important amino acids present (Figure 3.5).

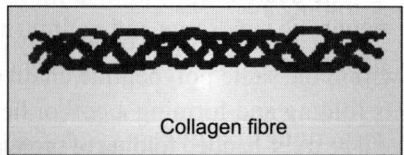

Collagen fibre

Figure 3.5: *Triple helical structure of collagen*

Denaturation of proteins

➤ Denaturation of protein may be defined as a disruption of the secondary, tertiary and wherever applicable quaternary organizations of protein molecule due to cleavage of noncovalent bonds.
➤ Primary structure is not affected during this process.
➤ Peptide bonds are not broken.
➤ Various agents bring about denaturation of protein are:
  • *Physical agents:* Heat, UV light, ultrasound, high pressure and even violent shaking can cause denaturation.
  • *Chemical agents:* Organic solvents, acids, alkalies, urea and various detergents cause protein denaturation.

Modification of protein after denaturation

1. *Physical changes:* Protein becomes more viscous and rate of diffusion decreases.
2. *Chemical changes:* Decreased solubility at pI and floccules may occur. Many chemical groups become inactive (for example –SH group).
3. *Biological changes:* Biologically enzymes and hormones become inactive.

Plasma proteins

The major six plasma proteins are:
1. Albumin
2. α_1-globulin
3. α_2-globulin

4. β-globulin
5. Fibrinogen
6. γ-globulin

They are separated using electrophoresis technique and also by precipitation methods. Fibrinogen is absent in serum.

Albumin

The name is derived from the white precipitate formed when egg is boiled (albus=white). It is present in high concentration that is about 60% of the total protein is albumin. It has one polypeptide chain with about 585 amino acids and 17 disulfide bonds having a molecular weight of 69000. Liver produces 12 g of albumin per day.

The decrease in serum albumin is called hypoalbuminemia. This will be seen in cirrhosis, nephrotic syndrome and malnutrition. In cirrhosis, the synthesis of albumin decreases and in nephrotic syndrome, the damaged nephrons lead to the excretion of more albumin in the urine.

Functions of albumin

Plasma albumin performs the following functions.
- Osmotic function
- Transport function
- Nutritive function
- Buffering function.

1. Osmotic function

Due to its high concentration and low molecular weight, albumin contributes to 80% of total plasma osmotic pressure (25 mm Hg). It plays a major role in maintaining blood volume and body fluid distribution. Decrease in plasma albumin level results in a fall in the osmotic pressure. This leads to enhanced fluid retention in tissue spaces leading to edema. Edema is seen in conditions where albumin level in blood is below 2 g/dL.

2. Transport function

Albumin is necessary for the transport of many hydrophobic substances such as:
Bilirubin,
Free fatty acids,
Drugs (like sulfa drugs, aspirin, salicylates, phenytoin dicoumarol),
Steroid hormones,
Thyroxin,
Calcium,
Copper, and
Heavy metals.

3. Nutritive function

Albumin serves as a source of amino acids for tissue protein synthesis, when it is broken down.

4. Buffering function

All proteins have buffering capacity. Since albumin is present in high concentration in blood, it shows maximum buffering capacity. The large number of histidine residues present in the albumin is responsible for buffering function of albumin.

Globulins

The different types of globulins present in plasma are $-\alpha_1$, α_2, β_1, β_2 and γ globulins. These proteins are glycoproteins with the molecular weight ranges from 90,000–1,30,000. The α- and β-globulins also function as transport proteins which transport hormones, vitamins, minerals, lipids, etc. The γ-globulins are known as immunoglobulins and they provide mainly immunity against any infections.

Fibrinogen

The fibrinogen is an acute phase protein. It is an essential factor in blood coagulation. The conversion of fibrinogen to fibrin occurs by cleaving of Arg-Gly peptide bonds of fibrinogen. It is synthesized by the liver. The fibrin monomers aggregate and precipitate to form a clot. Different types of plasma proteins and their concentrations in the blood are as follows:

Plasma protein	g/dL	%
Total protein	6.5–8	100%
Albumin	3.5–5	60%
Globulins	1.8–3	40%
α_1		3%
α_2		11%
β		11%
γ		16%
Fibrinogen	0.2–0.4	

Proteins belong to different globulins

(A) α_1-globulin

1. α_1-antitrypsin
2. α_1-acid glycoprotein
3. α_1-lipoproteins
4. Thyroxine binding globulin (TBG)

α₁-antitrypsin

- It is an acute phase reactant (APR) and protease inhibitor present in the extracellular fluid throughout the body.
- The level of certain proteins in blood may increase up to 1,000 folds in several inflammatory and neoplastic conditions. Such proteins are called as acute phase proteins. It neutralizes the lysosomal elastase, which is released during phagocytosis of particles by poly-morphonuclear leukocytes.
- Thus, α_1-antitrypsin has a protective role in the body.
- α_1-antitrypsin level is increased during any infection or inflammation because of this protective role. Hence, it is known as acute phase reactant.

(B) α_2-globulins

Important proteins under this group are:

1. *α₂-macroglobulins*
   - This has protective role in the body.
   - It is synthesized by hepatocytes.
   - It inactivates all the proteases, therefore, it is considered as in vivo anticoagulant.

2. *Haptoglobins*
   - The proteins, which bind with hemoglobin and help in the breakdown of hemoglobin to bilirubin.

3. *Ceruloplasmin*
   - It is a copper containing protein in the plasma.
   - It is known to have an antioxidant property.
   - It is thought that ceruloplasmin is involved in iron metabolism.
   - It is an acute phase reactive protein.
   - Its level is increased in the plasma in infections and malignant conditions, especially in Hodgkin's disease.
   - Ceruloplasmin levels are decreased in Wilson's disease and used in the diagnosis of this disease.

Bence Jones protein

➤ It is an abnormal protein, which occurs in blood and urine of multiple myeloma patient. It is a light chain of immunoglobulin.

➤ Simple heat test can detect its presence in urine. At 50–60°C these proteins specifically precipitate and on further heating the precipitate dissolves. Reverse process occurs upon cooling.

IMMUNOGLOBULIN (Ig)

The defense strategies of the body are collectively known as immunity.

Two types of immunity identified:

1. *Cellular immunity:* This is mediated by T-lymphocytes or T-cells (thymic origin).

2. *Humoral immunity:* Mediated by a specialized group of proteins known as immuno-globulins or antibodies.

> The B-lymphocytes or B-cells (mature in bone) are responsible for the production of immunoglobulins.
> The immunoglobulins are also known as γ globulins.
> Protective in function.
> Function as antibodies.
> Synthesized in response to a foreign substance called antigen.
> Provide immunity.
> There are five different types of immunoglobulins.
> They are IgA, IgG, IgM, IgD and IgE (remember it as Government (IgG) MADE).

Structure of immunoglobulin (Figure 3.6)

> All the immunoglobulin molecules consist of two identical heavy (H) chains MW = 53,000 –75,000 and two identical light (L) chains MW=23,000.
> They are held together by disulfide bridges.
> Heavy chains of immunoglobulins are linked to carbohydrates, hence, immunoglobulins are glycoproteins.
> Each chain (L or H) of Ig has two regions (domains), namely the constant and the variable.
> The amino terminal half of the light chain is the variable region (VL).
> The carboxy terminal half is the constant region (CL).
> There are 5 types of heavy chains: γ, α, μ, δ, ε.
> Light chains are of 2 types: kappa (κ) and lambda (λ).
> One quarter of the amino terminal region of heavy chain is variable (VH). Remaining three quarters constant (CH1, CH2, CH3).
> The amino acid sequence of variable regions of light and heavy chains is responsible for the specific binding of immunoglobulin (anti-body) with antigen.
> There are certain hypervariable regions within the variable regions of VL and VH.
> Light chains have 3 hypervariable regions.
> Heavy chains have 4 hypervariable regions.
> The hypervariable re-gions more speci-fically determine the antigen binding site.

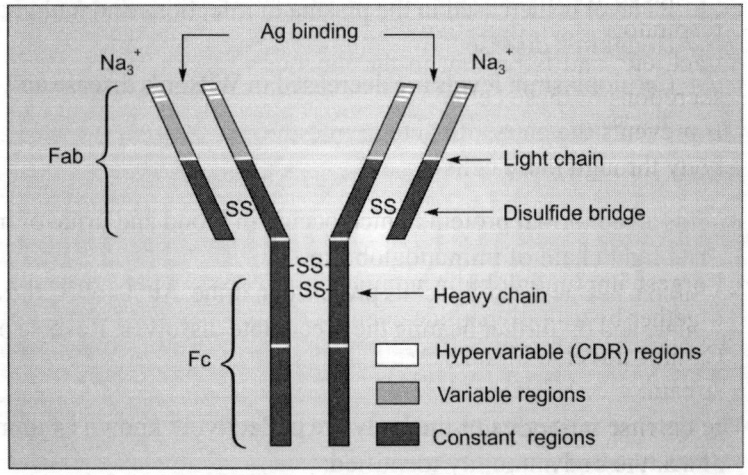

Figure 3.6: *Structure of immunoglobulin*

Type	Heavy chains	Light chains	Serum conc mg%	Placental transfer
IgG	γ	κ or λ	800–1500	+
IgM	μ	κ or λ	50–200	–
IgA	α	κ or λ	150–400	–
IgD	δ	κ or λ	1–10	–
IgE	ε	κ or λ	0.02–0.05	–

IgG

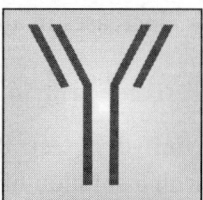

Figure 3.7

➤ Composed of a single unit (monomer).
➤ Major immunoglobulin present in the highest amount in plasma (75–80%).
➤ Produced in response to various infections and protects the body against infections.
➤ IgG can cross the placenta from the mother's blood to the fetus and provide immunity to the fetus.
➤ Triggers foreign cell destruction mediated by complement system.

IgA

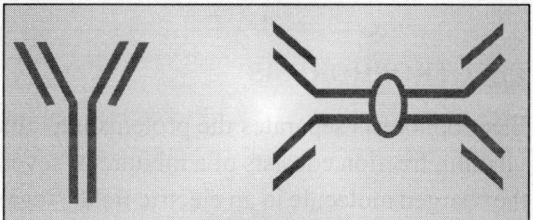

Figure 3.8

➤ Occurs as a single (monomer) or double unit (dimer) held together by J chain.
➤ Produced by the secretary cells of the respiratory tract, digestive tract, urinary tract, etc. and is present in the mucous secretions of these cells.
➤ It prevents the entry of bacteria into the body through these cells.

IgM

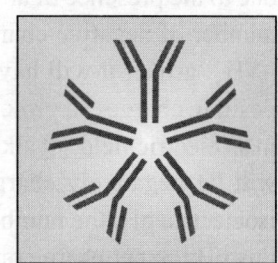

Figure 3.9

➤ Largest immunoglobulin composed of 5 Y-shaped units held together by a J polypeptide chain.
➤ Cannot traverse blood vessels, hence, it is restricted to blood stream.
➤ Is the first antibody to be produced whenever bacteria or viruses attack the body.
➤ It is also produced in the fetal stage of itself.

IgD

> Composed of single Y-shaped unit.
> It is present in very small amount.
> IgD molecules are present on the surface of B cells.
> The synthesis and function of this is still unknown.

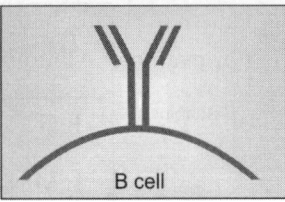

Figure 3.10

IgE

> Composed of single Y-shaped monomer.
> IgE molecules tightly bind with mast cells which release histamine and cause allergy.
> It is produced by the plasma cells of the respiratory tract.
> Increases in allergic diseases.

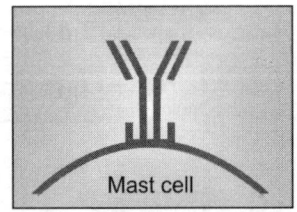

Figure 3.11

Tests for protein and amino acids

Ninhydrin test: It is a general test for amino acids and proteins. All amino acids, on heating with a solution of ninhydrin in acetone up to 100 °C give a purple-blue colored compound. Proline and hydroxy proline give yellow color with this test.

Biuret reaction: Proteins and long peptides answer this test. In alkaline medium (NaOH), the nitrogen atoms of the peptide bonds react with cupric ion (from copper sulfate) and gives violet colored complex. Exceptions are amino acids and dipeptide. They do not answer this test.

ELECTROPHORESIS

Electrophoresis separates the proteins into albumin, α_1, α_2, β_1, β_2 and globulins. Each of the globulin fraction consists of a mixture of several proteins. Electrophoresis is the migration of the charged molecule in an electric field. Negatively charged particles (anions) move towards anode (positively charged electrode). Positively charged particles (cations) move towards cathode (negatively charged electrode). Proteins in solution or plasma can be separated from one another by electrophoresis, because they are charged molecules. Proteins contain charges due to the presence of amino group (NH_3^+) and carboxyl group (COO^-). The presence of more number of negative charges depends on the number of $-COO^-$ group. If a protein has more $-NH_3^+$ group, it will have more positive charges. At acidic pH, the proteins will have more positive charges so proteins will be positively charged and moved towards negative electrode in an electric field. At alkaline pH, the proteins have more negative charges. Hence, the protein will be negatively charged and moved towards positive electrode in an electric field. At isoelectric pH, the number of positive charges is equal to the number of negative charges. At this pH the net charge on the protein is zero and it is electrically neutral.

Each protein has its own isoelectric pH.

Pattern of electrophoresis of serum of normal and abnormal conditions are shown in Figure 3.12. For example: Albumin has isoelectric pH of 4.7, globulin has 5.8–7.3.

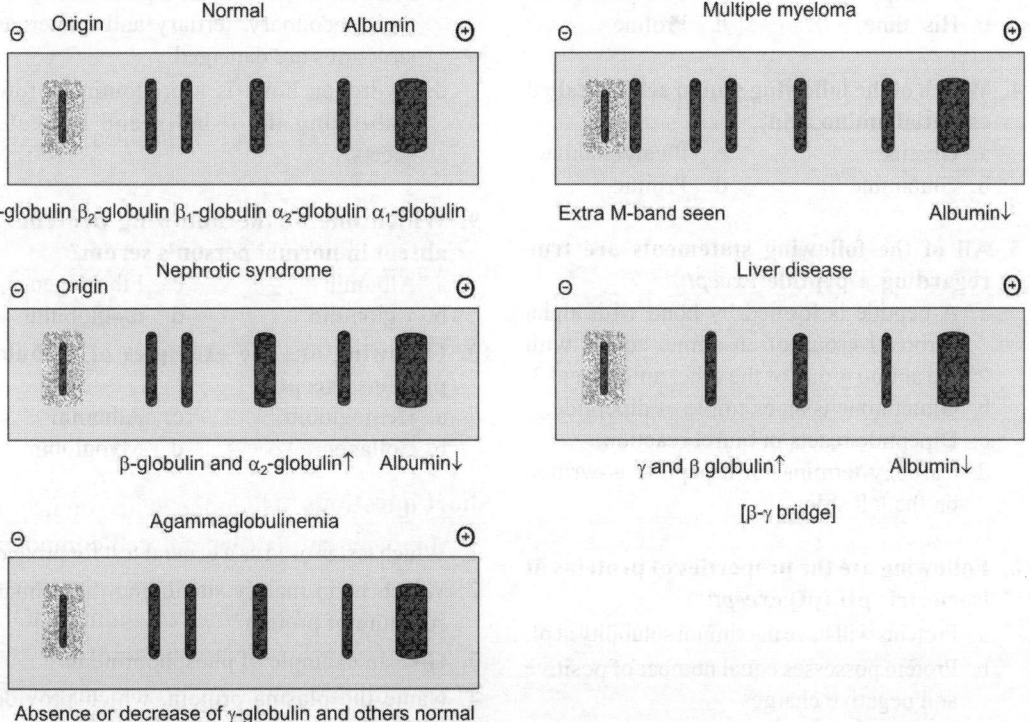

Figure 3.12: *Serum electrophoresis pattern of serum of normal and diseased conditions*

Self Test

Long questions

1. How will you classify proteins? Give one example to each class.
2. How will you classify amino acids? Give one example to each class.
3. Define essential amino acid. Give examples.
4. Give important functions of proteins in human body.
5. Explain the different levels of organization of protein structure.
6. What do you mean by denaturation of proteins? Give its consequences.
7. Name the proteins which belong to alpha-1-globulins and alpha-2-globulins.

Multiple choice questions

1. **All of the following statements are true regarding the amino acids *except*:**
   a. They contain an α-amino group and a carboxyl group.
   b. Proteins are made up of α-L-amino acids.
   c. They form peptide bond with each other to form a polypeptide.
   d. They react in alkaline medium with copper to form violet colour.

2. **Which of the following amino acids is a acidic amino acid?**
   a. Arginine   b. Aspartic acid
   c. Lysine   d. Leucine

3. **Which of the following amino acids is both neutral and aromatic in nature?**
   a. Alanine
   c. Phenylalanine
   b. Histidine
   d. Proline

4. **Which of the following amino acids is called essential amino acid?**
   a. Glycine
   c. Phenylalanine
   b. Glutamine
   d. Proline

5. **All of the following statements are true regarding a peptide** *except*:
   a. A peptide is formed by bond with alpha carboxyl group of an amino acid 1 with the amino group of the other amino acid 2.
   b. Glutathione is an example of dipeptide.
   c. Dipeptide reacts in biuret reaction.
   d. Carboxy terminal of a peptide is written on the left side.

6. **Following are the properties of proteins at isoelectric pH (pI)** *except*:
   a. Proteins will have maximum solubility at pI.
   b. Protein possesses equal number of positive and negative charges.
   c. Proteins exist in zwitterionic form.
   d. Below the isoelectric point, they possess net positive charge.

7. **Which one of the following proteins is not a conjugated protein?**
   a. Egg albumin
   c. Serum albumin
   b. Hemoglobin
   d. Casein

8. **Which one of the following statements is false regarding the structure of a protein?**
   a. Immunoglobulin possesses quaternary structure.
   b. Upon denaturation, primary structure is broken.
   c. Proteins lose their biological activity, if their secondary, tertiary and quaternary structures are damaged.
   d. Hydrogen bond is a predominant force stabilizing the α-helix and β-pleated sheets.

9. **Which one of the following proteins is absent in normal person's serum?**
   a. Albumin
   c. Fibrinogen
   b. γ-globulin
   d. α_2-globulin

10. **Following are the examples of globular proteins except.**
    a. Hemoglobin
    c. Albumin
    b. Collagen
    d. Myoglobin

Short questions

1. Which test is used as a general test for protein?
2. Which bond mainly stabilizing the primary structure of protein?
3. Give an example of phosphoprotein.
4. Name the plasma protein, which provides immunity to our body.
5. Mention the important function of albumin.
6. How many polypeptide chains are present in hemoglobin molecule?
7. Give an example for tertiary structure of a protein.
8. Name the sulfur containing amino acids.
9. What is the isoelectric pH of casein?
10. Name the urine protein which helps in diagnosis of multiple myeloma.
11. Give an example for acute phase proteins.
12. Give the reason for Wilson's disease.

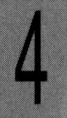

4

Metabolism of Amino Acids

Digestion and absorption of proteins

Proteins $\xrightarrow{\text{Proteolytic enzymes}}$ Amino acids $\xrightarrow{\text{Active transport}}$ (Sodium dependent) in intestinal epithelial tissue

Digestion in the stomach

The protein does not undergo any digestion in the mouth. When protein enters in the stomach the HCl content of the gastric juice unfolds the proteins and activates the proteolytic enzyme pepsin. This type of activation is called as zymogen activation.

Pepsin converts **protein polypeptides** into tripeptides, dipeptides and amino acids.

Digestion in the intestine: Trypsin, chymotrypsin, elastase, carboxypeptidase further digest the proteins and oligopeptides. The oligopeptidases act on the oligopeptides and convert them into tri and dipeptides. The enzymes like aminopeptidase, tripeptidase and dipeptidase finally convert these peptides into amino acids (Figure 4.1).

Absorption

The absorption of amino acids includes Na^+ dependent active transport mechanism, which requires ATP as energy source. After absorption, amino acids are utilized for the synthesis of protein but those, which are in excess and not required for protein synthesis are catabolized.

CATABOLISM OF AMINO ACIDS

Removal of Amino Groups

The α-amino group of amino acids is removed as ammonia (NH_3). The conversion of amino group to ammonia takes place in several tissues but liver is the major site for this conversion. The two major processes like transamination and deamination involved in the removal of amino groups.

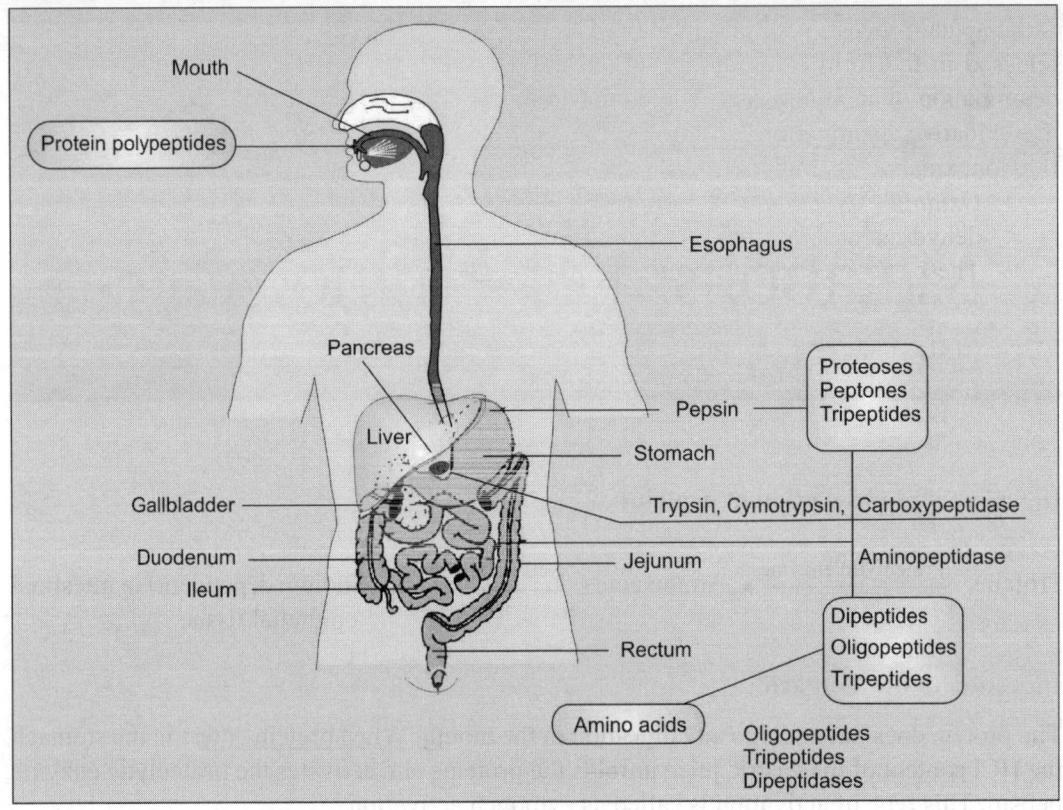

Figure 4.1

Transamination: Is the process of transfer of α-amino group of an amino acid to a keto acid forming a new amino acid and a keto acid. Enzymes, which catalyze the reversible set of reaction, are called as transaminases or aminotransferases and they require B_6 vitamin as coenzyme.

$$\alpha\text{-amino acid}_1 + \alpha\text{-keto acid}_2 \xrightleftharpoons{\text{Transaminase (PLP)}} \alpha\text{-keto acid}_1 + \alpha\text{-amino acid}_2$$

Liver contains two most important transaminases and they are:
1. Serum glutamate pyruvate transaminase (SGPT) or alanine transaminase (ALT)

$$\text{Alanine} + \alpha\text{-ketoglutarate} \xrightarrow{\text{SGPT/ALT}} \text{Pyruvate} + \text{glutamate}$$

Diagnostic significance: The level of this enzyme increases in liver disease.
2. Serum glutamate oxaloacetate transaminase (SGOT) or aspartate transaminase (AST)

$$\text{Aspartate} + \alpha\text{-ketoglutarate} \xrightarrow{\text{GOT/AST}} \text{Oxaloacetate} + \text{glutamate}$$

Diagnostic significance: The level of this enzyme increases in cardiac disorders (Myocardial infarction) as well as in liver diseases.

Deamination: Since transamination involves only the transfer of an α-amino group from one amino acid to a keto acid and as such there is no net loss of the amino group, deamination is the actual process, resulting in the removal of α-amino group of an amino acid, which is released in the form of ammonia. Liver and kidney are the main organs involved in the deamination of an amino acid. There are two types of deamination reactions.

I. Oxidative deamination

II. Nonoxidative deamination

    I. *Oxidative deamination:* L-amino acid oxidase, D-amino acid oxidase and glutamate dehydrogenase are the main enzymes involved in the deamination of amino acids. These enzymes remove electrons from the amino acids.

    1. L-amino acid

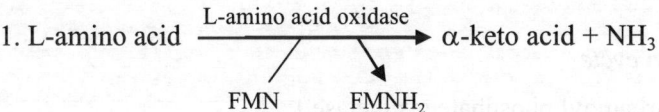

    2. D-amino acid or glycine

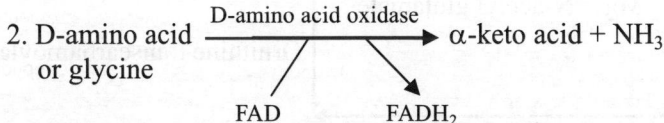

    3. Transdeamination using transaminase and glutamate dehydrogenase

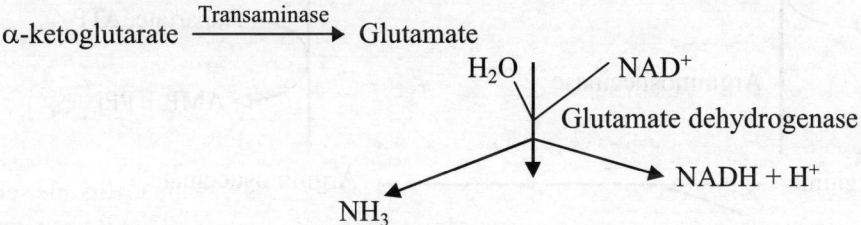

    II. *Nonoxidative deamination:* Deamination of some of the amino acids such as serine, cysteine and histidine is catalyzed by dehydratases, desulfhydrases and histidase enzyme respectively.

    Metabolic fate of ammonia: In human beings and primates, the ammonia is converted to urea in the liver mainly through urea cycle and it is excreted as such. Therefore, human beings and primates are called ureotilic.

UREA CYCLE (Krebs-Henseleit cycle)

Is the process, where the highly toxic substance ammonia, is converted to a less toxic excretory waste product urea ($NH_2–CO–NH_2$) in liver.

1. In the first step, ATP activates ammonia and it combines with CO_2 to form carbamoyl phosphate. This reaction is catalyzed by carbamoyl phosphate synthetase I enzyme, which requires N-acetyl glutamate as an activator.

2. Ornithine transcarbamoylase transfers the carbamoyl group from carbamoyl phosphate to ornithine and produces citrulline.

   These first two reactions occur in the mitochondria. Other reactions proceed in cytosol.

3. Citrulline combines with L-aspartate in the presence of argininosuccinate synthetase enzyme and ATP to form argininosuccinic acid.

4. Argininosuccinic acid is hydrolyzed by argininosuccinase to form arginine and fumaric acid.

5. In the last step, arginine is hydrolyzed by arginase to form ornithine and urea. Ornithine again enters to the urea cycle.

Schematic view of urea cycle

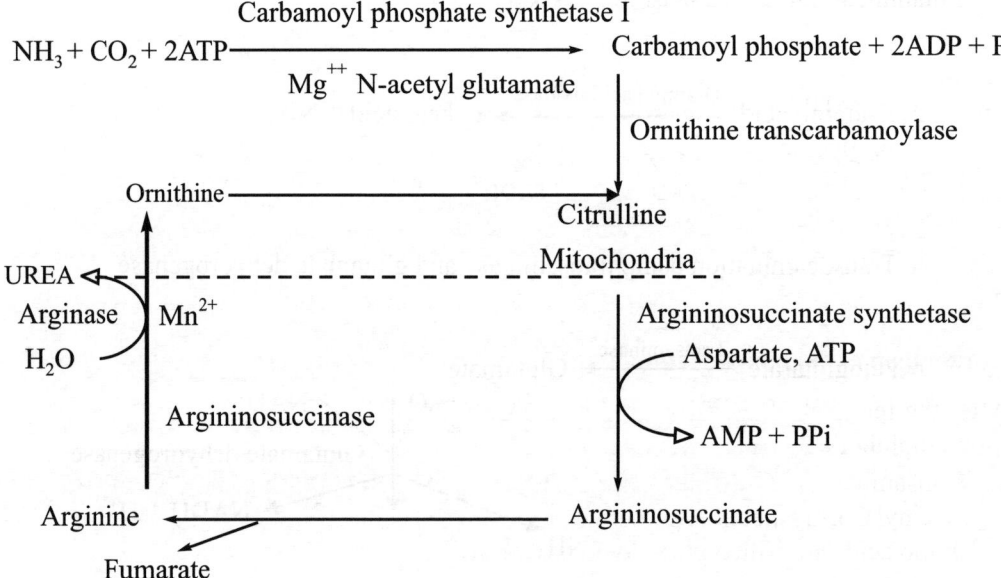

Table 4.1: *Inborn errors of urea cycle*

Defective enzyme	Disorder
Carbamoyl phosphate synthetase	Hyperammonemia type I
Ornithine transcarbamoylase	Hyperammonemia type II
Argininosuccinic acid synthetase	Citrullinemia
Argininosuccinase	Argininosuccinicaciduria
Arginase	Hyperarginemia

Clinical symptoms are vomiting, in infancy, lethargy, irritability, rejection of high protein diet and mental retardation.

Other fates of ammonia

1. Biosynthesis of nonessential amino acid: Ammonia is used in the amination of α-keto acids derived from carbohydrates, e.g.

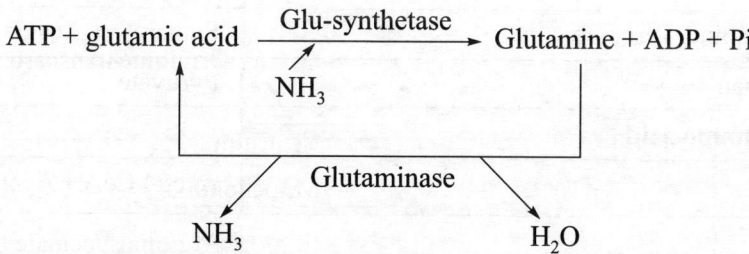

$$\text{α-ketoglutarate} + NH_3 \xrightarrow[\text{NADH} + H^+ \quad NAD^+]{\text{Glutamate dehydrogenase}} \text{L-glutamate}$$

2. Formation of glutamine: This is the main route of the disposal of ammonia from brain. Ammonia is converted into glutamine by glutamine synthetase. Glutamine is an important form for the transport of ammonia to kidney where glutaminase enzyme hydrolyses glutamine to glutamic acid and ammonia.

$$\text{ATP} + \text{glutamic acid} \xrightarrow[NH_3]{\text{Glu-synthetase}} \text{Glutamine} + \text{ADP} + \text{Pi}$$

Glutaminase

NH_3 H_2O

Catabolism of carbon skeleton of amino acids

After the removal of α-amino group as ammonia, the carbon skeletons of the amino acids form amphibolic intermediates are either converted into glucose or to fats and ketone bodies.

1. Transamination of alanine, glutamate and valine forms pyruvate, α-ketoglutarate and succinyl CoA respectively. These can be converted into glucose by gluconeogenesis. Such amino acids are called glucogenic amino acids.
2. Catabolism of phenylalanine also forms acetyl CoA or aceto acetyl CoA, which are the precursors of ketone bodies. Phenylalanine also forms fumaric acid, which is glucogenic. Hence, phenylamine is grouped under both glucogenic and ketogenic amino acids.
3. Leucine is the only amino acid whose end product of catabolism is acetoacetyl CoA. Hence, leucine is called ketogenic amino acid.

METABOLISM OF IMPORTANT AMINO ACIDS

1. Glycine
   - ➢ Simplest amino acid
   - ➢ Nonessential in the diet

Synthesis

$$\text{Serine} + FH_4 \xrightarrow[\text{(PLP)}]{\text{Serine transhydroxy methylase}} \text{Glycine} + N^5 \text{ methylene } FH_4$$

Table 4.2: *End product of catabolism of different amino acids and their amphibolic role*

Amino acids	End products
Glucogenic amino acids	
1. Glycine, Alanine, Serine, Threonine, Cysteine, OH-Proline	Pyruvate
2. Glutamic acid, Glutamine, Proline, Arginine, Histidine	α-ketoglutarate
3. Valine, Methionine	Succinyl CoA
Both glucogenic and ketogenic amino acids	
1. Isoleucine, leucine	Succinyl CoA + acetyl CoA
2. Phenylalanine, Tyrosine	Fumarate + Acetoacetyl CoA
3. Tryptophan	Pyruvate
Ketogenic amino acid	
1. Leucine	Acetyl CoA + Acetoacetyl CoA

Metabolic fate of glycine: Biologically, important compounds synthesized from glycine are:

1. Purine nucleotides
2. Glutathione (γ-glutamyl-cysteinyl-glycine)
3. Heme
4. Bile acid/salt
5. Creatine
6. Hippuric acid
7. 1-carbon metabolism
8. Serine

1. C_4, C_5, and N_7 of purine base present in adenine and guanine are contributed by glycine.
2. Six glycine molecules combine with succinyl CoA totally form heme group of heme proteins (viz. hemoglobin).
3. Bile acids (viz. cholic acid) get conjugated with glycine and forms glycocholic acid.
4. Glycine detoxifies benzoic acid in liver and forms hippuric acid.
5. Creatine constitutes about 0.5% of total muscle weight. It is synthesized from three amino acids, glycine, arginine and methionine.
6. Creatine phosphate, the phosphorylated derivative of creatine found in muscle, is a high energy compound that can reversibly donate a phosphate group to ADP to form ATP. This can be used to maintain the intracellular level of ATP during the first of a few minutes of intense muscular contraction.

$$\text{Creatine} + \text{ATP} \xrightarrow[\text{Creatine kinase}]{\text{Phosphorylated}} \text{Creatine phosphate} + \text{ADP}$$

$$\text{Arginine} + \text{glycine} \xrightarrow{\text{Arginine-glycine transaminidase}} \text{Guanidoacetic acid} + \text{ornithine}$$

In kidney, the guanidoacetic acid is methylated by SAM.

$$\underset{\text{(SAM)}}{\text{Guanidoacetic acid} + \text{S-adenosylmethionine}} \longrightarrow \underset{\text{(SAH)}}{\text{Creatine} + \text{S-adenosylhomocysteine}}$$

2. Glutamic acid

➤ Nonessential amino acid.
➤ It is synthesized by the action of glutamate dehydrogenase using α-ketoglutarate and NH_3.

$$\text{Amino acid} + \alpha\text{-ketoglutarate} \xrightarrow{\text{Aminotransferase}} \alpha\text{-keto acid} + \text{glutamic acid}$$

Metabolic fate of glutamate

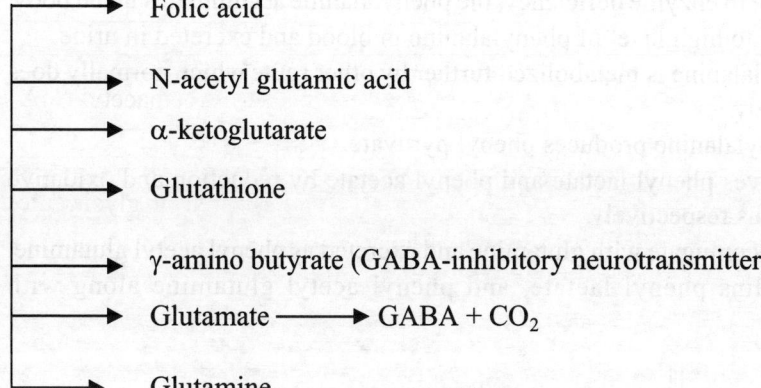

Folic acid

N-acetyl glutamic acid

α-ketoglutarate

Glutathione

γ-amino butyrate (GABA-inhibitory neurotransmitter)

Glutamate ⟶ GABA + CO_2

Glutamine

3. Phenylalanine

➤ It is not synthesized in human body (essential amino acid).
Normal condition: Proteins and tyrosine are formed from phenylalanine. Formation of tyrosine from phenylalanine requires phenylalanine hydroxylase enzyme. Defect in phenylalanine hydroxylase leads to phenylketonuria. Mental retardation and convulsions are the signs. The metabolite of phenylalanine like phenylpyruvate, phenyl lactate and acetate are excreted in urine.

The detection of these compounds help in the diagnosis of phenylketonuria.

4. Tyrosine

➤ It is synthesized from phenylalanine.

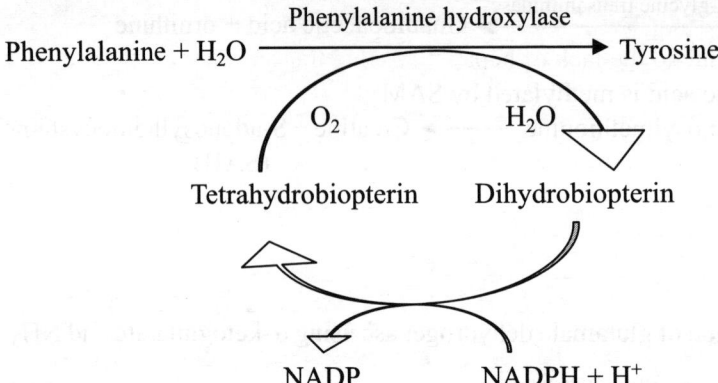

Phenylketonuria

- **Cause:** Deficiency of *phenylalanine hydroxylase.*
- Because of the block due to enzyme deficiency, the phenylalanine accumulates in the body.
- The accumulation leads to high level of phenylalanine in blood and excreted in urine.
- The accumulated phenylalanine is metabolized further by other route which normally does not take place in our body.
- Transamination of phenylalanine produces phenyl pyruvate.
- The phenyl pyruvate gives phenyl lactate and phenyl acetate by reduction and oxidative decarboxylation reactions respectively.
- The phenyl acetate may conjugate with glutamine and excreted as phenyl acetyl glutamine.
- So finally urine contains phenyl lactate, and phenyl acetyl glutamine along with phenylalanine.

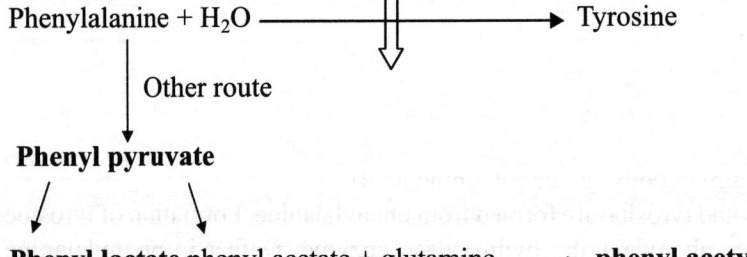

Metabolic fate

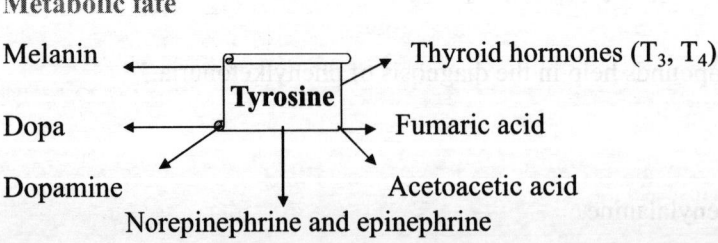

Tyrosinemia

This is a hereditary disease due to the lack of hepatic tyrosine transaminase enzyme.

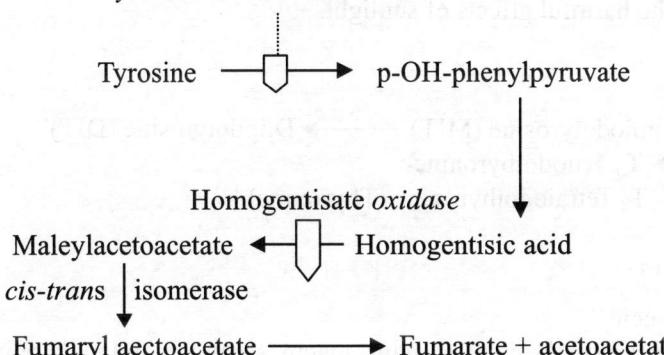

Alkaptonuria

Hereditary deficiency of homogentisate oxidase causes alkaptonuria. Homogentisic acid is excreted in urine. Urine turns black upon exposure to light. Black pigment is deposited in sclera, ear, nose and cartilages.

Sypmtoms of PKU, alkaptonuria and tyrosinemia are:

- Mental retardation
- Children have low IQ
- Low serotonin levels in brain

Synthesis of dopamine, epinephrine and norepinephrine

Tyrosine $\xrightarrow[\text{Tetrahydrobiopterin}]{\text{Tyrosine hydroxylase}}$ Dopa $\xrightarrow{\text{Dopa decarboxylase}}$ Dopamine $\xrightarrow[\text{Vitamin C}]{\text{Dopamine β-hydroxylase}}$ Norepinephrine

Norepinephrine $\xrightarrow[\text{N-methyl transferase CH}_3]{\text{S-Adenosyl methionine} \quad \text{S-Adenosyl homocysteine}}$ Epinephrine

Melanin

Tyrosine $\xrightarrow{\text{Tyrosinase}}$ Dopa $\longrightarrow$ Melanin

➢ Tyrosinase deficiency leads to **albinism.**
➢ Melanin is a pigment that occurs in the eye, hair and skin. In the epidermis, the pigment forming cells are called melanocytes. Here the melanin is synthesized to protect the underlying cells from the harmful effects of sunlight.

Synthesis of T_3 and T_4

Tyrosine + I^+ ⟶ Monoiodotyrosine (MIT) ⟶ Diiodotyrosine (DIT)

MIT + DIT ⟶ T_3 Triiodothyronine

DIT + DIT ⟶ T_4 Tetraiodothyronine (Thyroxine)

Metabolism of Tryptophan

➢ It is an essential amino acid.
➢ It is mainly required for the synthesis of proteins, niacin, serotonin and melatonin.

Metabolic fate of tryptophan

$$NAD^+$$
$$\uparrow$$
Serotonin ← tryptophan → **Niacin**
$$\downarrow$$
$$Melatonin$$

NAD$^+$ and NADP$^+$ are the acceptors of reducing equivalents (H^+) provided by various metabolic intermediates. Tryptophan (60 mg) form 1 mg niacin which is required for the formation of its coenzyme forms NAD$^+$ and NADP$^+$.

Synthesis of Serotonin

Tryptophan ⟶ 5-OH-tryptophan ⟶ 5-OH-tryptophamine (Serotonin)
$$CO_2$$

Serotonin is a vasoconstrictor and stimulator of smooth muscle contraction. The degradation product of serotonin is 5-hydroxy indoleacetic acid.

Hartnup's disease: Caused by a defect in the intestinal absorption and renal reabsorption of tryptophan. Tryptophan and its catabolic products, indoleacetic acid excreted in large amounts in the urine. Indoleacetic acid being excreted as indole acetyl glutamine after conjugation with glutamine.

Malignant carcinoid (Argentaffinoma): This is characterized by serotonin producing tumour cells in the argentaffin tissue of the abdominal cavity. Instead of 1%, the 60% of tryptophan is diverted to form serotonin. Pellagra like symptoms may be seen. Urine contains large amounts of 5-hydroxy indoleacetic acid.

Histidine metabolism

➤ It is a basic essential genetically coded amino acid.
➤ Histidine is also a precursor of histamine, a compound released by immune system cells during an allergic reaction.
➤ It is needed for growth and for the repair of tissue, as well as the maintenance of the myelin sheaths that act as protector for nerve cells.
➤ It is further required for the manufacture of both red and white blood cells, and helps to protect the body from damage caused by radiation and in removing heavy metals from the body.
➤ In the stomach, histidine is also helpful in producing gastric juices and people with a shortage of gastric juices or suffering from indigestion, may also benefit from this nutrient.

$$Histidine \xrightarrow[\text{PLP}]{\text{Decarboxylase}} Histamine + CO_2$$

➤ Histamine strongly stimulates the secretion of HCl by the parietal cells of the stomach.

FIGLU excretion test

Cause: Folic acid deficiency leads to deficiency of FH_4, which is required for the conversion of N-Formiminoglutamate to glutamic acid. Accumulation of FIGLU leads to excretion in the urine.

Megaloblastic anemia occurs in both folic acid and vitamin B_{12} deficiency. To differentiate the anemia due to folic acid deficiency from that of vitamin B_{12} deficiency FIGLU excretion test can be conducted.

Maple syrup urine disease

➤ It is an inborn error of branched chain amino acid metabolism.
Cause: Deficiency or complete absence of α-keto acid dehydrogenase. Accumulated α-keto acids excreted in the urine. These keto acids give a characteristic smell to the urine. It is similar to that of maple syrup. Mental retardation is the common symptom.

Methionine

Methionine is one of the essential amino acids (building blocks of protein), meaning that it cannot be produced by the body, and must be provided by the diet. It supplies sulfur and other compounds required by the body for normal metabolism and growth. Methionine also belongs to a group of compounds called lipotropics, or chemicals that help the liver process fats (lipids).

Methionine and cysteine are the only sulfur containing proteinogenic amino acids. The methionine derivative S-adenosyl methionine (SAM) serves as a methyl donor. Methionine plays a role in cysteine, carnitine and taurine synthesis by the transsulfuration pathway, lecithin production, the synthesis of phosphatidylcholine and other phospholipids. Improper conversion of methionine can lead to atherosclerosis.

Methionine is one of only two amino acids encoded by a single codon (AUG) in the standard genetic code (tryptophan, encoded by UGG, is the other).

S-adenosyl methionine (SAM)

It is an enzymatic cofactor involved in methyl group transfers. It methylates targets, many of which are in the brain. It deactivates dopamine by methylating a hydroxy group on the catechol.

$$\text{Methionine} + \text{ATP} \xrightarrow{\text{Methionine adenosyl transferase}} \text{SAM} + \text{PPi} + \text{Pi}$$

Formylmethionine

Formylmethionine (fMet) is a modified form of methionine in which a formyl group has been added to methionine's amino group. fMet is a starting residue in the synthesis of proteins in prokaryotes and, consequently, is located at the N-terminal of the polypeptide. fMet is delivered to the ribosome (30S)-mRNA complex by a specialized tRNA (tRNA.fMet) which has a 5'-CAU-3' anticodon that capable of binding with the AUG start codon located on the mRNA.

The addition of the formyl group to methionine is catalyzed by the enzyme transformylase. Transformylase will catalyze the addition of the formyl group to methionine only if methionine has been loaded onto tRNA.fMet and not onto tRNA.Met.

Synthesis of Creatine

Creatine is present in muscle, liver and kidney. Synthesis takes place in kidney and liver using three amino acids glycine, arginine and s-adenosyl methionine [SAM] (methyl donor).

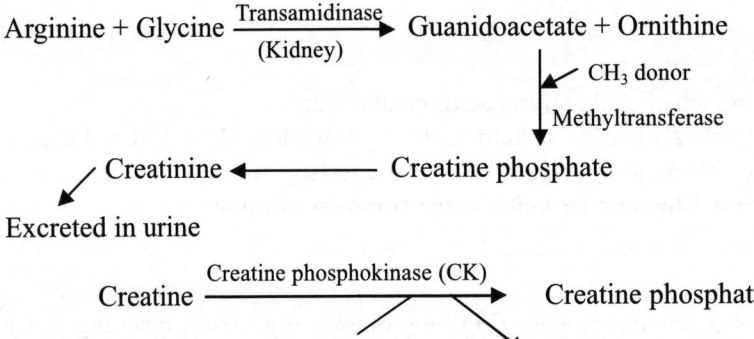

Creatinine excretion in urine is always constant in normal person. [1–1.5 g/day]. It varies in kidney disease and muscle diseases.

Methionine catabolism

S-adenosyl homocysteine undergoes hydrolysis to form homocysteine. Methionine without methyl group is homocysteine.

$$SAH \xrightarrow{\text{Hydrolase}} \text{Homocysteine} + \text{Adenosine}$$

Formation of methionine from homocysteine:

For the conversion of methionine to homocysteine, the source of methyl group is N^5-methyl FH^4. It is transferred to vitamin B_{12} to form methyl cobalamine, it's a coenzyme. The methyl group from this is transferred to homocysteine to form methionine.

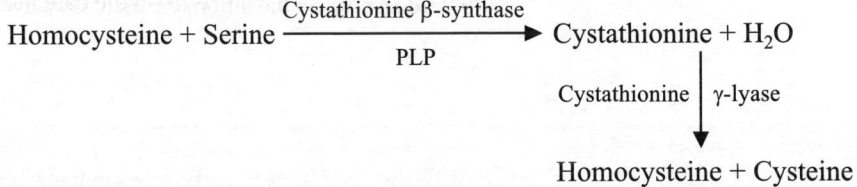

$$\text{Homocysteine} + \text{Serine} \xrightarrow[\text{PLP}]{\text{Cystathionine } \beta\text{-synthase}} \text{Cystathionine} + H_2O$$

$$\text{Cystathionine} \mid \gamma\text{-lyase}$$

$$\downarrow$$

$$\text{Homocysteine} + \text{Cysteine}$$

Special compounds formed from other amino acids.

Table 4.3

Amino acids	Special compounds
Histidine	Histamine, Carnosine, Anserine, Formiminoglutamic acid (FIGLU)
Cysteine	Taurine, Glutathione
Methionine	Cysteine, S-adenosyl methionine (SAM) 1 carbon donor

Self Test

1. Outline the urea cycle and note the site of synthesis.

2. What is the need for urea synthesis in our body?

3. Describe the process of removal of ammonia from amino acids.

4. Explain the specialised compounds formed from gly, phe, and trp.

5. Name the enzymes required for the following reactions.

   a. $NH_3 + ATP + CO_2 \rightarrow$ Carbamoyl phosphate

   b. Phenylalanine $\longrightarrow$ Tyrosine

   c. Creatine $\longrightarrow$ Creatine phosphate

   d. Tyrosine $\longrightarrow$ Dopa

6. Describe the synthesis of creatine in our body.

7. Write a note on inborn errors of amino acid metabolism.

8. What are glucogenic, both glucogenic and ketogenic and ketogenic amino acids?

9. Write the metabolic fate of tryptophan.

10. What are the compounds formed from tyrosine?

11. How tyrosine is formed from phenylalanine?

12. Write the cause for the following inborn errors of metabolism.

    a. Alkaptonuria

    b. Phenylketonuria

    c. Maple syrup urine disease

    d. Albinism

13. Draw the flowchart to show the synthesis of serotonin from tryptophan.

14. Which amino acid is responsible for the synthesis of niacin in our body?

15. What is FIGLU excretion test and what is its significance?

16. Write the importance of glycine.

17. Name the compounds formed from glutamate.

18. Briefly discuss the transamination and oxidative deamination processes.

19. What is the fate of ammonia?

20. Add a note on the inborn errors of urea cycle.

5

Chemistry of Carbohydrates

Carbohydrates are organic substances containing C, H and O usually in the ratio of 1:2:1. They are defined as polyhydroxy aldehyde or ketone derivatives.

Classification: They are classified into four major groups.

1. **Monosaccharides:** These are simple sugars and cannot be hydrolyzed further into simpler forms.

Monosaccharides are further classified on the basis of number of carbon atoms present as well as on the presence of functional groups (Table 5.1).

Table 5.1

Number of carbon atoms	Examples	Functional groups present
Trioses (3 carbons)	Glyceraldehyde Dihydroxy acetone	Aldehyde (aldotriose) Ketone (ketotriose)
Tetroses (4 carbons)	Erythrose	Aldehyde (aldotetrose)
Pentoses (5 carbons)	Ribose Xylose Xylulose	Aldehyde (aldopentose) Aldehyde (aldopentose) Ketone (ketopentose)
Hexoses (6 carbons)	Glucose Galactose Fructose	Aldehyde (aldohexose) Aldehyde (aldohexose) Ketone (ketohexose)

2. **Disaccharides:** They contain two molecules of same or different monosaccharide units. On hydrolysis, they yield two monosaccharide units. Two monosaccharide units are joined by glycosidic bond (Table 5.2).

3. **Oligosaccharides:** They contain 3–6 molecules of monosaccharide units.

For example, Maltotriose (Glucose + Glucose + Glucose)

4. **Polysaccharides:** They contain more than 6 molecules of monosaccharide units.

Table 5.2

Examples	Product formed upon hydrolysis	Glycosidic linkage	Sources
Maltose	glucose + glucose	α 1-4	Malt
Lactose	galactose + glucose	β 1-4	Milk
Sucrose	glucose + fructose	β 1-2	Sugarcane
Isomaltose	glucose + glucose	α 1-6	Digestion of amylopectin

They are further classified into homopolysaccharides and heteropolysaccharides.

a. **Homopolysaccharide:** They are polymer of same monosacchraide units.

There are several examples for homopolysaccharides, they are:

Table 5.3

Examples	Monosaccharide unit	Sources
Starch	Glucose	plant, rice
Dextrin	Glucose	from starch hydrolysis
Glycogen	Glucose	liver, muscle
Cellulose	Glucose	plant fibers
Inulin	Fructose	dahlia roots
Chitin	N-acetyl glucosamine	shells of arthropod

Starch

Starch is a mixture of two polysaccharides: 1. Amylose, 2. Amylopectin.

The major differences between amylose and amylopectin are:

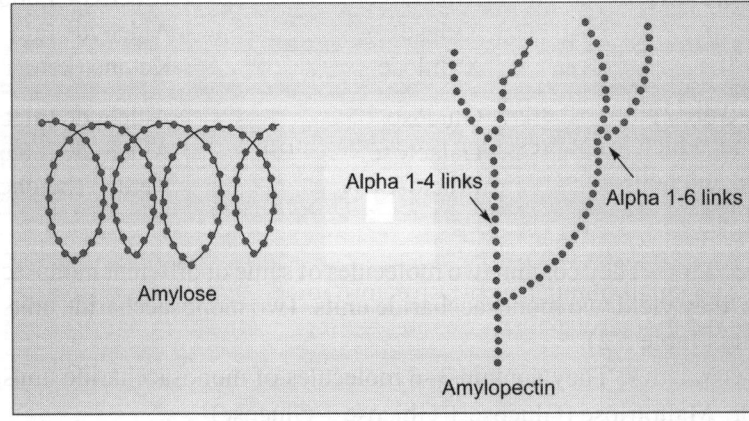

Figure 5.1: *Structure of starch*

Table 5.4

	Amylose	*Amylopectin*
1. Amount present in starch	15–20%	80–85%
2. Structure	Unbranched, linear	Highly branched. Branch point appears after every 24–30 glucose in straight chain form.
3. Molecular weight	60 kDa	500 kDa
4. Linkage	250 to 300 glucose residues are joined by α 1-4 glycosidic links	Mainly formed by α 1-4 linkages between glucose residues. Branch point occurs by forming α 1-6 glycosidic links.
5. Reaction with iodine solution	Blue color forms because the iodine molecules are trapped inside the helical structure. Color disappears upon heating. Reappears upon cooling!	Reddish violet colour.

Glycogen: Glycogen is stored in liver and muscle. It is a polymer of glucose units. It is also called as animal starch. It is similar to the amylopectin component of starch. But it has more branches than starch. There are 11 to 18 glucose residues between any branch points.

Dextrin

These are partially hydrolyzed product of starch.

Cellulose

It is made up of β-D-glucose joined by β 1-4 glycosidic bonds. Cellulose is digested by cellulase enzyme, which is not present in human body. But cellulose acts as dietary fiber, adds bulk to the food and helps in peristalsis.

Inulin

Inulin consists of a small number of β-D-fructose joined by β 2-1 glycosidic linkages. It is used to measure the glomerular filtration rate, a test to assess the function of kidney.

b. **Heteropolysaccharide:** They are polymer of different monosaccharide units or their derivatives.

For example, Mucopolysaccharides (MPS) and blood group substances.

Mucopolysaccharides (MPS) are hyaluronic acid, chondroitin sulfate, heparin, keratan sulfate, heparan sulfate and dermatan sulfate.

Mucopolysaccharides are heteropolysaccharides, which remain when protein is removed from proteoglycan. Mucopolysaccharides are also known as glycosaminoglycans.

Table 5.5

Mucopolysaccharide	*Composition*	*Occurence*
1. Chondroitin sulfate	Glucuronic acid + N-acetyl galactosamine	Cartilage
2. Dermatan sulfate	Glucuronic acid or iduronic acid and N-acetyl galactosamine	Animal tissue
3. Keratan sulfate	Galactose and N-acetyl glucosamine	Cornea and helps in corneal transparency
4. Heparan sulfate (Highly sulfated)	Glucuronic acid and N-acetyl glucosamine	Liver, lungs, arterial wall, blood anticoagulant
5. Hyaluronic acid (Sulfate free)	Glucuronic acid and N-acetyl glucosamine	Synovial fluid of joint, vitreous humour of eye, umbelical cord, cell membrane and skin

Biomedical importance of mucopolysaccharides

1. Mucopolysaccharides are acidic in nature because of their polyanionic property. They are the components of ground substances throughout the extracellular space. They are attached to proteins and form proteoglycans.

2. Hyaluronic acid acts as a barrier in tissues against the penetration of bacteria. Hyaluronidase present in bacteria can digest hyaluronic acid and acts as a "spreading factor". Hyaluronidase present in testicular secretions helps in fertilization by favoring the entry of spermatozoa into the ovum.

3. Heparin acts as anticoagulant in vitro as well as in vivo. It inhibits thrombin.

ISOMERISM IN CARBOHYDRATES

The presence of asymmetric carbon atoms (A carbon atom to which four different atoms or groups attached is known as asymmetric carbon) in a compound produces following effect:

1. Formation of the sterioisomerism of the compound.

2. Confers optical activity to the compound.

1. Sterioisomerism

Such compounds which are identical in composition and structural formula but differ in spatial configuration are called sterioisomers. These include:

a. *Enantiomer:* D- and L-sugars are referred to as enantiomers. Their structures are the mirror images of each other. Only D-glucose or D-sugar is utilized by humans.

   D- and L-glucoses are termed D and L forms depending on the arrangement of H and OH on the penultimate carbon atom. When the sugar has –OH group on right, this form is D-isomer. If –OH group is on left side then it is L-isomer.

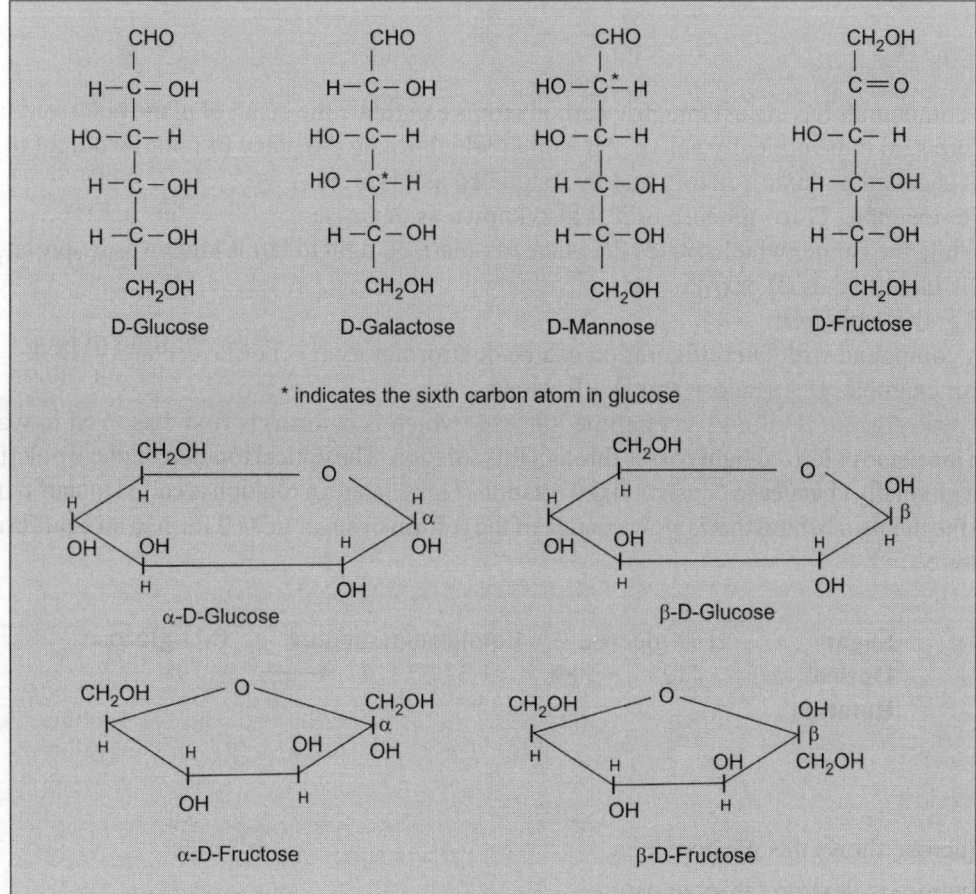

Figure 5.2: *The structure of important hexoses. Glucose and fructose are shown in their respective pyranose and furanose ring structure forms, α and β carbons represent anomeric carbon atoms*

b. *Anomerism:* Sugars in solution exist in ring form and not in straight chain form. Aldosugar forms mainly pyranose ring and ketosugar forms furanose ring structure.

   Carbon 1, after ring formation becomes asymmetric and it is called anomeric carbon atom.

If the two sugars which differ in the configuration at only C1 in case of aldoses and C2 in ketoses are known as anomers and represented as alpha and beta sugars.

For example, (1) α-D-glucose and β-D-glucose, (2) α-D-fructose and β-D-fructose.

c. *Epimerism*: The isomers formed due to variations in the configuration of –H and –OH groups around a single carbon atom in a sugar molecule is called epimers.

Mannose is 2-epimer of glucose because these two have different configuration only around C2.

Similarly, galactose is 4-epimer of glucose because these two have different configuration only around at C4.

2. Optical activity

The compounds having asymmetric carbon atoms can rotate the beam of plane polarized light and are said to be optically active. An isomer which rotate the plane of polarized light to the right is called as dextrorotatory and is designated as (d) or +.

For example, D-(d)-glucose or it is also known as dextrose.

While the isomer which rotates the plane of polarized light to left is known as levorotatory, and is identified as (l) or (–).

E.g. D-(l)-fructose.

A compound with D-configuration can be dextrorotatory (D+) or levorotatory (D–).

For example, D + glucose and D – fructose.

Mutarotation: Ordinary crystalline glucose (which is α form) is first dissolved in water, then the plane polarized light passes through this solution. The optical rotation of plane polarized light gradually changes to constant fixed rotation. This change in rotation is called mutarotation. The mechanism behind this is slow change of the α form of sugar to its β form to an equilibrium mixture.

Sugar	α-D-glucose	Equilibrium mixture	β-D-glucose
Optical Rotation	+ 112° ⟶	+ 52.5° ⟵	+ 19°

Inversion

- Sucrose shows this phenomenon.
- Sucrose is dextrorotatory in nature.
- After hydrolysis, it gives mixture of glucose and fructose.
- The hydrolyzed mixture shows levorotatory activity.
- This phenomenon is called inversion.
- This is because optical activity of fructose is –92° and glucose is 52.5°. The sum is negative.
- The enzyme that digests sucrose is sucrase, it is also known as invertase.
- The sucrose is the example for invert sugar.

Glycosidic bond

It is the linkage formed between –OH group of anomeric carbon of one sugar with any –OH group of another sugar (or alcohol) resulting in the loss of a water molecule. This linkage is involved in the formation of disaccharide and polysaccharides.

Reduction tests

Due to the presence of a free aldehyde or ketone group, carbohydrates are readily oxidized and behave as the reducing agents. These sugars have the capacity to reduce cupric ion (Cu^{2+}) to cuprous ion (Cu^+). Therefore, only the reducing sugars like sucrose will give positive reactions. Nonreducing sugars like sucrose will respond to these tests provided, it is first hydrolyzed into its reducing components like glucose and fructose.

Benedict's test

When 0.5 ml solution containing reducing sugar is boiled with 5.0 ml Benedict's reagent (blue color) for five minutes, brick red or green or yellow colored precipitate appears. This indicates the presence of reducing sugar in the given sample. This test is applied for the detection of reducing sugars in urine in case of diabetes and galactosemia [Benedict's reagent contains sodium citrate, sodium carbonate and copper sulfate].

Special carbohydrates

1. Amino sugars

Sugars containing an –NH_2 group in their structure are called amino sugars, e.g. D-glucosamine. N-acetyl derivative of D-glucosamine and D-galactosamine occur as constituent of mucopolysaccharides. It is also present in some antibiotics.

2. Glycosides

Glycosides are compounds containing a carbohydrate and a noncarbohydrate part, aglycone. Carbon 1 of carbohydrate is attached to aglycone part, e.g. cardiac glycosides; used in cardiac insufficiency. Ouabain; a sodium pump inhibitor.

3. Sialic acid

Sialic acid is N-acetyl neuraminic acid (NANA). It is present in mucopolysaccharide and glycolipid, ganglioside.

4. Deoxy sugar

It lacks one O atom in II or III carbon atoms of a carbohydrate.

For example, deoxy ribose. It is present in nucleic acid DNA. 6-deoxy L-galactose or fucose. It is present on cell membrane.

Glycoprotein and proteoglycan

Glycoproteins

They are proteins to which carbohydrates are covalently attached.
For example, Immunoglobulin, egg albumin.

Proteoglycans

They are also proteins to which carbohydrates are covalently attached, but the carbohydrates differ chemically from those attached to glycoproteins. The carbohydrates may be glucosamine or galactosamine and or their acetyl derivatives, uronic acids and sulfate groups.

Self Test

Answer the following questions

1. Define carbohydrates.
2. Classify the carbohydrates with a suitable example for each class.
3. Explain the stereoisomerism of carbohydrates.
4. How monosaccharides are further classified?
5. What are the two types of polysaccharides?
6. Define the asymmetric carbon atom.
7. Explain the term mutarotation.
8. What are disaccharides? Give example and composition.
9. What are proteoglycans and mucopoly-saccharides?
10. Write briefly on mucopolysaccharide. Write their biomedical importance.
11. Discuss on the structures of starch and glycogen.
12. Differentiate between amylose and amy-lopectin.
13. If the two monosaccharides differ in the configuration around a single carbon atom, are called as what?
14. Name the nonreducing disaccharide.
15. What do you call for the α and β cyclic form of D-glucose?
16. Name the non-carbohydrate moiety present in glycoside.
17. Give an example for a glycoside.
18. Name the polysaccharide employed for the assessment of kidney function tests.
19. Mention the glycosaminoglycan that serves as a lubricant and shock absorbent of joints.

Multiple choice questions

1. **One of the following is not an aldose   [d]**
   a. Glucose
   b. Galactose
   c. Mannose
   d. Fructose

2. **Which among the following glycosamino-glycans serves as an anticoagulant   [a]**
   a. Heparin
   b. Hyaluronic acid
   c. Chondroitin sulfate
   d. Keratan sulfate

3. **The polysaccharide containing β glycosidic linkage   [c]**
   a. Starch
   b. Glycogen
   c. Dextrin
   d. Cellulose

4. In general, the carbon atoms involved in reducing action involves   [a]
   a. 1 and 2
   b. 2 and 3
   c. 3 and 4
   d. 5 and 6

5. Which of the following is not true regarding glucose?   [d]
   a. It is an aldohexose
   b. It is a reducing sugar
   c. It is present in starch and cellulose
   d. It is an epimer of fructose

6. The glycosaminoglycan which does not contain uronic acid   [d]
   a. Heparin
   b. Hyaluronic acid
   c. Chondroitin sulfate
   d. Keratan sulfate

7. Which of the following is a deoxy sugar?   [a]
   a. Ribose
   b. Fructose
   c. Glucosamine
   d. Xylulose

8. Which of the following is not found in glycosaminoglycan?   [c]
   a. L-iduronic acid
   b. D-glucuronic acid
   c. Ribose
   d. N-acetyl galactosamine

9. Which of the following is a hetero-polysaccharide?   [d]
   a. Dextrin
   b. Chitin
   c. Inulin
   d. Heparin

10. Which of the following statements is wrong regarding starch?   [b]
   a. Starch is made of both linear and branched polysaccharides.
   b. Starch gives red colour with I_2 reactions.
   c. Starch can be hydrolysed to glucose in the body.
   d. Glycogen is known as animal starch.

11. Which of the following is an example for invert sugar?   [c]
   a. Glucose
   b. Fructose
   c. Sucrose
   d. Maltose

12. All the following are the examples for monosaccharides except   [c]
   a. glucose
   b. fructose
   c. sucrose
   d. galactose

13. The bond which links the monosaccharide units is   [d]
   a. ester bond
   b. phosphate bond
   c. disulfide bond
   d. glycosidic bond

14. All of the following polysaccharides contain glucose as the monosaccharide units except   [b]
   a. starch
   b. inulin
   c. glycogen
   d. dextrin

15. Regarding amylopectin component of starch the following statements are true except   [b]
   a. it is highly branched
   b. it is unbranched
   c. it gives reddish violet color with iodine
   d. its amount present in starch is 80–85%

16. Glycogen is   [c]
   a. a polymer of glucose
   b. stored in liver and muscle
   c. stored in liver and brain
   d. having 11–18 glucose residues between any branching points.

17. **Cellulose** [b]
    a. contains β-D glucose and β 1-4 glycosidic bonds
    b. digested by sucrase enzyme
    c. acts as dietary fibre
    d. digested by cellulase enzyme

18. **Regarding the heteropolysaccharides the following statements are correct** *except* [d]
    a. polymer of different monosaccharide units
    b. heparin and chondroitin sulfates are the examples
    c. components of ground substances throughout the extracellular space
    d. glycogen and starch are the examples

19. **All the following are the functions of heteropolysaccharides** *except* [c]
    a. Hyaluronic acid acts as a barrier in tissues against the penetration of bacteria.
    b. Hyaluronidase present in testicular secretions helps in fertilisation by favouring the entry of spermatozoa into the ovum.
    c. Chondroitin sulfate acts anticogulant.
    d. Heparin acts as anticoagulant in vitro as well as in vivo. It inhibits thrombin.

20. **The following statements are true** *except* [a]
    a. D- and L-sugars are referred to as enantiomers.
    b. D-sugars are utilised by humans.
    c. When the sugar has –OH group on right, it is D-isomer.
    d. When the sugar has –OH group on left, it is L-isomer.

21. **Anomerism means** [d]
    a. Carbon 1, after ring formation becomes asymmetric and it is called as anomeric carbon atom.
    b. Carbon 6, after ring formation becomes asymmetric and it is called as anomeric carbon atom.
    c. Carbon 2, after ring formation becomes asymmetric and it is called as anomeric carbon atom.
    d. Mirror images.

22. **Regarding epimerism following statements are true** *except* [d]
    a. The isomers formed due to variations in the configuration of –H and –OH groups around a single carbon atom in a sugar molecule is called as epimers.
    b. Mannose is 2-epimer of glucose.
    c. Galactose is 4-epimer of glucose.
    d. Fructose is a 4-epimer of glucose.

23. **Which one of the following is not a reducing sugar?** [b]
    a. Glucose
    b. Sucrose
    c. Fructose
    d. Mannose

24. **Carbohydrates** [d]
    a. are most abundant dietary source of energy for all organisms
    b. are precursors for many organic compounds like fats and amino acids
    c. participate in the structure of cell membrane and cellular functions
    d. build the muscle mass

6

Digestion and Absorption of Carbohydrates

Digestion is the process of hydrolysis of naturally occurring foodstuffs into simpler forms. However, before discussing the digestion and absorption, it is essential to know the digestive enzymes and other chemicals secreted from the gastrointestinal tract.

The saliva of mouth contains salivary amylase and its action on foodstuffs is very limited.

Gastric juice

➢ Pepsinogen, inactive form of the enzyme pepsin, which is secreted by chief cells of stomach.
➢ HCl secreted from parietal cells.
➢ Intrinsic factor from parietal cells.
➢ Mucin from mucus cells.

Pancreatic juice

➢ Trypsinogen, inactive form of trypsin
➢ Chymotrypsinogen, inactive form of chymotrypsin and then converted to its active form
➢ Procarboxypeptidase, inactive form of carboxypeptidase
➢ Amylase
➢ Lipase
➢ Ribonuclease

Intestinal

➢ Aminopeptidase
➢ Dipeptidase
➢ Nucleotidase
➢ Maltase
➢ Sucrase
➢ Lactase
➢ Isomaltase

Digestion of carbohydrates

- The diet of human beings contains carbohydrates, fat and proteins, which are high molecular weight complex compounds.
- They are absorbed only when they are hydrolyzed to simpler forms.
- The major carbohydrates of our diet are starch and glycogen, are the polysaccharides. These polysaccharides are hydrolyzed to maltose and glucose by the action of number of enzymes.
- The digestion of carbohydrates starts at the mouth.
- Salivary amylase hydrolyzes α-1, 4-glycosidic linkages randomly within the polysaccharide chain and produce disaccharides and monosaccharides.
- After the food reaches to the duodenum, pancreatic amylase also helps in the digestion of polysaccharides.
- The further digestion takes place in small intestine by the intestinal enzymes, which hydrolyze terminal α-1, 4-glycosidic linkage.
- At the same time, disaccharidases like maltase, lactase and sucrase digest disaccharides like maltose, lactose and sucrose respectively into their respective monosaccharide units (Figure 6.1).

Digestion of important food products

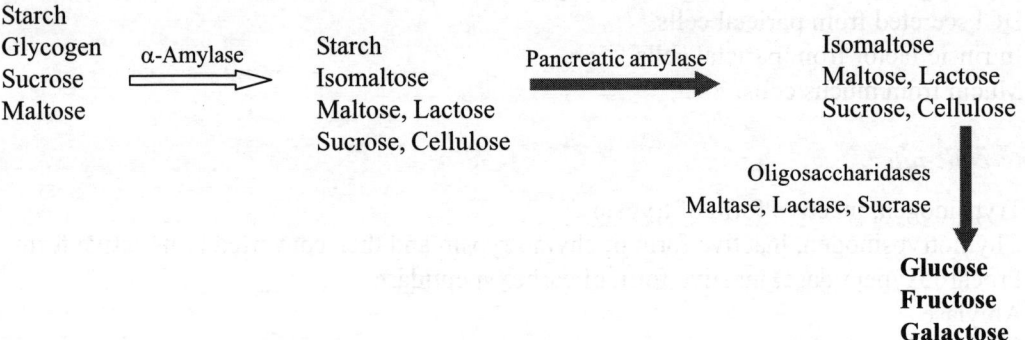

- Cellulose is not digested further but it helps in the easy peristaltic movement of food and provides bulk to the feces.
- Lactase deficiency leads to lactose intolerance.

Absorption of monosaccharides

- After digestion, all monosaccharides are almost completely absorbed from the small intestine.
- The **galactose** and **glucose** are absorbed very rapidly by the **active process**, which is linked to the transport of sodium and requires energy in the form of hydrolysis of high-energy phosphate bond ATP (Figure 6.2).

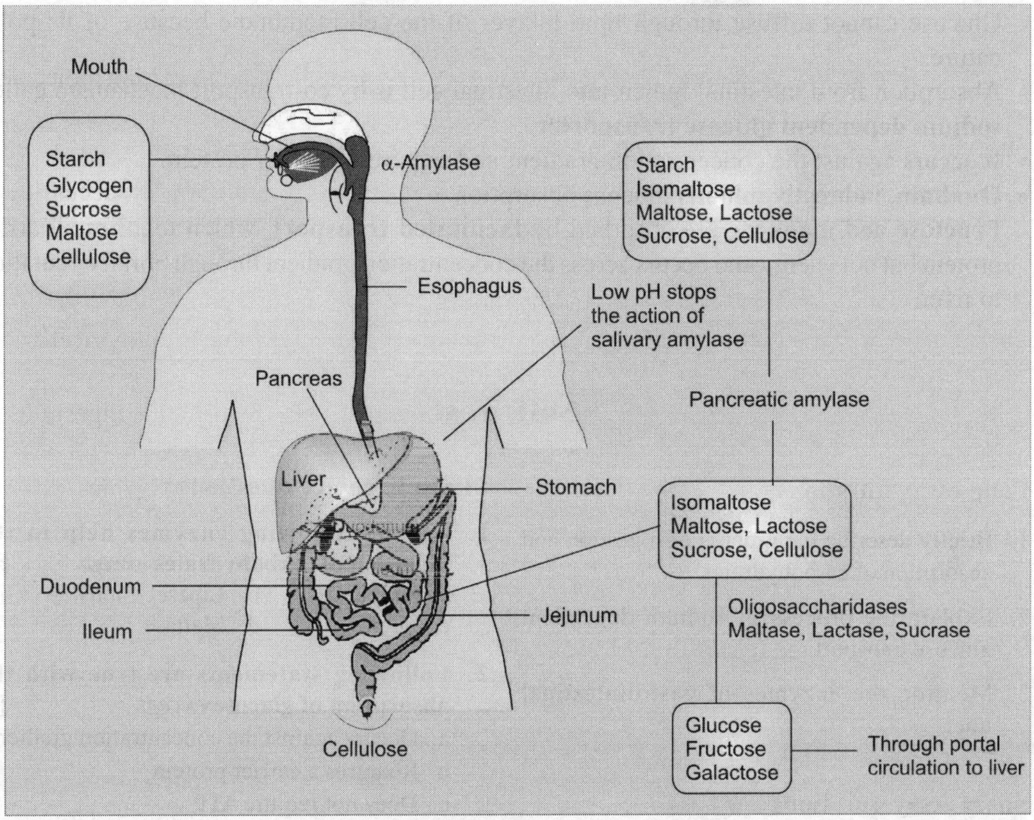

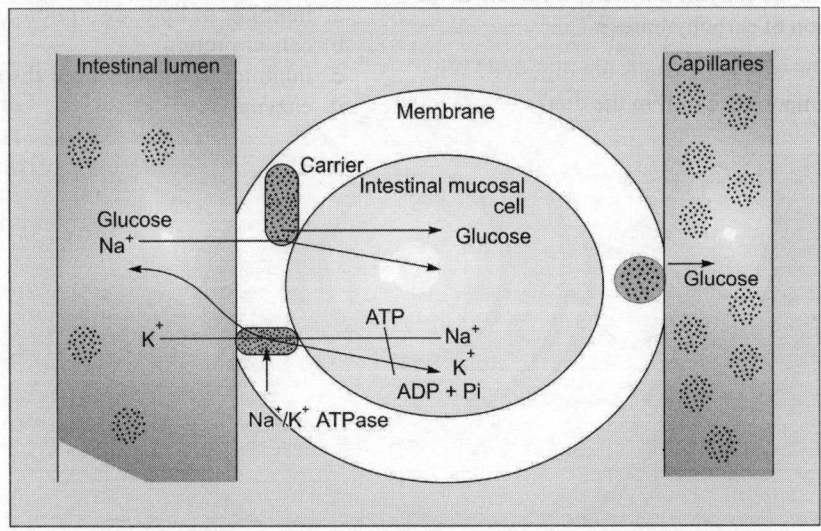

Mouth

Starch
Glycogen
Sucrose
Maltose
Cellulose

α-Amylase

Starch
Isomaltose
Maltose, Lactose
Sucrose, Cellulose

Esophagus

Low pH stops
the action of
salivary amylase

Pancreas

Pancreatic amylase

Liver

Stomach

Isomaltose
Maltose, Lactose
Sucrose, Cellulose

Duodenum

Ileum

Jejunum

Oligosaccharidases
Maltase, Lactase, Sucrase

Cellulose

Glucose
Fructose
Galactose

Through portal
circulation to liver

Figure 6.1

Intestinal lumen

Capillaries

Membrane

Carrier

Intestinal mucosal
cell

Glucose
Na⁺

Glucose

Glucose

ATP

Na⁺

K⁺

K⁺

ADP + Pi

Na⁺/K⁺ ATPase

Figure 6.2

- Glucose cannot diffuse through lipid bilayer of the cell membrane because of its polar nature.
- Absorption from intestinal lumen into intestinal cell is by co-transport mechanism called **sodium dependent glucose transporter**.
- It occurs against the concentration gradient and requires a carrier protein.
- **Ouabain,** indirectly inhibits glucose absorption.
- **Fructose** and **mannose** are absorbed by **facilitated transport**, which requires a carrier protein but not energy and occurs across the concentration gradient through portal circulation to liver.

Self Test

Long essay questions

1. Briefly describe the process of digestion and absorption of carbohydrates.
2. Explain the process of sodium dependent glucose transport.
3. Mention the enzymes of gastrointestinal tract.

Short essay questions

1. Add a brief note on absorption of glucose.
2. Mention the enzymes, which play a role in the digestion of carbohydrates?
3. Describe why cellulose is not digested? What is the importance of it in the diet?

Multiple choice questions

1. **All the following enzymes help in the digestion of carbohydrates** *except*   [b]
   a. Amylase   b. Lipase
   c. Sucrase   d. Maltase

2. **Following statements are true with the absorption of glucose** *except*   [c]
   a. Occurs against the concentration gradient
   b. Requires a carrier protein
   c. Does not require ATP
   d. Sodium dependent transport mechanism

3. **The ouabain is the**   [c]
   a. inhibitor of lipid absorption
   b. carrier protein
   c. inhibitor of carbohydrate absorption
   d. enzyme

7

Metabolism of Carbohydrates

Glucose is the main source of energy to our body. When glucose is oxidized, the free energy released is converted into energy in the form of ATP.

The energy currency of our body is ATP. If the glucose is oxidized without trapping the free energy then much of the energy will be wasted. Hence, the body preserves the energy in the form of ATP just as a battery cells.

In our body glucose can be obtained from:
1. the digestion of dietary carbohydrates.
2. glycogen breakdown.
3. gluconeogenesis.

Different pathways, which involve glucose, are:

Glycolysis: It is a process of oxidation of glucose either to pyruvate or lactate.

Glycogenesis: The synthesis of glycogen from glucose in liver or muscle for the purpose of storing glucose for energy is called glycogenesis.

Glycogenolysis: The formation of glucose or glucose-1-phosphate by breaking glycogen in liver or muscle respectively is called glycogenolysis.

Gluconeogenesis: Synthesis of glucose in liver and kidney using noncarbohydrate sources like pyruvate, lactate, glycerol, propionic acid or from the carbon skeleton of glucogenic amino acids like alanine, aspartic acid, etc.

Other pathways, which involve glucose, are:
1. Hexose monophosphate shunt
2. Uronic acid pathway
3. Interconversion of glucose, galactose and fructose.

GLYCOLYSIS

- The pathway of breakdown of glucose to yield energy is called as glycolysis.
- This pathway is also called as Embden-Meyerhof pathway.

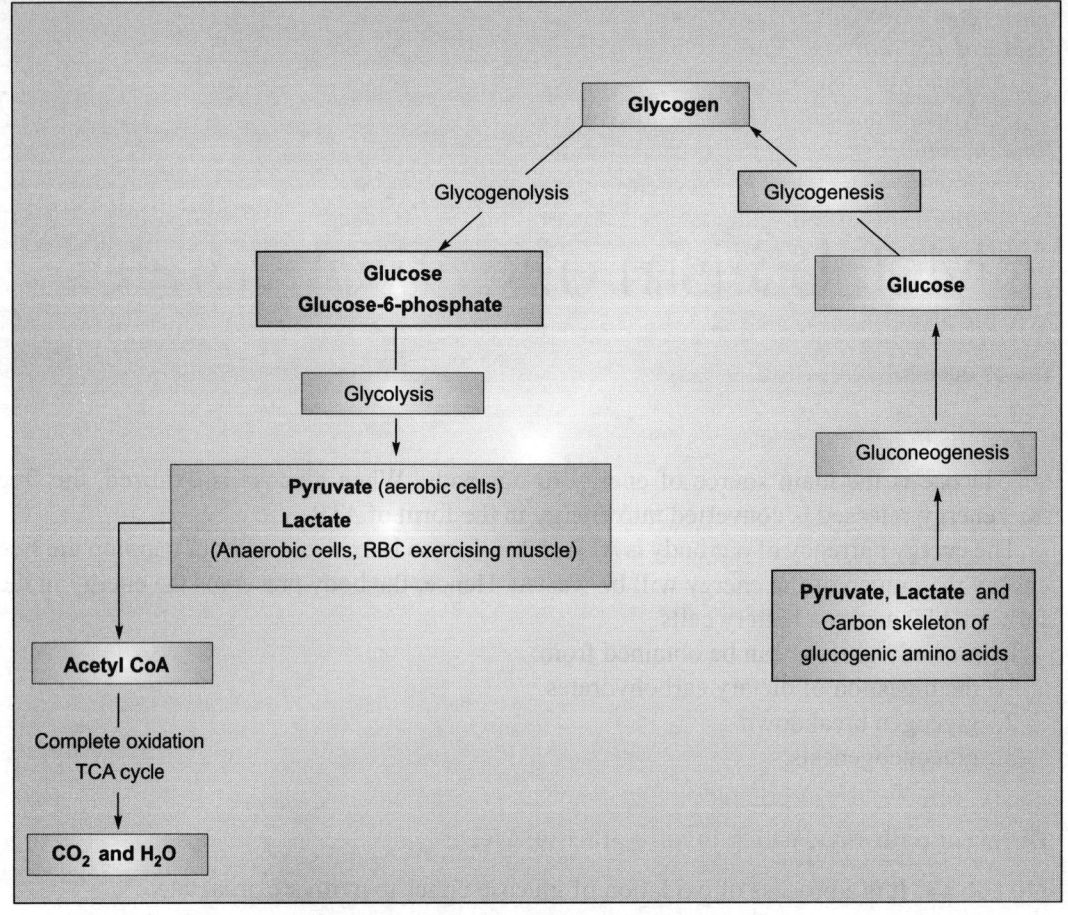

Chart 7.1: *Different pathways involving glucose*

- This pathway occurs in all types of living cells.
- Pathway takes place in all the cells of the body.
- Is the source of energy in erythrocytes.
- Anaerobic glycolysis forms the major source of energy for muscle during exercise.
- Provide carbon skeletons for the synthesis of nonessential amino acids.
- Most of the reactions are reversible.
- The entry of glucose from ECF (Extracellular fluid) to cell, is under the control of insulin.
- Glycolysis occurrence is prerequisite for the aerobic oxidation of carbohydrates.
- Aerobic oxidation takes place in cells possessing mitochondria.
- Is the major pathway for ATP synthesis in tissues lacking mitochondria, e.g. erythrocytes, cornea, lens, etc.

There are two types of glycolysis.

1. *Aerobic glycolysis:* This occurs in cells function in the presence of oxygen. They are cells containing mitochondria actively using oxygen. Here glucose is broken down to 2 molecules of pyruvate and net ATP formed is equal to 8 ATP.

2. *Anaerobic glycolysis:* Occurs in cells under hypoxic conditions. During severe exercises, there will be depletion of oxygen in the tissues. Also RBC gets its energy by anaerobic glycolysis. Two molecules of lactate are formed as the end product. In this type only 2 molecules of ATP are formed.

Aerobic glycolysis

Site of occurence: Cytosol.

Reactions of aerobic glycolysis (Figure 7.1)

1. In the first step the glucose is irreversibly activated to glucose-6-phosphate in the cell. The step is catalyzed by *hexokinase* enzyme. This requires Mg^{2+} and ATP. In liver, *glucokinase* is a specific enzyme, also catalyzes this reaction at higher concentration of glucose.

Table 7.1	
Glucokinase	**Hexokinase**
Present in liver	Present in all tissues
Phosphorylation of Glu	Phosphorylation of hexoses
High K_m for glucose	High affinity for substrates
Not inhibited by Glu-6-P	Inhibited by Glu-6-P

Glucose-6-P: Impermeable to the cell membrane. Central molecule with a variety of metabolic fates; glycolysis, glycogenesis, gluconeogenesis and HMP (Hexose Mono Phosphate) shunt.

2. Next the glucose-6-phosphate is isomerised to fructose-6-phosphate by *phosphohexose isomerase* enzyme.

3. Fructose-6-phosphate is then irreversibly phosphorylated by *phosphofructokinase* enzyme to fructose-1, 6-bisphosphate. Fructose-1, 6-bisphosphate contains two phosphoric acid groups at C1 and C6 of fructose via phosphate ester bond.

4. Later fructose-1, 6-bisphosphate molecule (six carbon sugar) is cleaved by *aldolase* enzyme to yield glyceraldehyde-3-phosphate and dihydroxy acetone phosphate (two 3 carbon sugars-trioses).

5. Dihydroxy acetone phosphate formed in the above step is converted back to glyceraldehyde-3-phosphate by *phosphotriose isomerase* enzyme.

6. Now we have two molecules of glyceraldehyde-3-phosphate molecules, which get oxidized to 1, 3-bisphosphoglycerate by the action of *glyceraldehyde-3-phosphate*

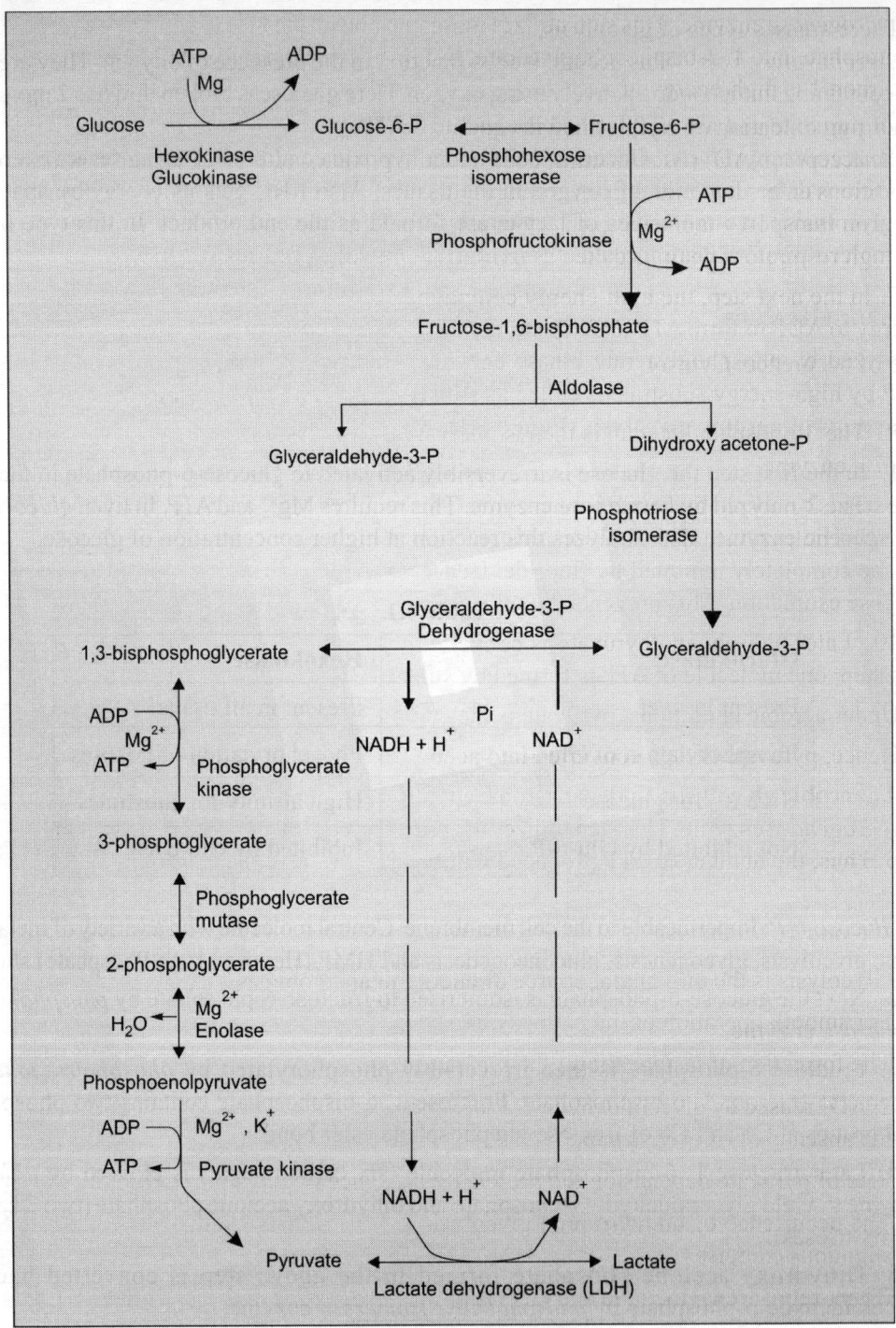

Figure 7.1: *Glycolysis*

dehydrogenase enzyme. This step utilizes inorganic phosphate (P_i) to convert glyceraldehyde-3-phosphate into 1, 3-bisphosphoglycerate. In 1, 3-bisphosphoglycerate, the phosphate group at carbon 1 is high-energy group.

During oxidation of glyceraldehyde-3-phosphate, the reducing equivalents are transferred to the acceptor NAD^+ (Nicotinamide adenine dinucleotide). The reduced NADH under aerobic conditions enters into mitochondria and produces 3 molecules of ATP through its passage into electron transport chain or respiratory chain. This type of formation of energy currency ATP through respiratory chain is called as **oxidative phosphorylation**.

7. In the next step, the high-energy compound 1, 3-bisphosphoglycerate transfers its high energy to ADP to form ATP resulting in the formation of 3 phosphoglycerate. This reaction is catalyzed by phosphoglycerate kinase enzyme. This type of formation of energy currency ATP by high-energy substrate is called as **substrate level phosphorylation**.

8. The 3-phosphoglycerate is then isomerised to 2-phosphoglcerate by *phosphoglycerate mutase* enzyme.

9. The 2-phosphoglycerate is then converted to one more high-energy compound called as phosphoenolpyruvate. This reaction is catalyzed by *enolase* enzyme. The activity of this enzyme can be completely inhibited by fluoride. Hence, fluoride is used during blood collection for glucose estimation. This prevents the utilisation of glucose by RBC.

10. Later phosphoenolpyruvate is converted to pyruvate by pyruvate *kinase* enzyme. In this step, one molecule of ATP is formed by **substrate level phosphorylation**.

Under aerobic conditions, pyruvate is the end product of glycolysis.

Hence, pyruvate is then converted into acetyl CoA or oxaloacetate in the mitochondria.

Anaerobic glycolysis: Under anaerobic condition, pyruvate is reduced to lactate-by-lactate *dehydrogenase* enzyme. This step utilizes the reducing equivalent NADH formed in the earlier step. Thus, the number of ATP produced will be less in anaerobic condition.

Steps 5 and 10 are linked

➢ Glycolysis is the only major source of energy in anaerobiosis.

➢ For smooth operation of the pathway, NADH is to be converted to NAD^+.

➢ The formation of lactate allows the regeneration of NAD^+.

➢ NAD^+ reused by glyceraldehyde-3-P-dehydrogenase. So that glycolysis proceeds even in the absence of oxygen to supply ATP.

➢ Fate of pyruvate depends on the presence or absence of oxygen in the cells.

➢ The occurrence of uninterrupted glycolysis is very important in skeletal muscle during strenuous exercise.

➢ Brain, retina, renal medulla and GI (Gastrointestinal) tract derive energy from glycolysis.

➢ Glycolysis in the erythrocytes leads to lactate production, since the mitochondria, the centres for oxidation are absent.

Energetics of aerobic glycolysis per glucose molecule

1. Energy consuming steps of glycolysis are
   Step 1 and Step 3 $\longrightarrow$ 2 ATP

2. Energy yielding steps of glycolysis are
   a. Oxidative phosphorylation
      Step 6 $\longrightarrow$ NADH $\times$ 2 $\longrightarrow$ 3 ATP $\times$ 2 = 6 ATP
   b. Substrate level phosphorylation
      Step 7 and Step 10 $\longrightarrow$ 2 ATP $\times$ 2 = 4 ATP

   Total number of ATP produced = 10 ATP
   Net ATP production (10 – 2) = 8 ATP

Energetics of anaerobic glycolysis per glucose molecule

1. Energy consuming steps of glycolysis are
   Step 1 and Step 2 $\longrightarrow$ 2 ATP

2. Energy yielding steps of anaerobic glycolysis are
   Substrate level phosphorylation
      Step 7 and Step 10 $\longrightarrow$ 2 ATP $\times$ 2 = 4 ATP

   Total number of ATP produced = 4 ATP
   Net ATP production (4 – 2) = 2 ATP

Shuttle pathways

If the cytosolic NADH uses malate-aspartate shuttle, 3 ATPs are produced. If it uses glycerol phosphate shuttle produces 2 ATPs.

Regulation

Insulin favors glycolysis by activating key glycolytic enzymes like glucokinase, phospho-fructokinase (PFK) and pyruvate kinase.

Glucocorticoid inhibits glycolysis and favors gluconeogenesis.

Glu-6-P inhibits hexokinase. This enzyme prevents the accumulation of Glu-6-P.

PFK is the most important regulatory enzyme.

ATP, citrate and H^+ ions are the important allosteric inhibitors.

Fructose-2, 6-bisphosphate, AMP and Pi are the allosteric activators of PFK.

Role of fructose-2, 6-bisphosphate (F2, 6BP)

It is the most regulatory factor for controlling PFK and ultimately glycolysis in the liver.

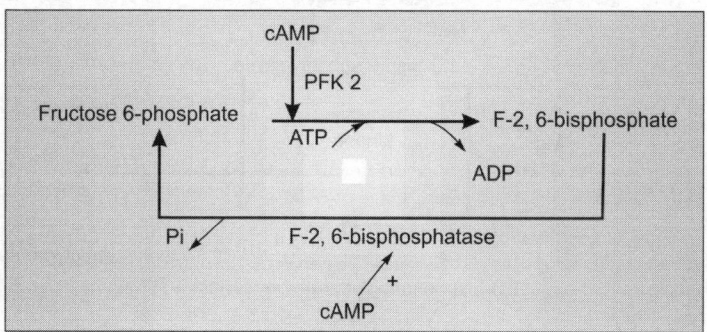

Figure 7.2

The function of synthesis and degradation of F2, 6BP is brought out by a single enzyme (with two active sites), which is bifunctional or tandem enzyme. The activity of these enzymes is controlled by covalent modification, which in turn regulated by cyclic AMP. The cAMP brings about the phosphorylation of the tandem enzyme, resulting in the inactivation of active site responsible for the synthesis of F2, 6BP but activation of the active site responsible for the hydrolysis of F2, 6BP.

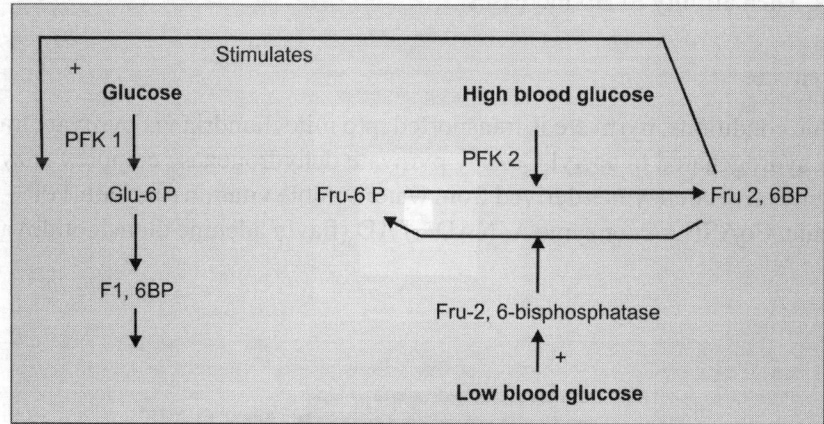

Figure 7.3

There is no stimulation when Fru-2, 6-bisphosphate decreases, with low **glucose** the PFK1 remains inactive.

Rapaport leubering cycle (BPG shunt)

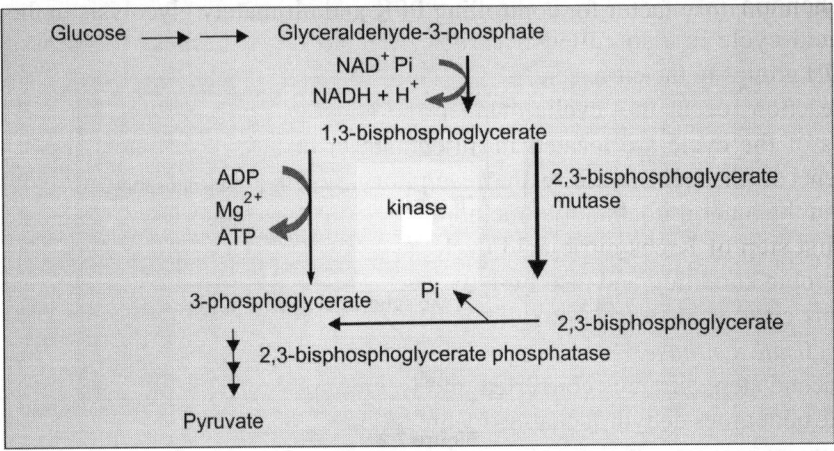

Figure 7.4

- Kinase reaction is bypassed in the erythrocytes.
- No energy is trapped from 2, 3-BPG.
- BPG when combines with Hb, reduces the affinity of Hb towards oxygen. In the presence of 2, 3-BPG, oxyhemoglobin will unload oxygen more easily in tissues.
- The 2, 3-BPG increases in hypoxic condition.
- 15 to 25% of the lactate formed goes through this pathway.
- In hexokinase deficiency, phosphorylation does not takes place further. So 2, 3-BPG decreases. Then affinity to Hb increases.

Fates of pyruvate

Under aerobic conditions, pyruvate is transported into mitochondria via pyruvate transporter. Then it is dehydrogenated to acetyl CoA by pyruvate dehydrogenase complex enzyme. This enzyme requires five coenzymes derived from water soluble vitamin (they are TPP = thiamine pyrophosphate, CoASH = coenzyme A, NAD$^+$, FAD (flavin adenine dinucleotide) and lipoic acid.

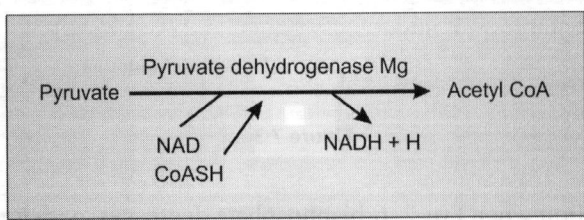

Figure 7.5

Krebs citric acid cycle (Figure 7.6)

Site: Mitochondria

➢ Citric acid cycle is also called tricarboxylic acid cycle because of the presence of 3 –COOH groups in the citric acid.

➢ These reactions occur in a cyclic manner and generate large amounts of ATP since the enzymes of the cycle are located in mitochondria facilitating the transfer of reducing equivalents from Krebs cycle to the respiratory chain, the enzymes of which are also located in the inner mitochondrial membrane.

➢ In the first step of Krebs citric acid cycle, acetyl CoA which is formed from pyruvate under aerobic condition and also by fatty acid oxidation combines with oxaloacetic acid and forms citric acid (a tricarboxylic acid). The reaction is catalyzed by a condensing enzyme *citrate synthase.*

➢ In the second step, citrate is converted into isocitrate by the action of *aconitase* enzyme. Isocitrate undergoes dehydrogenation by the *isocitrate dehydrogenase* enzyme in the third step to oxalosuccinate. Molecule of NADH formed enters into electron transport chain and forms 3 ATPs.

➢ This is followed by decarboxylation to form α-ketoglutarate with the help of *isocitrate dehydrogenase* enzyme.

➢ Then the α-ketoglutarate undergoes decarboxylation to form succinyl CoA in a manner similar to the conversion of pyruvate to acetyl CoA. This is catalyzed by *α-ketoglutarate dehydrogenase* enzyme. One molecule of NADH formed enters into electron transport chain and forms 3 ATPs.

➢ Succinyl CoA is then converted into succinate by the enzyme *succinate thiokinase.* In this step, a high-energy phosphate is produced by **substrate level phosphorylation**.

➢ In the next step, the dehydrogenation of succinate is catalyzed by mitochondrial inner membrane enzyme *succinate dehydrogenase.* This step produces 2 ATPs because of production of one molecule of $FADH_2$.

➢ *Fumarase* catalyzes the addition of water molecule to fumarate and forms malate.

➢ Malate is converted into oxaloacetate by *malate dehydrogenase* enzyme with production of one molecule of NADH, which is equivalent to 3 ATPs (step 8).

Cis-acontitate is a transient one with very short half-life. Immediate H_2O added to it and forms isocitrate.

$$\text{Isocitrate} \longleftrightarrow \text{oxalosuccinate} \xrightarrow{\text{CO}_2} \text{α-ketoglutarate.}$$

It is an oxidative decarboxylation.

Oxalosuccinate is unstable so it undergoes spontaneous decarboxylation to from α-KG.

Twelve ATPs are formed per turn of TCA cycle

Step 3, 4, 8 (3 NADH⁺)	$\longrightarrow$	3×3 ATP = 9 ATP
Step 6 (1 FADH₂)	$\longrightarrow$	2 ATP = 2 ATP
Step 5 (1 ATP)	$\longrightarrow$	1 ATP = 1 ATP
		12 ATP

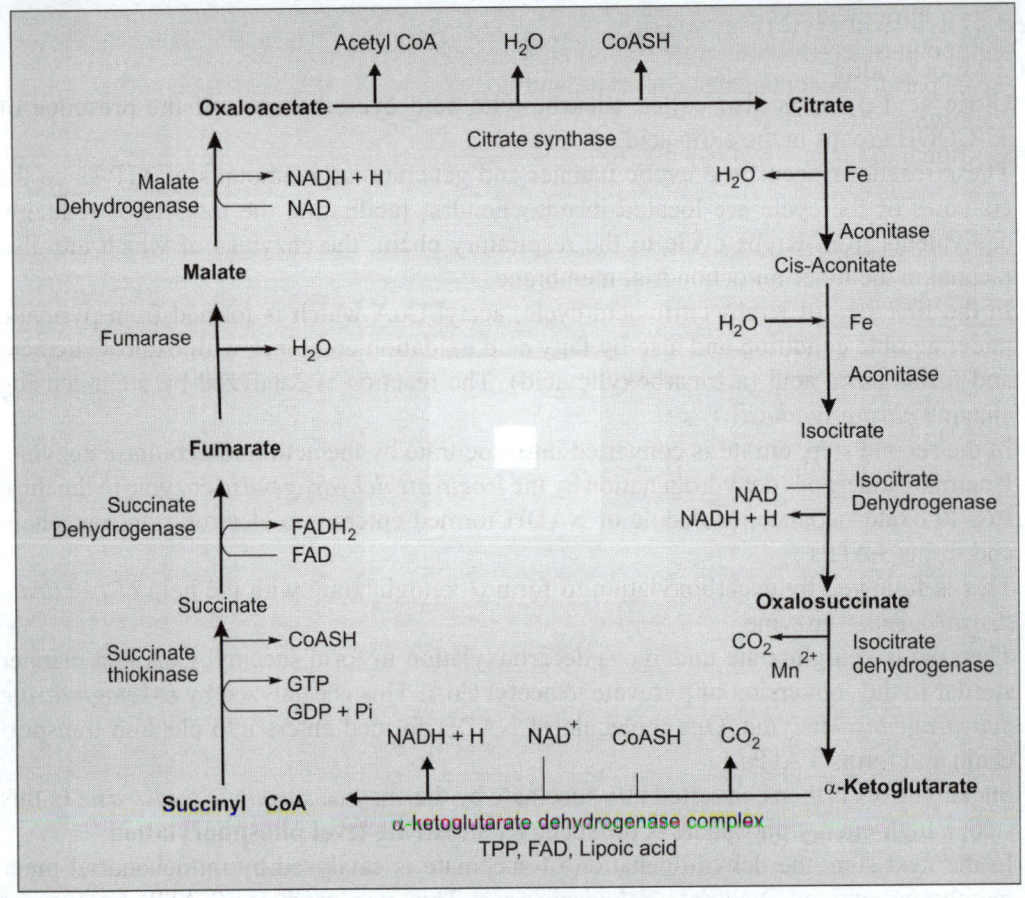

Figure 7.6

Total number of ATPs formed by the complete oxidation of glucose = 38 ATP

1. From aerobic glycolysis	= 10 ATP
2. Action of pyruvate dehydrogenase (3 × 2)	= 6 ATP
3. TCA cycle (2 mole pyruvate) 12 ATP × 2	= 24 ATP
	40 ATP
Number of ATPs utilized = 2 ATP	– 2 ATP
	Total = 38 ATP

Role of TCA cycle

1. It is the energy producing final pathway for the oxidation of glucose; acetyl CoA formed from fatty acid breakdown and amino acids.
2. It also provides citrate for fatty acid synthesis.
3. The intermediates of TCA cycle are used for the synthesis of amino acids, glucose by gluconeogenesis.

4. Since citric acid cycle is involved in the synthesis as well as breakdown of biological compounds, it is called as amphibolic pathway (i.e. both anabolic and catabolic). TCA cycle takes part in gluconeogensis, transamination, deamination and synthesis of fatty acids.

Regulation of citric acid cycle: TCA cycle is controlled by respiratory rate, which is proportional to the energy consumption. The level of NAD^+ also stimulates the TCA cycle.

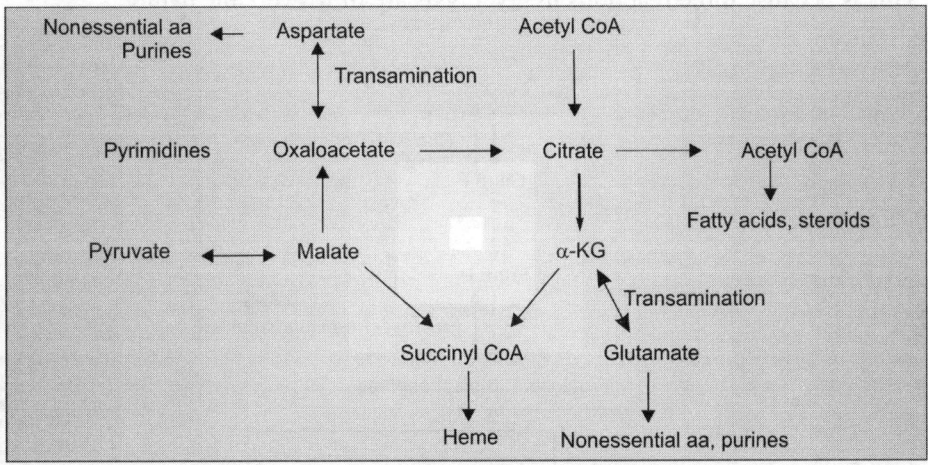

Figure 7.7

Inhibitors that inhibit the enzymes of TCA cycle:

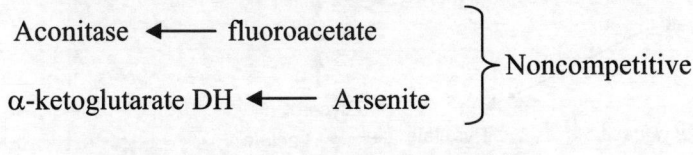

Succinate DH ◄─── Malonate} Competitive

Regulation of TCA cycle

1. Citrate synthase: Inhibited by ATP, NADH, acyl CoA and succinyl CoA.
2. Isocitrate dehydrogenase: Inhibited by ATP and NADH and activated by ADP.
3. α-KG inhibited by NADH and succinyl CoA.
    *   The availability of ADP: Important to proceeding the TCA cycle, if not oxidation of NADH and $FADH_2$ through election chain stops. Accumulations of NADH and $FADH_2$, inhibit the enzymes of TCA cycle.

Gluconeogenesis (Figure 7.8)

Gluconeogensis is the process of formation of glucose from various noncarbohydrate sources such as glucogenic amino acids (refer chemistry of amino acids), lactate, pyruvate, glycerol or propionate.

Gluconeogensis occurs in the fasting state or on a low carbohydrate diet particularly in liver and some other tissues, which are solely dependent on glucose for their energy demand. The major metabolic significance of gluconeogensis is to maintain the blood glucose level and to supply glucose for brain and cardiac muscle.

Glycolysis is the breakdown of glucose, whereas gluconeogensis is the synthesis of glucose from noncarbohydrate sources. But both these processes are not exactly reciprocal to each other. This is because three reactions in glycolysis are of irreversible nature.

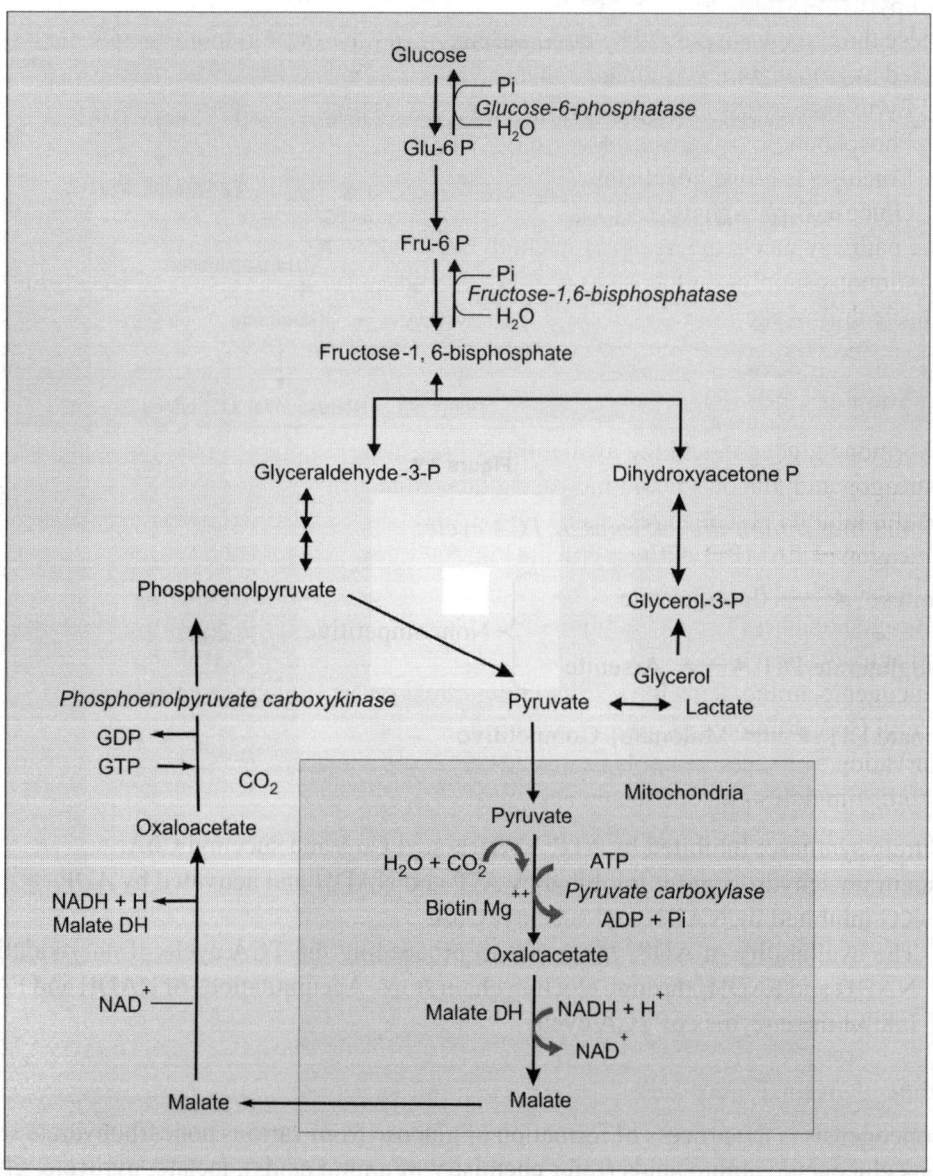

Figure 7.8

- Mainly occurs in cytosol.
- Some precursors are produced in mitochondria.
- Takes place in liver and kidney.
- Synthesis of glucose or glycogen from noncarbohydrates like pyruvate, lactate, glucogenic amino acids, glycerol and propionic acid.
- Pathway involves steps of TCA cycle and reversal of glycolysis.
- The "3" irreversible steps of glycolysis are catalyzed by hexokinase, phosphofructokinase and pyruvate kinase.
- These three stages bypassed by alternate enzymes specific to gluconeogenesis and they are called as key enzymes of gluconeogenesis.
  1. Pyruvate carboxylase
  2. Phosphoenolpyruvate carboxykinase (PEPCK)
  3. Fructose-1, 6-bisphosphatase
  4. Glucose-6-phosphatase
- The pathway meets the needs of the body for glucose.
- Continuous supply of glucose as a source of energy for the CNS, brain, RBC and skeletal muscle during starvation.

Regulation of gluconeogenesis

The hormone glucagon and the availability of substrates mainly regulate gluconeogenesis.
  Glucagon and glucocorticoid increase gluconeogenesis.
  Insulin inhibits gluconeogenesis.
- Glucagon → cAMP→ active pyruvate kinase → inactive pyruvate kinase → phosphoenol-pyruvate → reduced → pyruvate ↓
- Glucagon reduces the concentration of fructose-2, 6-bisphosphate so, PFK1 remains inactive and activates fructose-1, 6-bisphosphatase that favors gluconeogenesis.
- Glucogenic amino acids have stimulating effect on key gluconeogenic enzymes.
- Acetyl CoA promotes gluconeogenesis.
- Starvation → excessive lipolysis in adipose tissues and acetyl CoA accumulates in the liver, which stimulates gluconeogenic enzymes.

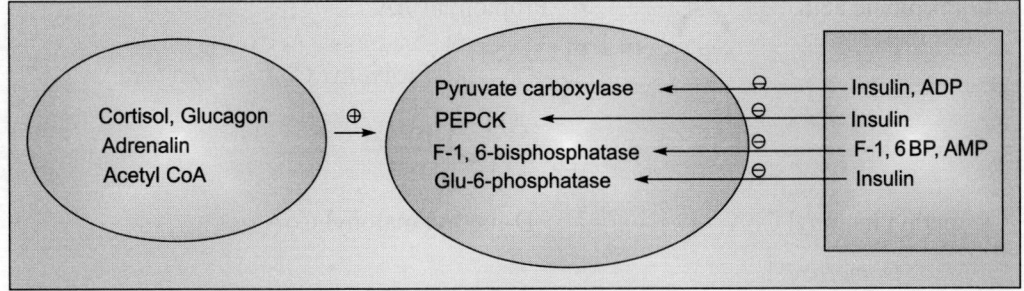

Figure 7.9

Substrates for Gluconeogenesis

Gly, Ala, Ser, Thr, Cys, Trp → pyruvate → oxaloacetate

Arg, His, Glu, gln, pro → α-KG →→→ oxaloacetate →→ Glucose

   Phe, Tyr, Asp, Asn → fumarate

   Val, isoleucine, Met → succinyl CoA

Propionyl CoA →→ succinyl CoA → oxaloacetate

1. Lactate and glucogenic amino acids are the most important substrates

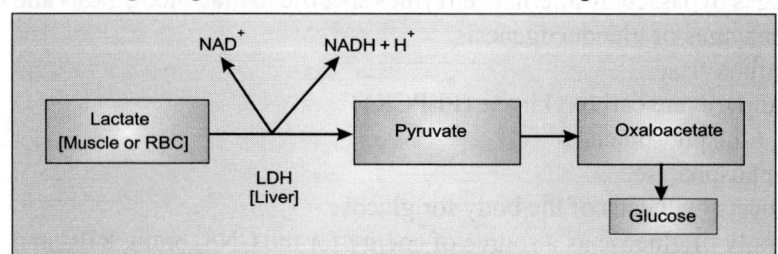

Figure 7.10

2. Glucose-alanine cycle

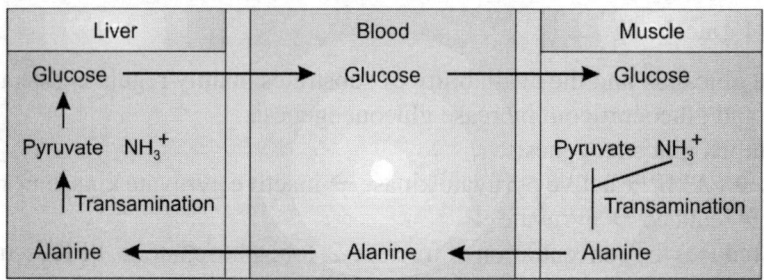

Figure 7.11

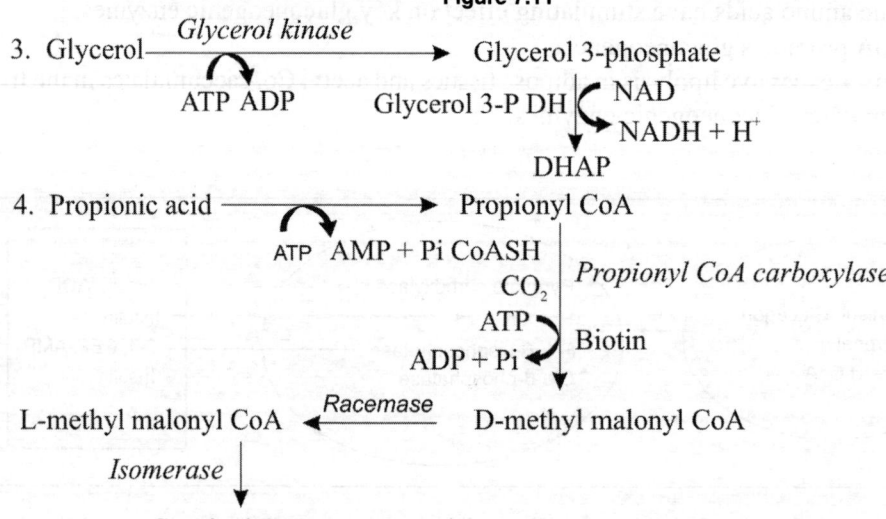

3. Glycerol —*Glycerol kinase*→ Glycerol 3-phosphate
   ATP ADP   Glycerol 3-P DH ⟨ NAD
                                    ⟩ NADH + H⁺
                              DHAP

4. Propionic acid ——→ Propionyl CoA
   ATP AMP + Pi CoASH
           CO₂ *Propionyl CoA carboxylase*
           ATP ⟩ Biotin
   ADP + Pi

L-methyl malonyl CoA ←*Racemase*— D-methyl malonyl CoA

Isomerase ↓

   Succinyl CoA

Cori's cycle

It is the process of conversion of glucose/glycogen to lactate in the muscle and this lactate is converted back to glucose in liver.

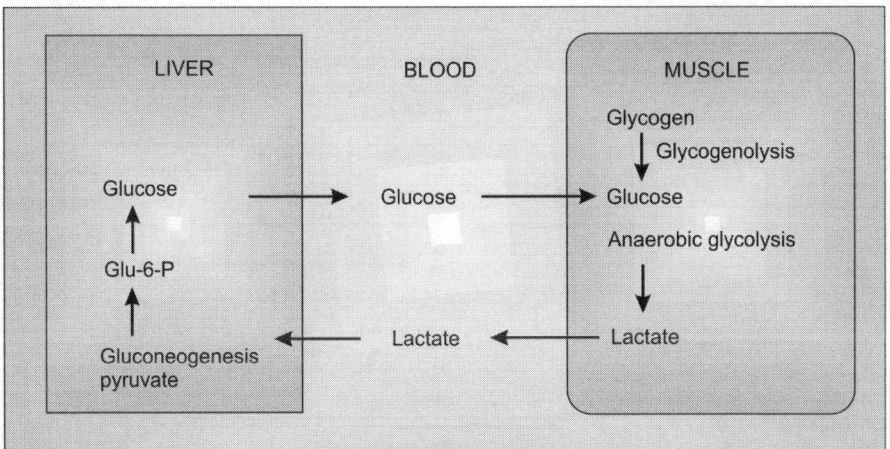

Figure 7.12: *Cori's cycle*

- During active muscle contraction glycogen breaks down and glucose-6-p formed, enters anaerobic glycolysis to form lactate → blood → liver → → glucose → blood → tissues.

Metabolism of glycogen

- Glycogen is the storage form of glucose in our body.
- Glycogen is mainly stored in muscle and liver.
- Stored glycogen of liver is used for maintaining blood glucose level during hypoglycemia. The muscle glycogen is used for providing energy during exercise.

Glycogenesis (Figures 7.13 and 7.14)

The synthesis of glycogen from glucose is called glycogenesis.

It is operative in several tissues but liver and muscle are the main organs for the synthesis of glycogen.

1. For its conversion to glycogen, glucose is firstly phosphorylated to form glucose-6-phosphate by the enzyme *hexokinase*, which also requires ATP and Mg^{2+}. In the fed state another enzyme *glucokinase*, present in the liver, converts most of the glucose into glycogen.
2. Glucose-6-phosphate is then epimerised to form glucose-1-phosphate by *phosphoglucomutase* enzyme.
3. Glucose-1-phosphate reacts with UTP and is converted to uridine diphosphate glucose (UDP-Glucose). This reaction is catalyzed by *UDP-glucose pyrophosphorylase* enzyme. Pyrophosphate released during this process is hydrolyzed to inorganic phosphate.
4. From UDP-glucose, glucose is transferred to preexisting glycogen molecule called as glycogen primer. The incoming glucose is linked to the precursor glycogen by α 1-4 glycosidc linkages resulting in the elongation of preexisting branches.

5. When the chain length is increased by 10–12 glucose molecules, a minimum length of six glucose molecules, is transferred from this by the branching enzyme onto the neighboring chain in such a way that, it forms a new branching point (α 1-6 linkage).

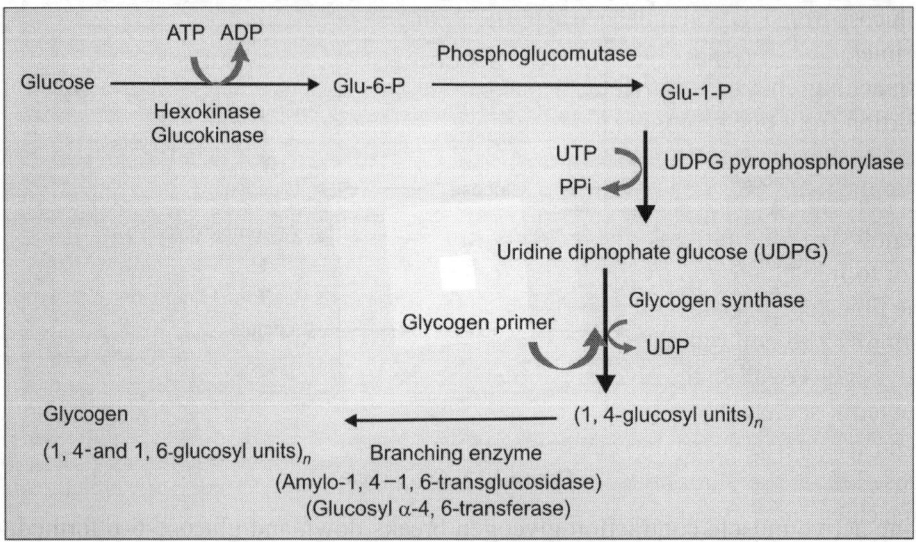

Figure 7.13: *Glycogenesis*

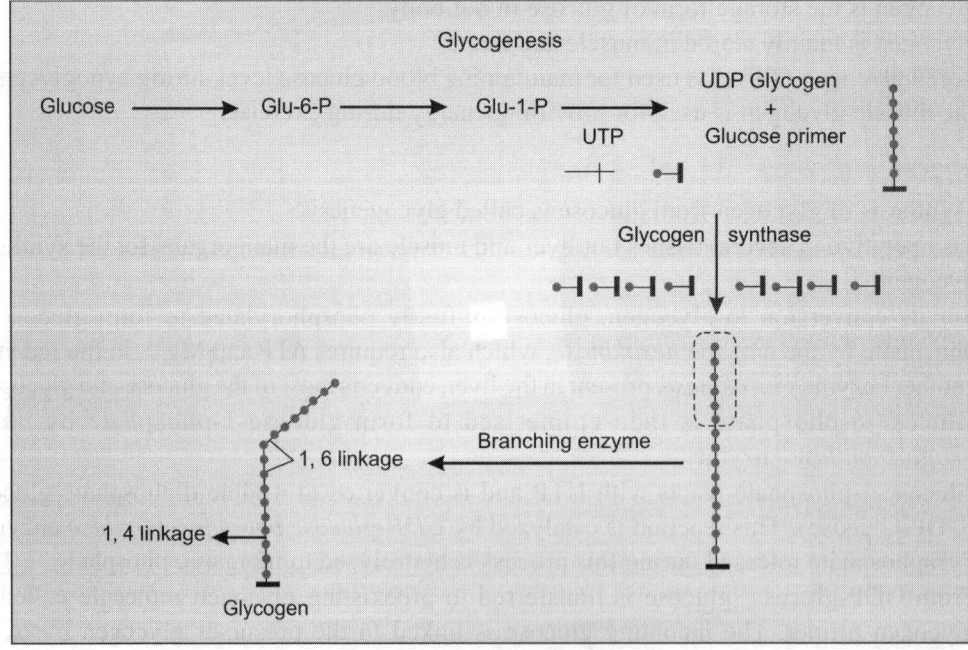

Figure 7.14: *Glycogenesis*

6. The branch again grows by the addition of the glucose molecules at the α 1-4 linkage. With the further branching it results in the formation of a highly branched polymer of glucose called glycogen.
   • UDPG is the carrier of glucose.
   • Glucose from UDPG is attached at the nonreducing end of glucose molecules of glycogen primer.
   • Branching enzyme (Amylo 1, 4 –1, 6 transglucosidase transfers 6 glucose residues portion from one chain to a neighboring chain to form a α-1, 6 linkage.

Glycogenolysis (Figure 7.15 and 7.16)

Glycogenolysis is the process of breakdown of glycogen either to glucose-6-phosphate in muscle or to free glucose in liver.

1. In the first step, glucose molecules are sequentially removed as glucose-1-phosphate. This reaction is rate controlling step and is catalyzed by *glycogen phosphorylase* enzyme. It removes glucose from the glycogen molecule until nearly four glucose residues are left on the outermost chain.
2. *Glucan transferase* enzyme transfers a trisaccharide unit out of the four molecules of glucose left on the outer branch to the neighboring exposed branch point.
3. Debranching enzyme removes the glucose molecule present at the branch point as free glucose.
4. Thus with the combined action of glycogen phosphorylase, glucan transferase and debranching enzyme; the glycogen molecule is hydrolyzed to glucose-1-phosphate and free glucose.
5. Glucose-1-phosphate formed is converted into glucose-6-phosphate by *phosphoglucomutase* enzyme.
6. In liver and kidney, glucose-6-phosphate further hydrolyzed to glucose by the action of glucose-6-phosphatase enzyme. This enzyme is absent in muscle. Hence, muscle glycogen cannot be converted in to glucose. Liver glycogen is mainly used to maitain the level of blood glucose.

$$\text{Glycogen} \xrightarrow[\text{Phosphorylase}]{\text{Pi}} \text{Glu-1-P} \xrightarrow{\text{Phosphoglucomutase}} \text{Glu-6-P} \xrightarrow[\text{Glu-6-phosphatase}]{\text{H}_2\text{O Pi}} \text{Glucose}$$

• Phosphorylase phosphorolytically splits α-1, 4 glucoside bonds from the outermost chains of glycogen until 4 residues remain on either side of α-1, 6 branch point [limit dextrin].
• α-1, 4 glucan transferase transfers 3 glucose residue portions from one side chain to the other exposing α-1, 6 branch points.
• Amylo 1, 6-glucosidase splits the 1, 6 linkages.

Muscle glycogenolysis

Glycogen → Glu-1-P → Glu-6-P → glycolysis → lactate

Regulation of glycogenesis and glycogenolysis.
• The glycogen synthase and phosphorylase exist in active and inactive forms.
• The dephosphorylated form of glycogen synthase is active.

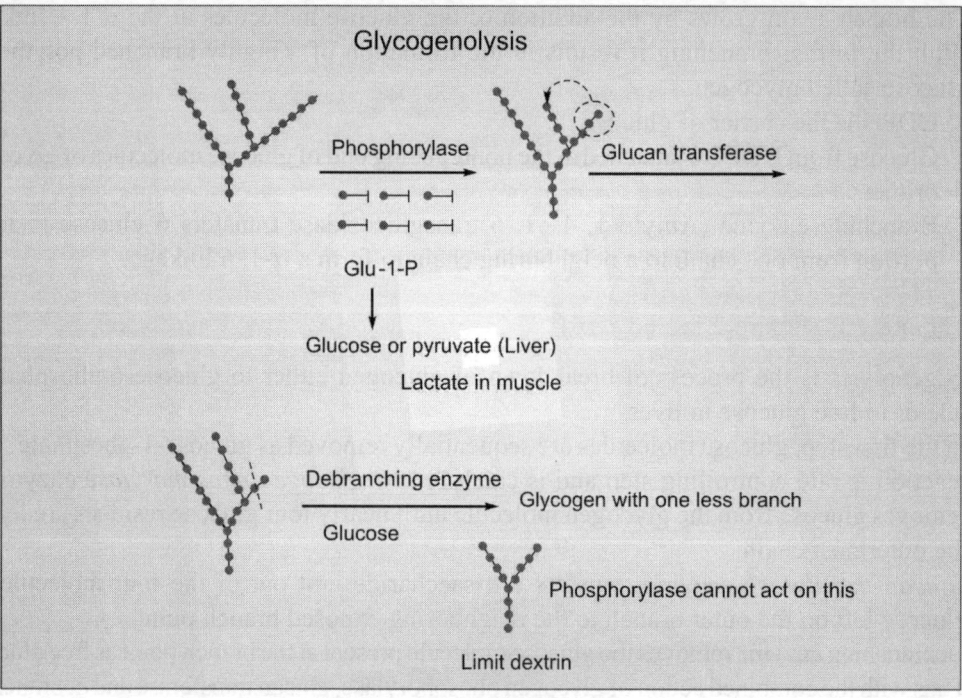

Figure 7.15: *Glycogenolysis*

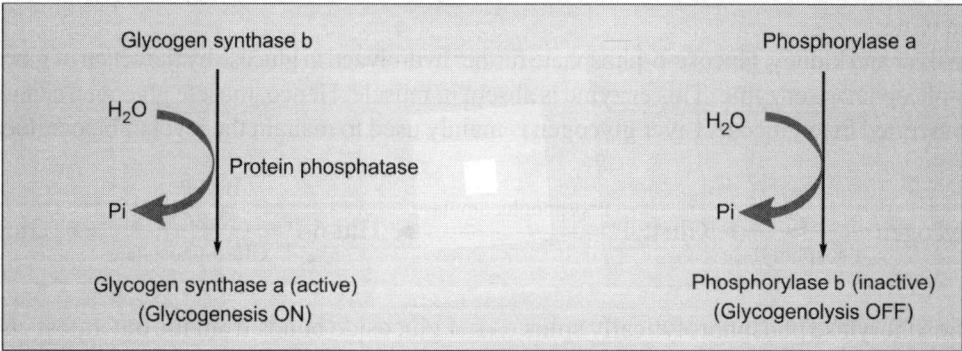

Figure 7.16: *Regulation of glycogen metabolism*

- Phosphorylated form of phosphorylase is active.
- The activation of phosphorylase depends on high cAMP level. At the same time high cAMP level inactivates glycogen synthase.

Allosteric regulation

- In a well fed state, glu-6-P level is high which activates glycogen synthase.
- On the other hand, glu-6-P and ATP allosterically inhibit phosphorylase.
- Free glucose also acts, as inhibitor to phosphorylase.

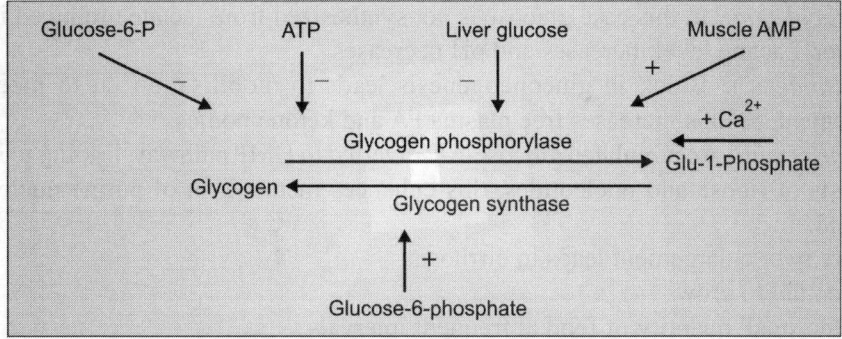

Figure 7.17: *Regulators of glycogen metabolism*

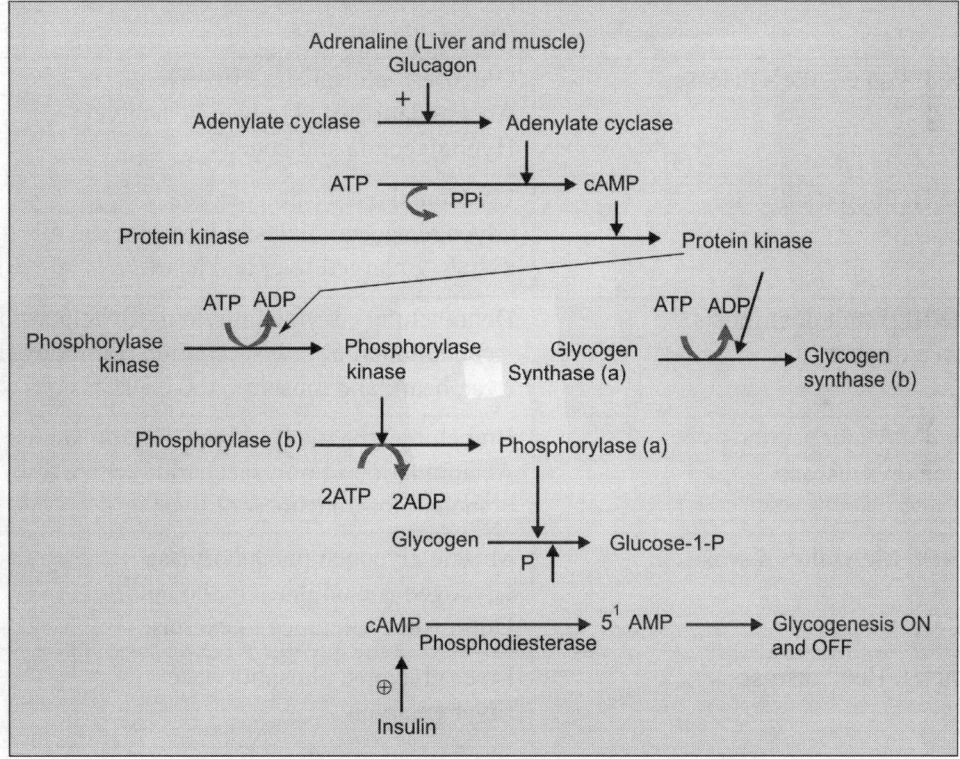

Figure 7.18: *Regulation of glycogen synthase and phosphorylase*

GLYCOGEN STORAGE DISEASES

- Genetic diseases [may be inherited].
- Deposition of abnormal type or abnormal quantity of glycogen in the tissues.

Von Gierke's Disease

1. Fasting hypoglycemia.

2. *Lactic acidemia:* In this case glucose is not synthesized from lactate produced in muscle and liver. Lactate level increases and pH decreases.

3. *Hyperlipidemia:* Block in gluconeogenesis leads to mobilisation fat to meet energy requirement. So this increases free plasma FA and ketone bodies.

4. *Hyperuricemia:* Accumulated glucose-6-P diverted to HMP pathway, leading to increased synthesis of ribose and nucleotides, this enhances metabolism of purine nucleotides to uric acid.

5. Massive liver enlargement leads to cirrhosis.

6. Children fail to grow.
   ➤ Given small quantity of food at frequent intervals.

Table 7.2	
Diseases	*Defect and features*
Type I. von Gierke's disease	Glucose-6-phosphatase [liver] Accumulation of glycogen in the liver Hypoglycemia and ketosis
Type II. Pompe's disease	Lysosomal α-1, 4-glucosidase Glycogen accumulates in lysosomes in all tissues. Enlarged liver and heart
Type III. Limit dextrinosis [Cori's disease]	Debranching enzyme [amylo α-1, 6-glucosidase Accumulation of polysaccharide [limit dextrin] liver, heart, and muscle
Type IV. Amylopectinosis or Anderson's disease	Branching enzyme [glucosyl 4, 6 transferase] Accumulation of polysaccharide with a few branch points, cirrhosis of liver
Type V. McArdle's disease	Muscle glycogen phosphorylase Glycogen accumulates in the muscle Diminished tolerance to exercise
Type VI. Hers' disease	Liver glycogen phosphorylase Liver enlarged

HMP Shunt or Pentose phosphate pathway or phosphogluconate pathway

An alternative pathway to glycolysis and TCA cycle for the oxidation of glucose.

Location: Cytosol—liver, adipose tissue, adrenal gland, RBC, testes and lactating mammary gland are highly active in HMP shunt.

These tissues except RBC, are involved in the biosynthesis of fatty acids, which are dependent on the supply of NADPH.

$$\text{Glucose-6-P} + H_2O + 2\ NADP^+ \rightarrow \text{Ribulose-5-P} + CO_2 + 2NADPH + 2\ H^+$$

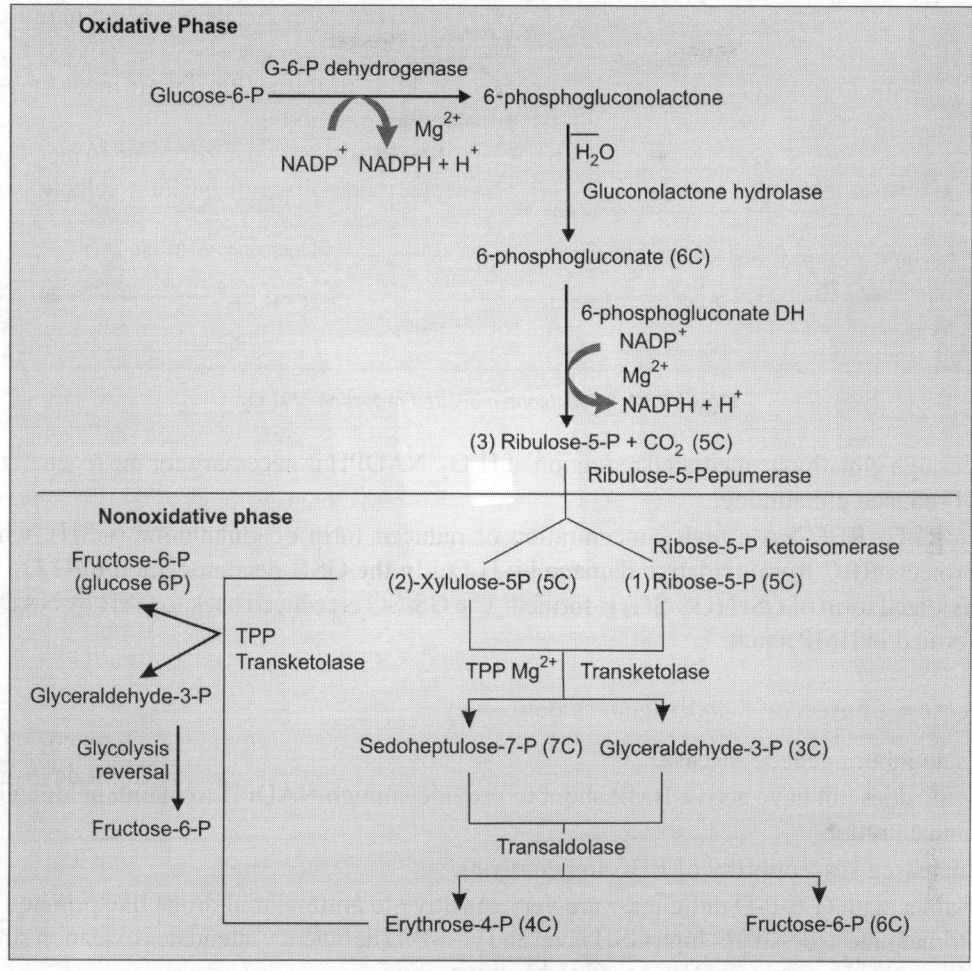

Figure 7.19: *HMP shunt*

Three molecules of Ribulose-5-P are required in the nonoxidative phase multiplying the above step.

3 mol. G-6-P + 3 H_2O = 6 $NADP^+$ → 3 mol. Ribulose-5-P + $3CO_2$ + 6NADPH + 6 H^+

Significance of HMP Shunt

➤ Generating pentoses and NADPH.
➤ The pentoses or its derivatives (Ribose-5-P) are useful for the synthesis of nucleic acids and nucleotides like ATP, NAD^+, FAD.
➤ NADPH is required for the biosynthesis of FA, steroids and synthesis of glutamic acid.
➤ The continuous production of H_2O_2 in living cells can chemically damage unsaturated lipids, proteins. This is prevented through antioxidant reactions involving NADPH that is

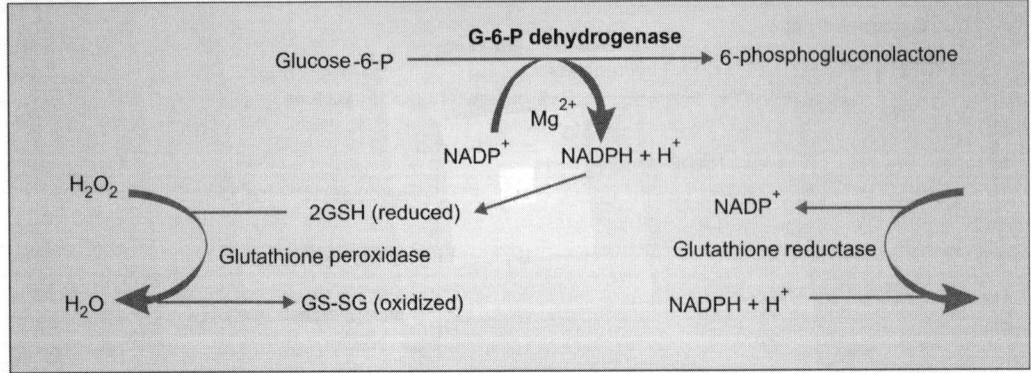

Figure 7.20: *Glutathione mediated reduction of H_2O_2*

through glutathione mediated reduction of H_2O_2. NADPH is necessary for the regeneration of reduced glutathione.

➤ In RBC: RBC has a high concentration of reduced form of glutathione (GSH), which protects RBC from oxidative damage by H_2O_2. In the GSH decomposition of H_2O_2, the oxidized form of GSH (GS-SG) is formed. The GS-SG is reduced back to GSH by NADPH formed in HMP shunt.

Glucose-6-phosphate dehydrogenase deficiency

➤ Is an inborn genetic disease.
➤ RBC does not have active HMP shunt to provide enough NADPH to maintain high GSH concentration.
➤ Increased susceptibility of RBC to hemolysis.
➤ Babies with G-6-P-D deficiency are very sensitive to antimalarial drugs like primaquine.
➤ Primaquine necessitates high GSH level and G-6-P-D deficiency attenuates oxidation stress.
➤ When the drugs given, RBCs tend to hemolyze.
➤ Drugs like aspirin and sulfa drugs also cause hemolysis of RBCs.
➤ The G-6-P-D estimation is useful when:
  • The patient is suffering from severe hemolytic anemia.
  • Treating the patient with antimalarial drugs.

Galactose metabolism

Galactosemia

• Due to the deficiency of galactose 1-phosphate uridyltransferase.
• Is a rare congenital disease in infants.
• Galactose accumulated   → galactosemia (blood)
                            → galactosuria (urine)
• High level of galactose in blood is reduced by aldose reductase in the eye to galacitol, which accumulated causing cataract.

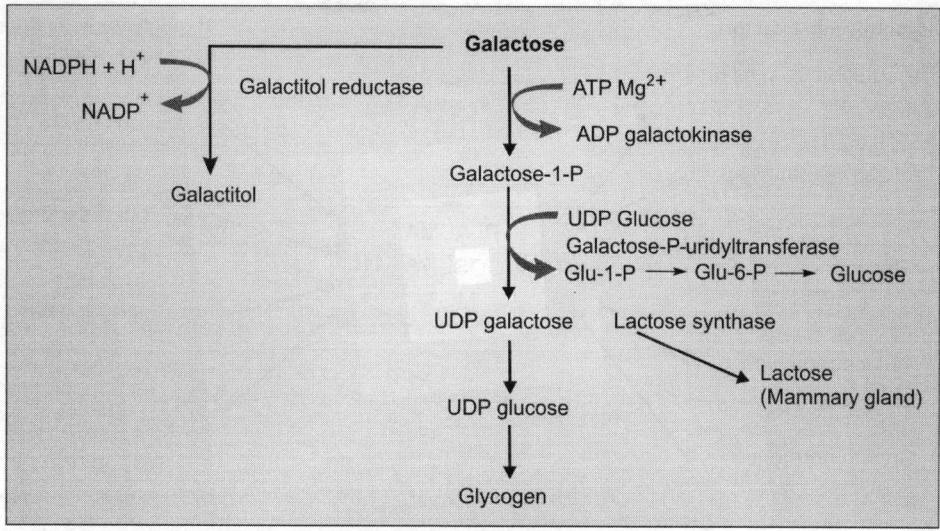

Figure 7.21: Galactose metabolism

- The accumulation of gal-1-p and galactitol in tissues like liver, nervous tissue, lens and kidney lead to impaired functions.

    Symptoms: Weight loss in infants, hepatosplenomegaly, jaundice, mental retardation, etc. in severe conditions, cataract aminoaciduria and albuminuria are observed.

    Treatment: Withdrawal of the diet containing galactose and lactose.

Fate of galactose

1. In liver, most of the galactose is converted into UDP-galactose and then to liver glycogen.
2. It is also used for the synthesis of glycolipid in brain and nervous tissue.

    In lactating mammary gland, galactose is converted into lactose by *synthase* enzyme.

BLOOD GLUCOSE REGULATION

The concentration of glucose in the blood is regulated by several metabolic pathways which are mainly modulated by several hormones. The major metabolic pathways are glycogenesis, glycogenolysis, gluconeogenesis, glycolysis, TCA cycle, HMP shunt, lipogenesis, lipolysis and protein synthesis.

During a brief fast: The decrease in the blood glucose level is avoided by breakdown of glycogen stored in the liver. After a meal, the absorbed glucose is converted to glycogen or fat.

Postprandial blood sugar regulation: After the meal, absorption of glucose from the intestine increases the glucose level in the blood. The increased blood glucose stimulates the β cells of pancreas to secrete insulin.

Fasting blood sugar regulation: In normal conditions after 4–5 hour of a meal, blood glucose level decreases near to fasting levels. Further decrease in the blood glucose is prevented by the hyperglycemic hormones.

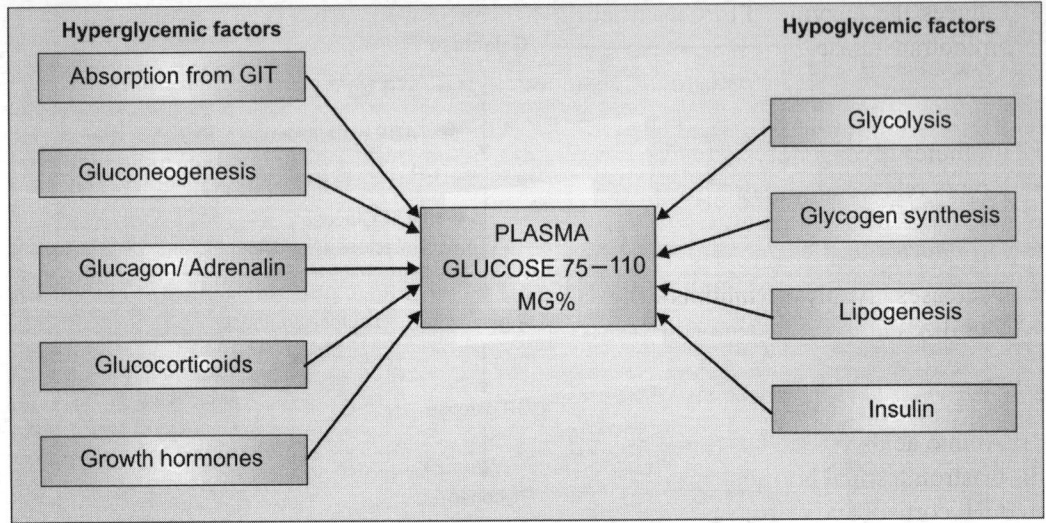

Figure 7.22: *Hyperglycemic and hypoglycemic factors*

Normal levels

Fasting: After 12 hr of fasting, the sugar estimated 70–110 mg%.

PPBS: After 2 hr of normal breakfast or lunch, sugar estimated 90–140 mg%.

RBS: At any time, sugar estimated 90–150 mg%.

Regulation by hormones

Insulin (Hypoglycemic hormone)

- Insulin lowers blood glucose
- Favors glycogen synthesis
- Promotes glycolysis
- Inhibits gluconeogenesis

Glucagon

- Promotes gluconeogenesis
- Enhances glycogenolysis
- Decreases glycogen synthesis
- Inhibits glycolysis
- Promotes fatty acid oxidation, energy production and ketone body synthesis
- Amino acid uptake by the liver promotes glycogenolysis

Cortisol

- Increases glycogenolysis
- Enhances release of amino acids by the muscle

- Induces the enzymes PEPCK, fructose-1, 6-bisphosphatase, glucose-6-phosphatase and aminotransferase

Adrenaline

- Promotes glycogenolysis
- Favors release of glucose

Growth hormone

- Decreases glycolysis (inhibits PFK)
- Mobilizes fatty acids from adipose tissues

Factors stimulating insulin secretion

 i. Amino acids
 ii. Gastrointestinal hormones
iii. GH, cortisol and estrogens
iv. Glucose is the important stimulus for the insulin release.

Factors inhibiting insulin secretion

 i. Epinephrine suppresses insulin secretion and promotes energy metabolism by mobilizing energy yielding compounds like glucose from liver and fatty acids from adipose tissue.

DIABETES MELLITUS

It is a clinical condition characterized by increased blood glucose level due to absence or insufficient insulin.

It is broadly divided into two types namely:
Type I: Insulin-dependent diabetes mellitus (IDDM).
Type II: Noninsulin-dependent diabetes mellitus.

Type I or juvenile onset diabetes: (12–15 years age) Characterized by total deficiency of insulin due to destruction of cells of pancreas.
Patient usually develops:
Polyuria: Large amount of glucose and water excretion.
Polydypsia: Loss of fluid stimulates the thirst center. Person drinks more and more water.
Polyphagia: Lipid and protein breakdowns, more weight loss. Person eats more frequently.
Patient may show boils, abscesses, cellulites. Complications of this type are retinopathy neuropathy and nephropathy.

Noninsulin-dependent diabetes mellitus

This type comprises 90% of all diabetic population. The patients have minimum symptoms.
- Not dependent on insulin.
- Obesity is common with NIDDM.
- Usually occurs after the age of 40 years. Sometimes in young person also.

Diagnosis: Type I can be known by serious metabolic disturbances with increased blood glucose.

Criteria for the diagnosis
- All adults older than 45 years of age should have a measurement of fasting blood glucose for every three months.
- Person with BMI of 27 kg/m^2.
- Persons with family history of diabetes mellitus.
- Individual with history of gestational diabetes mellitus or delivery of large baby.
- With HDL < 35 mg.
- Persons with impaired glucose tolerance.
- Elevated fasting glucose on more than one occasion.

Diabetes due to secondary causes
- Pancreatic disease
- Cushing's syndrome
- Acromegaly (increased GH)
- Increased secretion of glucagon (tumour of pancreas)
- Hyperaldosteronism

Metabolic changes in diabetes mellitus
Carbohydrate metabolism
- Hyperglycemia (↓ or impaired transport and uptake of glucose in muscles and adipose tissue)
- Key glycolytic enzymes decrease
- Increased gluconeogenesis
- Glycogen synthesis decreases
- Glycosylated Hb increases in uncontrolled diabetes mellitus
- Sorbitol pathway: hyperglycemia → glucose → sorbitol
- Increased amino acids breakdown
Protein metabolism: Protein synthesis decreases
Fat metabolism: Fatty acid synthesis decreases
Lipid breakdown increases
FA → acetyl CoA → cholesterol syntheis or ketone body formation.

Clinical complications of diabetes mellitus are:

Retinopathy
- Hyperglycemia leads to sorbitol formation.
- This may lead to retinal microvascular abnormalities—leads to retinopathy and blindness.

Neuropathy
- A common complication.
- Identified by symptoms like pain, numbness, tingling or burning sensation in extremities.

Angiopathy

- Damage of basement membrane of blood vessels.
- It increases risk of stroke and coronary artery disease.
- It may cause atherosclerosis in medium sized cerebral arteries (leading to paralysis) and coronary arteries. (Leading to myocardial information) or peripheral vessels (Leading to gangrene of limbs).
- If small vesicles are affected, it is called microaniopathy.
- Microangiopathy leads to diabetic retinopathy and nephropathy.

Nephropathy

- Damages to the glomerulus of nephron of kidney and associated capillaries.
- This leads to ↓ filtering capacity.
- Capillary damage is caused by angiopathy. Urinary protein detection is useful in the diagnosis of nephropathy.

Hyperlipidemia and atherosclerosis

- Serum triglyceride, cholesterol and VLDL levels increase in type II
- HDL decreases
- These factors increased the risk of atherosclerosis.

Diabetic ketoacidosis

Deficiency of insulin increases the lipid breakdown → increased acetyl CoA → increased cholesterol and ketone bodies. In this condition, acetone smell of breath, ketonuria and ketonemia seen. Whole condition is called as ketosis. This leads to the decreased in blood pH.

Metabolic acidosis seen due to diabetes, so it is called as diabetic ketoacidosis.

Hyperglycemic hyperosmolar non-ketotic Coma (HHNC)

Characterised by glu > 600 mg %.

Blood pH slightly decreases or normal. Serum osmolality > 350 mosm/kg. Osmotic diuresis due to glycosuria causes severe H_2O and electrolyte depletion.

Coma results from dehydration of cerebral cells.

HHNC primarily seen in type II.

Lactic Acidosis

Cause: Accumulation of lactic acid due to over production or under utilisation.

If diabetic patients treated with hypoglycemic drugs (phenformins), lactic acidosis seen.

Infection: Susceptible to infection.

Pregnancy: Fetal abnormalities, premature birth, bag babies, chances of absorption, if they are not treated for diabetes.

Self Test

Long essay questions

1. Outline the reactions of anaerobic glycolysis. Give its energetics.
2. Briefly discuss the aerobic glycolysis under the following headings.
   a. reactions
   b. energetics
   c. regulation
3. Explain the steps involved in TCA cycle. Give the energetics.
4. Mention the importance of TCA cycle.
5. Describe how glycogen is formed and utilised in human body.
6. Discuss the metabolism which follows the strenuous exercise.
7. Explain the significance of HMP shunt.
8. Give the key reactions of gluconeogenesis.
9. How pyruvate is converted to acetyl CoA?

Short essay questions

1. Which pathway is referred to as amphibolic pathway?
2. Name the linkage present in glycogen at branching point.
3. Glucose-6-phosphatase deficiency leads what?
4. Which enzyme converts glucose to glucose-6-phosphate during fed state?
5. What do call if conversion of muscle lactates into liver glucose?
6. Which pathway helps in the detoxication of bilirubin?
7. Which enzyme deficiency leads to galactosemia?
8. Name the deficient enzyme in von Gierke's disease.
9. Which enzyme deficiency leads to McArdle's disease?
10. Name the enzyme, which is deficient in lactose intolerance.

Multiple choice questions

1. **All of the following are inhibitors of the TCA cycle EXCEPT**
   a. aconitase
   b. malonate
   c. fluoroacetate
   d. fluoride

2. **One of the following enzymes catalyzes substrate level phosphorylation**
   a. hexokinase
   b. enolase
   c. phosphoglycerate kinase
   d. succinate dehydrogenase

3. **The non-competitive inhibitor that inhibits glyceraldehyde-3-P dehydrogenase is**
   a. fluoride
   b. bromohydroxy acetone-P
   c. malonate
   d. arsenite

4. **The number of ATP molecules produced on complete oxidation of glucose under aerobic condition is**
   a. 38 ATP
   b. 10 ATP
   c. 2 ATP
   d. 8 ATP

5. **All of the following are the rate limiting enzymes of gluconeogenesis EXCEPT**
   a. pyruvate kinase
   b. glucose-6-phosphatase
   c. fructose-6-phosphatase
   d. phosphoenol pyruvate carboxykinase

6. **All of the following organs contain glucose-6-phosphatase EXCEPT**
   a. kidney
   b. liver
   c. muscle
   d. intestine

7. One of the following is NOT a symptom of von Gierke's disease is
   a. liver enlargement
   b. fasting hypoglycemia
   c. ketosis
   d. hypouricemia

8. The hexose monophosphate shunt is located in
   a. cytosol   c. lysosome
   b. mitochondrion   d. golgi apparatus

9. Hexokinase
   a. is present in all the tissues
   b. phosphorylates hexoses
   c. is not inhibited by glucose-6-phosphate
   d. has high affinity for substrates

10. The end product of muscle glycolysis is
    a. pyruvate
    b. fructose-6-P
    c. glyceraldehyde-3-phosphate
    d. lactate

11. Regarding 2, 3 BPG, the following statements are true EXCEPT
    a. it binds to oxyhemoglobin and helps in unloading of oxygen
    b. it reduces the affinity of hemoglobin to oxygen
    c. it does not bind to hemoglobin
    d. its concentration increases in hypoxic conditions

12. All of the following enzymes catalyze irreversible steps in glycolysis EXCEPT
    a. pyruvate kinase
    b. hexokinase
    c. enolase
    d. phosphofructokinase

13. All of the following inhibit the enzyme glycogen phosphorylase EXCEPT
    a. glucose-6-phosphate
    b. ATP
    c. AMP
    d. liver glucose

14. The pathway that predominantly produces NADPH is
    a. TCA cycle   b. glycolysis
    c. HMP shunt   d. gluconeogenesis

15. A classical example of exergonic reaction is the hydrolysis of
    a. ADP   b. GMP
    c. ATP   d. GTP

16. The end product of anaerobic glycolysis is
    a. pyruvate
    b. fructose-6-P
    c. glyceraldehyde-3-phosphate
    d. lactate

17. The glycolytic enzyme inhibited by fluoride is
    a. pyruvate kinase
    b. enolase
    c. glyceraldehyde-3-phosphate dehydrogenase
    d. hexokinase

18. One of the following hormones inhibits gluconeogenesis
    a. glucagon   b. insulincytosol
    c. adrenaline   d. cortisol

19. The fate of pyruvate in aerobic condition is its conversion to
    a. lactate   b. cholesterol
    c. acetyl CoA   d. ribose

20. The final and common pathway for the oxidation of carbohydrates, fats and proteins is
    a. the gluconeogenesis
    b. the tricarboxylic acid cycle
    c. the hexose monophosphate shunt
    d. the glycogenesis

21. **One molecule of glucose on complete oxidation yields**
   a. 30 molecules of ATP
   b. 24 molecules of ATP
   c. 10 molecules of ATP
   d. 38 molecules of ATP

22. **Cori's cycle involves in the conversion of**
   a. pyruvate to lactate in muscle
   b. muscle lactate to glucose in the liver
   c. pyruvate to glucose in the liver
   d. liver glucose to lactate

23. **A hormone that stimulates the activation of glycogen phosphorylase is**
   a. glucagon
   b. insulin
   c. progesterone
   d. estrogen

24. **McArdle's disease is due to the deficiency of**
   a. liver glycogen phosphorylase
   b. liver glycogen synthase
   c. lysosomal glucosidase
   d. muscle glycogen phosphorylase

25. **Glucose-6-phosphate dehydrogenase catalyzes the conversion of glucose to**
   a. fructose-6-phosphate
   b. 6-phosphogluconolactone
   c. xylulose-5-phosphate
   d. ribulose-5-phosphate

26. **One of the following is not a significant function of the HMP shunt**
   a. pentose production
   b. NADH production
   c. NADPH production
   d. ribose-5-P production

27. **All of the following inhibit the enzyme citrate synthase EXCEPT**
   a. ATP
   b. NADH
   c. acyl CoA
   d. ADP

28. **One of the following enzymes catalyzes substrate level phosphorylation in the TCA cycle**
   a. fumarase
   b. malate dehydrogenase
   c. succinate thiokinase
   d. α-ketoglutarate dehydrogenase

29. **The noncompetitive inhibitor that inhibits glyceraldehyde-3-P dehydrogenase is**
   a. fluoride
   b. bromohydroxy acetone-P
   c. malonate
   d. iodoacetate

30. **The complete oxidation of one molecule of acetyl CoA in the TCA cycle generates**
   a. 12 ATPs
   b. 10 ATPs
   c. 38 ATPs
   d. 8 ATPs

31. **Malonate is a competitive inhibitor of**
   a. aconitase
   b. α-ketoglutarate dehydrogenase
   c. succinate dehydrogenase
   d. fumarase

32. **During glycogenesis, the α-1, 6 linkage is introduced by**
   a. amylo-1, 4–1, 6 transglucosidase
   b. 1, 4 glucan transferase
   c. phosphorylase
   d. glycogen synthase

33. **Glucose-6-phosphatase is absent in**
   a. kidney   c. muscle
   b. liver   d. intestine

34. **von Gierke's disease is the result of a deficiency of**
   a. liver phosphorylase
   b. liver glucose-6-phosphatase
   c. glycogen synthase
   d. muscle phosphorylase

35. **One of the following processes does not require NADPH**
    a. synthesis of fatty acids
    b. reduction of glutathione
    c. synthesis of glycogen
    d. synthesis of steroids

36. **One of the following conditions supports the formation of fructose 2, 6-bisphosphate**
    a. high blood glucose
    b. low blood glucose
    c. normal blood glucose
    d. high blood cholesterol

37. **Regarding glucokinase, all of the following statements are true EXCEPT**
    a. it is present in all the tissues
    b. it is present in liver
    c. it is not inhibited by glucose-6-phosphate
    d. it has high K_m for glucose

38. **The synthesis of glucose from non-carbohydrate sources is called**
    a. gluconeogenesis   c. glycolysis
    b. glycogenesis   d. glycogenolysis

39. **Hers' disease is due to the deficiency of**
    a. liver phosphorylase
    b. liver glucose-6-phosphatase
    c. glycogen synthase
    d. muscle phosphorylase

40. **All the following are the examples for non-competitive inhibitors EXCEPT**
    a. iodoacetate   c. malonate
    b. arsenite   d. fluoride

41. **Total number of ATPs formed during aerobic glycolysis is**
    a. 10   c. 4
    b. 8   d. 2

42. **Net ATP formed during anaerobic glycolysis**
    a. 8   c. 2
    b. 4   d. 10

43. **Hormone which stimulate glycolysis is**
    a. Glucagon   c. Throxine
    b. Insulin   d. Cortisol

44. **TCA cycle operates in**
    a. Cytosol   c. Ribosomes
    b. Mitochondria   d. Nucleus

45. **Number of ATPs formed in TCA from acetyl CoA, formed from a molecule of glucose is**
    a. 30   c. 38
    b. 32   d. 40

8

Lipid Chemistry

L ipid or fat is characterized by their physical property with water, it says, "touch me not" but, it goes well into solution with organic solvents. To the tongue, it is tasteful; within limits, it is good for the life but makes it danger when it is in excess.

Definition

Lipids are heterogeneous group of naturally occurring compounds, which are relatively insoluble in water but freely soluble in nonpolar organic solvents like, benzene, chloroform, ether and alcohol.

➢ Coming from animals and plants living or fossilized.

➢ Formed of long-chain hydrocarbon groups (carbon and hydrogen) but may also contain oxygen, phosphorus, nitrogen and sulfur.

Functions of lipids

1. Triglycerides are the major storage form of energy.

2. They provide essential fatty acids; phospholipids, hormones (prostaglandins) and they form important constituents of cell membrane.

3. Absorption of vitamins A, D, E and K depends on the presence of lipids in the diet.

4. The basic unit of lipids, i.e. acetyl CoA (the active form of acetic acid) is used for the synthesis of cholesterol and hence steroid hormones.

5. The lipids maintain the membrane structure and integrity.

6. Since lipids are hydrocarbon organic compounds, their insulating effect have been utilized in the body for protecting internal organs from shock.

7. They help in blood coagulation.

8. Dipalmitoyl lecithin, a phospholipid acts as a surfactant and is required for the normal functioning of the lung alveoli.

Classification of Lipids

I. Simple lipids

They are esters of fatty acids with glycerol or higher alcohols.

These include fats and waxes.

Fats: Esters of fatty acids with glycerol. A fat in the liquid state is known as oil. Fat is also called as triglyceride or triacylglycerol.

Triacylglycerol (Triglyceride):

- Nearly all the commercially important fats and oils of animal and plant origins consist almost exclusively of the simple lipid class triacylglycerols (often termed "triglycerides").
- They consist of a glycerol moiety with each hydroxyl group esterified to a fatty acid. In nature, they are synthesised by enzyme systems, which determine that a centre of asymmetry is created about carbon-2 of the glycerol backbone, so they exist in enantiomeric forms, i.e. with different fatty acids in each position.
- They are esters of fatty acids with the trihydric alcohol glycerol.
- Glycerol with one molecule of fatty acid is called monoacyl glycerol.
- Glycerol with two molecules of fatty acid is called diacyl glycerol.

$$CH_2OH$$
$$|$$
$$R''COO–CH$$
$$|$$
$$CH_2OH$$

2-monoacyl glycerol

- Glycerol with three fatty acids is called *triglyceride*.

$$\alpha_1 CH_2–OH$$
$$|$$
$$\beta CH–OH \quad + 3 \text{ fatty acids} \quad \longrightarrow \quad \beta CH–O–CO–R_2$$
$$|$$
$$\alpha_2 CH_2–OH$$

Glycerol

$$\alpha_1 CH_2–O–CO–R_1$$
$$\alpha_2 CH_2–O–CO–R_3$$

Triacylglycerol

R_1, R_2 and R_3 indicate the fatty acids. The fatty acids may be same or different type. Usually R_2 is an unsaturated fatty acid.

Waxes: Esters of fatty acids with monohydric long chain alcohols.

In their most common form, wax esters consist of fatty acids esterified to long-chain alcohols with similar chain-lengths. The latter tend to be saturated or have one double bond only. Such compounds are found in animal, plant and microbial tissues and they have a variety of functions, such as acting as energy stores, waterproofing and lubrication.

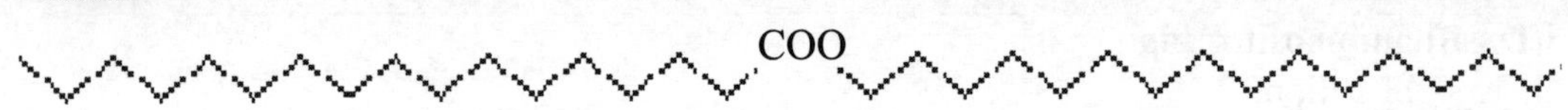

$$\text{\textasciitilde\textasciitilde\textasciitilde\textasciitilde\textasciitilde COO \textasciitilde\textasciitilde\textasciitilde\textasciitilde\textasciitilde}$$

In some tissues, such as skin, avian preen glands or plant leaf surfaces, the wax components can be much more complicated in their structures and compositions. They can contain aliphatic diols, free alcohols, hydrocarbons (e.g. squalene), aldehydes and ketones.

II. Compound lipids

They are esters of fatty acid with one of the various alcohols and in addition, it contains other groups (nonlipid component). The subclasses are:

A. Phospholipid

Phospholipids are compound lipids containing alcohol, fatty acid, phosphoric acid and a nitrogenous base or other alcoholic group. These are derivatives of phosphatidic acid and include lecithin, cardiolipin, cephalin, plasmalogen and sphingomyelin.

$$CH_2-O-CO-R_1$$
$$|$$
$$CH-O-CO-R_2$$
$$|$$
$$CH_2-O-\text{phosphoric acid}$$

Phosphatidic acid

$$CH_2-O-CO-R_1$$
$$|$$
$$CH-O-CO-R_2$$
$$|$$
$$CH_2-O-\text{phosphoric acid–choline}$$

Lecithin (phosphatidyl choline)

1. **Lecithin:** Contains alcohol, fatty acid, phosphoric acid and choline. The fatty acid part of R_1 is a saturated fatty acid and R_2 at β position is an unsaturated fatty acid. Lecithin is present in brain, nervous tissue, and sperm and egg yolk. Lecithins are surface-active agents and help in emulsification of fats. Dipalmitoyl lecithin is a lung surfactant (lowers surface tension) prevents the collapse of lung alveoli. Absence of dipalmitoyl lecithin in premature infants may produce respiratory distress syndrome or hyaline membrane disease.

2. **Cephalins:** Contain alcohol, fatty acid, phosphoric acid and ethanolamine or serine as a nitrogenous base instead of choline present in lecithin. Cephalins are present in brain, erythrocytes and many other tissues.

3. **Phosphatidyl inositol:** It is a phospholipid containing phosphatidic acid bound to the alcohol inositol instead of a nitrogenous base. They are important components of cell membrane. The action of certain hormones (e.g. oxytocin, vasopressin) is mediated through phosphatidyl inositol (PI). In response to hormonal action, PI is cleaved to diacyl glycerol

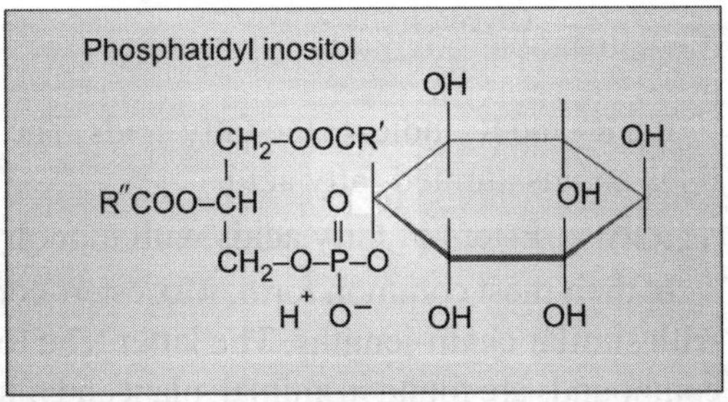

Phosphatidyl inositol

Figure 8.1

(DAG) and inositol triphosphate (IP_3). Both these compounds act as second messenger for hormonal action.

4. Plasmalogen: They differ from lecithin or cephalin in α_1 position (see Figure 8.1) of glycerol where the fatty acid is replaced by a long chain unsaturated aliphatic aldehyde such as palmitic or stearic aldehyde. Plasmalogens are present in large quantities in the skeletal muscle, cardiac muscle and in semen.

5. Cardiolipin: It is a diphosphatidyl glycerol. It contains two molecules of phosphatidic acid held by glycerol. It is present in the inner mitochondrial membrane and has antigenic properties.

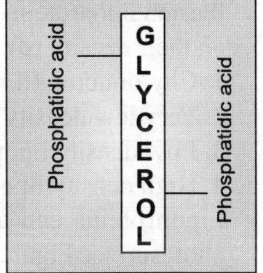

Figure 8.2

6. Ceramide: It is formed by the esterification of sphingosine (an amino alcohol) with a fatty acid of high molecular weight. Principally found in white matter of brain in myelin sheath and medullated nerves. Ceramide is common for all glycolipid and sphingomyelin.

7. Sphingomyelin: This is a sphingophospholipid. It does not contain glycerol but an unsaturated amino alcohol, i.e. sphingosine. They contain a molecule of choline, phosphoric acid and a fatty acid. Sphingomyelin makes up a large part of the myelin sheath. These are also present in brain, lungs, nerves and other tissues.

Deposition of sphingomyelin in liver, lymph nodes, bone marrow and central nervous system results in Niemann-Pick disease. It may be due to the deficiency of sphingomyelinase enzyme in these tissues.

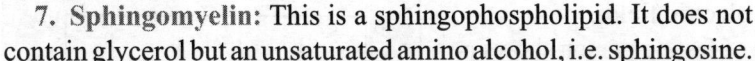

$$R.CHOH.CH.CH_2-O-P-O-CH_2CH_2N^+(CH_3)_3$$

B. Glycolipids

They contain fatty acid, sphingosine (alcohol), carbohydrate or carbohydrate derivative.

For example, cerebroside, ganglioside.

1. Cerebrosides: They contain a molecule of fatty acid, an amino alcohol sphingosine and a sugar (ussually galactose). They are present in white matter of brain and myelin sheath of nerves. Their level is increased in Gaucher's disease in tissues like reticuloendothelial cells in spleen, liver, lymph node and bone.

2. Gangliosides: They are designated as GM_1, GM_2, etc. and are found in grey matter of the brain and contain N-acetylneuraminic acid (sialic acid), fatty acid, alcohol sphingosine and three molecules of hexoses (such as glucose or galactose). In Tay-Sach's disease, ganglioside level increases.

C. Lipoproteins

- The different types of lipoproteins are high density lipoprotein (HDL), low density lipoprotein (LDL), very low density lipoprotein (VLDL) and chylomicron.

- Since lipids are water insoluble, they are present in the blood in the form of lipoproteins which are water soluble.
- Lipoproteins (also belong to conjugated protein class) are composed of triglyceride and cholesterol ester core surrounded by a shell of proteins (also called as apoproteins), phospholipid and free cholesterol.
- They have an outer polar surface, which makes them water soluble.
- Plasma lipoproteins can be separated by ultracentrifugation into four distinct groups based on their density (d).
  1. Chylomicron (d < 0.96)
  2. Very low density lipoprotein (VLDL, d = 0.96 to 1.006)
  3. Low density lipoprotein (LDL, d = 1.006 to 1.063)
  4. High density lipoprotein (HDL, d = 1.063 to 1.21)
- Lipoproteins can also be separated by electrophoresis (see Figure 8.3) based on the difference in their mobilization in an electric field.
- Normally, serum sample of fasting person shows no chylomicron band at the point of sample application.

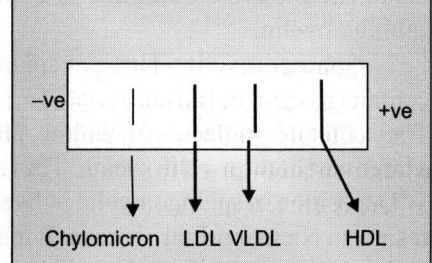

Figure 8.3

Functions

Chylomicron: Transports dietary triglyceride and cholesterol esters from intestine to peripheral tissues and liver.

VLDL: Transports endogenous triglyceride from liver to extrahepatic tissues.

LDL: Transports cholesterol from liver to extrahepatic tissues.

HDL: Transports cholesterol from extrahepatic tissues back to the liver in an esterified form.

The characteristic apoproteins present in chylomicron is apo B 48 and in LDL and VLDL, it is apo B 100.

Hyperlipoproteinemias

The presence of excessive amounts of VLDL (excess of TG), LDL (excess of cholesterol) or chylomicron in plasma following 12–14 hours of fasting is collectively called as hyperlipoproteinemia or hyperlipidemia. The elevation of lipids in plasma leads to deposition of cholesterol in the intima of the arterial walls leading to atherosclerosis.

The hyperlipidemias are of several types they are:

Hyperlipoproteinemia Type I: Presence of chylomicron, high TG, VLDL and normal cholesterol.

Hyperlipoproteinemia Type II a: Normal TG, high LDL and, therefore, high cholesterol.

Hyperlipoproteinemia Type II b: High LDL, high VLDL, high cholesterol and high TG.

Hyperlipoproteinemia Type IV: High VLDL and, therefore, increased TG and normal cholesterol.

III. Derived lipid

Substances derived from the above groups by hydrolysis.
For example, fatty acid, glycerol, alcohol and cholesterol.

Fatty acid

Definition: Fatty acids are aliphatic monocarboxylic organic acids with chain length usually ranging from C-4 to C-24 and these are the constituents of lipid. The fatty acids have the general formula R–CO–OH.

Nomenclature: Fatty acids are named after the name of the hydrocarbon with the same number of carbon atoms, with suffix -*oic* acid for saturated fatty acid and the suffix -*enoic* acid for the unsaturated fatty acid.

Numbering of a fatty acid

The carbon atoms of the fatty acids are numbered from the –COOH group (carboxyl group). Carboxyl group carbon atom is C1, and then next carbon atom is C2. The carbon atom adjacent to the –COOH group is also called as α-carbon atom, next carbon atom is β and so on. The last carbon atom or CH_3 group is designated as ω carbon atom. For example, oleic acid is written as 18:1; 9 or Δ^9, 18:1.

$$\omega \qquad\qquad\qquad\qquad\qquad \beta \quad\ \alpha$$
$$CH_3\text{–}(CH_2)_7\text{–}CH=CH\text{–}(CH_2)_5\text{–}CH_2\text{–}CH_2\text{–}COOH$$
$$10 \quad 9 \qquad\qquad 3 \quad 2 \quad 1$$

Oleic acid (18:1; 9) or Δ^9, 18:1 indicates fatty acid having 18 carbons with one double bond at carbon atom 9. The position of the double bond can also be indicated by the symbol 'Δ' followed by the position of the double bond in superscript.

The fatty acids are numbered from the ω-carbon.

The linoleic acid is called ω-series because of the presence of first double bond from ω-carbon at the 6th carbon.

$$18 \quad 17 \qquad 13 \quad 12 \quad 11 \quad 10 \quad 9 \quad 8 \qquad 1$$
$$CH_3\text{–}(CH_2)_4\text{–}CH=CH\text{–}CH_2\text{–}CH=CH\text{–}(CH_2)_7\text{–}COOH$$
$$\omega \quad\ 5 \qquad 6$$

Likewise linolenic acid is ω-3 series

$$18 \qquad\qquad\qquad\qquad\qquad\qquad\qquad\qquad 1$$
$$CH_3\text{–}CH_2\text{–}CH=CH\text{–}CH_2\text{–}CH=CH\text{–}CH_2\text{–}CH=CH\text{–}(CH_2)_7\text{–}COOH$$
$$\omega \quad 2 \quad 3$$

Arachidonic acid is ω-series

$$20 \qquad\qquad 14 \qquad\qquad 11 \qquad\qquad 8 \qquad\qquad 5 \qquad\qquad 1$$
$$CH_3\text{–}(CH_2)_4\text{–}CH=CH\text{–}CH_2\text{–}CH=CH\text{–}CH_2\text{–}CH=CH\text{–}CH_2\text{–}CH=CH\text{–}(CH_2)_3\text{–}COOH$$
$$\omega \quad\ 5 \quad 6$$

Classification of fatty acid

Saturated fatty acid

Do not have a double bond.
For example, acetic acid (2 carbon atoms), butyric acid (4 carbon atoms), palmitic acid (C16), stearic acid (C18) and lignoceric acid (C24).

Unsaturated fatty acid

The fatty acids, which have double bonds, are called unsaturated fatty acids. They are further classified into monounsaturated fatty acid [MUFA] contains one double bond.
    For example, palmitoleic acid (C16, Δ^9), oleic acid (C18, Δ^9).
    Polyunsaturated fatty acids [PUFA]: Contains more than one double bond.
    For example, linoleic acid, linolenic acid and arachidonic acid.

Essential fatty acids or PUFA

Fatty acids, which are not sythesised in the body and should be supplied through diet, are called essential fatty acids. They contain more than one double bond. For example, linoleic acid, linolenic acid and arachidonic acid (PUFA). These fatty acids are not synthesised in human body because of lack of the desaturase enzyme, which introduces double bonds beyond 9th and 10th carbon atoms.

1. Linoleic acid represented as (18:2; 9, 12) or [$\Delta^{9, 12}$; 18]. It means that this fatty acid contains 18 carbon atoms and two double bonds at position C9 and C12.

$$CH_3-(CH_2)_4-CH=CH-CH_2-CH=CH-(CH_2)_7-COOH$$

2. Linolenic acid, represented as (18:3; 9, 12, 15) or [$\Delta^{9, 12, 15}$; 18]

$$CH_3-CH_2-CH=CH-CH_2-CH=CH-CH_2-CH=CH-(CH_2)_7-COOH$$

3. Arachidonic acid represented as (20:4; 5, 8, 11, 14) or [$\Delta^{5, 8, 11, 14}$, 20]

$$CH_3-(CH_2)_4-CH=CH-CH_2-CH=CH-CH_2-CH=CH-CH_2-CH=CH-(CH_2)_3-COOH$$
$$20 \qquad\qquad 14 \qquad\qquad 11 \qquad\qquad 8 \qquad\qquad 5$$

Functions of fatty acids

1. Essential fatty acids are involved in the esterification of cholesterol and thus, help in its transport and metabolism. So essential fatty acid lowers cholesterol level and hence, decreases the risk of heart disease.
2. Essential fatty acids are the constituents of the cell membrane and membranes of cell organelle (e.g. mitochondria).
3. They are essential for maintaining normal growth and health.
4. Fatty acids are components of simple and compound lipids, which are present in various tissues like adipose tissue.

5. They are responsible for the hydrophobic nature of the compounds. They provide energy when they are oxidized in human body.
6. Prostaglandins and luekotriens are formed from PUFA (arachidonic acid). They act as local hormones.
7. They protect the liver from accumulation of fat (prevent fatty liver).
8. Essential fatty acids help to prevent skin disease.

Glycerol

It is a trihydric alcohol as it contains three hydroxyl groups.

It is a gluconeogenic substance because on lipolysis of dietary lipid releases glycerol, which is converted into glucose in liver.

Steroids and cholesterol

Steroids are often found in association of lipids. They are compounds having special ring called cyclopentanoperhydrophenanthrene nucleus.

For example, Steroid hormone, bile acid, vitamin D.

Cholesterol

- It is one of the important steroids present in the body. It has 27 carbons, an –OH group, a double bond, two methyl groups at C_{10} and C_{13} and a side chain at C_{17}.
- It is the precursor of various compounds such as vitamin D_3, bile acids and adreno-cortical and sex hormones.
- Cholesterol is widely distributed in all cells of the body but nervous tissue is rich in cholesterol.
- Steroids containing one or more –OH groups are known as sterols.
- Normal fasting serum cholesterol level is 150–200 mg/dL.
- It is synthesised in our body using acetyl CoA as precursor (1g/day).

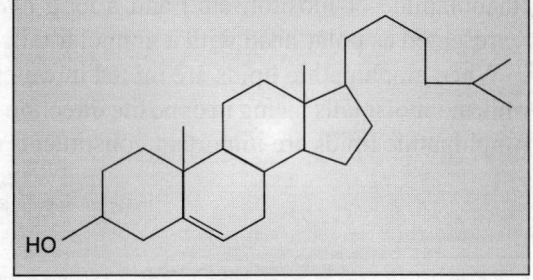

Figure 8.4

- Cholesterol exists in free and ester form. Cholesterol gets esterified through esterase enzymes.
- Excess cholesterol is harmful to body in that it gets deposited in the intima of the arteries producing atherosclerosis. This can narrow the lumen of blood vessel impeding blood flow, which cause thrombosis.

Functions of cholesterol

Cholesterol, if maintained in normal level, has number of good effects. They are:
1. It is a precursor for the synthesis of bile acids in liver.

2. The steroid hormone in adrenal cortex and sex hormones in gonads are mainly synhesized from cholesterol.
3. Cholesterol form 7 dehydrocholesterol in skin, is converted to vitamin D_3 by UV rays.
4. Cholesterol is a poor conductor of heat and hence acts as an insulator.
5. Cholesterol is a poor conductor of electricity. Cholesterol is abundant in brain and nervous tissue where it functions as an insulating covering for structure, which generates and transmits electrical impulse.

Properties of Lipids

Physical properties

Oils and fats (lipids) are similar in nature. Oils and lipids are different only in their physical properties. Triglycerides, which contain a higher proportion of unsaturated fatty acid or short chain fatty acid, are liquid at 20°C and are usually called as oils, e.g. vegetable oils.

Fats, on the other hand, are solid at room temperature and contain saturated long chain fatty acid, e.g. animal fat, dalda.

Amphipathic nature of lipids

The lipid that possesses both hydrophobic (nonpolar) and hydrophilic (polar) groups is known as an amphipathic lipid. These include fatty acid, phospholipids (e.g. lecithin), sphingolipid and bile salts.

Phospholipids have a hydrophilic head (phosphate group) attached to choline or ethanolamine or inositol, etc.) and a long hydrophobic tail. The general structure may be represented as polar head with a nonpolar tail.

When amphipathic lipids are mixed in water, the polar heads face towards aqueous phase while nonpolar tails facing in opposite direction. This nature leads to the formation of a micelle. Amphipathic lipids are important constituents of the lipid bilayer of biological membranes.

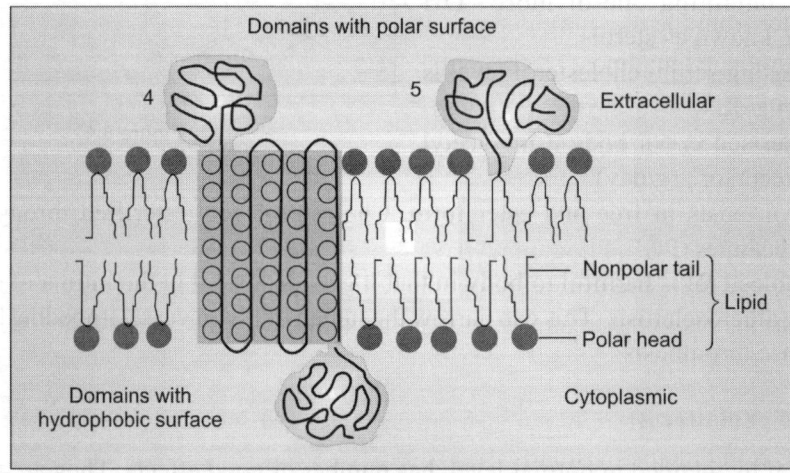

Figure 8.5

Triglycerides (triacylglycerol): Can be hydrolyzed by acids, alkalies or enzymes such as lipases.

For example,   Triacylgylcerol $\xrightarrow{\text{Acid/alkali/lipase}}$ Glycerol + 3 palmitic acid
                    + (Tripalmitin)   (Sodium salt)

Prostaglandins (PGs) and related compounds

- Prostaglandins and their related compounds are prostacyclins (PGI), thromboxanes (TXA) and leukotrienes (LT) are collectively known as eicosanoids.
- Eicosanoids are considered as locally acting hormones with a wide range of biochemical functions.
- Prostaglandins are derivatives of a hypothetical 20-carbon fatty acid namely prostanoic acid.
- The various prostanoids are:
  a. Prostaglandins, e.g. PGE_1, PGE_2, PGE_3
  b. Prostacyclins, e.g. PGI_2, PGI_3
  c. Thromboxanes, e.g. TXA_1, TXA_2
- Prostaglandins are named as PG plus a third letter (E, F, A, D), which corresponds to the type, and arrangement of functional group in the molecule and the subscript indicates number of double bonds [PGE_1].
- Prostaglandins are synthesized from arachidonic acid, which is released from membrane bound phospholipids.
- Corticosteroid and aspirin inhibit the prostaglandin synthesis.

Biochemical actions of prostaglandins

- Prostaglandins act as local hormones.
- They differ from the true hormones in many ways.
- PGs are produced in almost all the tissues.
- PGs are not stored and they are degraded to inactive products at the site of their production.
- PGs are produced in small amounts with low half-lives.

1. *Regulation of blood pressure*
   - PGs' mediates (PGE, PGA and PGI_2) are vasodilator in function, this results in increase in the blood flow and decreased peripheral resistance to lower the BP.
   - Serve as agents in the treatment of hypertension.

2. *Inflammation*
   - The PGs (PGE_1 and PGE_2) induce the symptoms of inflammation (redness, swelling, edema, etc.) due to arteriolar vasodilation.
   - Corticosteroids are usually used to treat inflammation which inhibits PG synthesis.

3. *Reproduction*

- PGE_2 and PGF_2 are used for the medical termination of pregnancy and induction of labor.

4. *Pain and fever*

- Pyrogens (fever producing agents) may promote PG synthesis leading to the formation of PGE_2 in the hypothalamus, the site of regulation of body temperature.
- PGE_2, along with histamine and bradykinin cause pain. The cause for migraine is increased PGE_2 level.
- Aspirin and other nonsteroidal drugs inhibit PG synthesis and thus control fever and pain.

5. *Prevention of gastric ulcer*

- Inhibits gastric HCl recretion.

6. *Effects on respiratory function*

- PGE is a bronchodilator whereas PGF act as constrictor of smooth muscles. PGE_1 and PGE_2 are used in the treatment of asthma.

7. *Influence on renal function*

- PGE increases GFR and promotes urine output.
- PGE increases the excretion of sodium and potassium.

8. *Metabolism*

PGE:
- Decreases lipolysis.
- Increases glycogenesis.
- Promotes mobilization of calcium from the bone.

9. *Platelet aggregation and thrombosis*

- The prostaglandins, namely prostacyclins (PGI_2), inhibit platelet aggregation.
- Thrombaxanes (TXA_2) and PGE_2 promote platelet aggregation and blood clotting that might lead to thrombosis.
- Thus, they are antagonistic in their action.
- In the overall effect, PGI_2 acts as a vasodilator, while TXA_2 is a vasoconstrictor.
- Thromboxane (TXA_2) and prostaglandin (PGE_1) promote platelet aggregation and prostacyclin (PGI_2) inhibits the platelet aggregation.
- Inhibitors of prostaglandin synthesis (aspirin, ibuprofen) are used in controlling fever, pain, migraine and inflammation.

- Prostaglandins are found in seminal fluid, plasma and other tissues. They have pharmacological and biochemical actions and act on smooth muscle, blood vessel and adipose tissue.

Leukotriens

- These are the mediators of allergic reactions and inflammation.
- They also cause bronchoconstriction, increase vascular permeability and mucus secretion. (e.g. LTA_3, LTA_4).
- Certain fish foods contain an unsaturated fatty acid namely eicosapentanoic acid (EPA) (20 carbon atoms and 5 double bonds), which inhibits the synthesis of thromboxanes (TXA_2), thus decreases platelet aggregation and thrombosis and, therefore, lowers the risk of myocardial complications as seen in the Eskimos.

Self Test

Long essay questions

a. Write an account of classification of lipids with suitable example.
b. Define lipids. What are their biomedical importance?
c. Describe the structure, classification and functions of phospholipids.
d. Discuss the saturated and unsaturated fatty acids of biological importance.
e. Describe the structure of steroids. Add a note on functions of cholesterol.
f. What are lipoproteins? How they are separated? What is the significance of their level in blood?

Write short notes on

a. Structure of triacyl glycerol (TG)
b. Glycolipids
c. Essential fatty acids
d. Rancidity
e. Saponification number
f. Iodine number
g. Lecithin
h. Sphingomyelin
i. Prostaglandins
j. Lipoproteins
k. Lipotropic factors
l. Amphipathic nature of the lipids.

Short questions

a. Which lipid serves as fuel reserve in animals?
b. The number of mg of KOH required to hydrolyse 1 gm of fat or oil is known as what?
c. Name the phospholipid that produces second messenger in hormonal action is.
d. Name the glycolipid containing N-acetyl neuraminic acid.
e. What do you call it, if the steroids contain a cyclic ring?
f. Give an example for an antioxidant.

Multiple choice questions

1. **The nitrogenous base present in lecithin is**
   a. Ethanolamine
   b. Inositol
   c. Serine
   d. Choline

2. **The number of double bonds present in arachidonic acid is**
   a. 1
   b. 2
   c. 3
   d. 4

3. **Which of the following is an amphipathic lipid?**
   a. Phospholipid
   b. Fatty acid
   c. Bile salts
   d. all the three

4. **Name of the test employed to check the adulteration of butter.**
   a. Iodine number
   b. Saponification number
   c. Zak's method
   d. Reichert-Meissl number

5. **All the following alcohols are present in phospholipids *except***
   a. Sphingosine
   b. Inositol
   c. Mannitol
   d. Glycerol

6. **Which of the following is not a phospholipid?**
   a. Plasmalogen
   b. Lecithin
   c. Sphingomyelin
   d. Ganglioside

7. **Which of the following is a essential fatty acid?**
   a. 1-oleic acid
   b. Arachidic acid
   c. Linoleic acid
   d. Palmitic acid

8. **Sphingomyelin contains which of the following components?**
   a. Glycerol, phosphoric acid, 2 fatty acids and choline
   b. Sphingosine, phosphoric acid, 1 fatty acid and choline
   c. Sphingosine, phosphoric acid and 2 fatty acids
   d. Glycerol, phosphoric acid and 2 fatty acids.

9. **The plasma lipoprotein which is least dense**
   a. VLDL
   b. LDL
   c. HDL
   d. Chylomicron

10. **The plasma lipoprotein which moves fast towards the anode during electrophoresis is**
    a. VLDL
    b. LDL
    c. HDL
    d. Chylomicron

11. **The polyunsaturated fatty acids (PUFA) are richly present in**
    a. Sunflower oil
    b. Butter
    c. Ghee
    d. Coconut oil

12. **Deficiency of which phospholipid causes respiratory distress syndrome**
    a. Cardiolipin
    b. Phosphatidic acid
    c. Dipalmitoyl lecithin
    d. Cephalin

Explain the following
1. Vegetable oils are liquid at room temperature whereas aniaml fat is solid.
2. Lecithin is an amphipathic molecule.
3. Butter becomes rancid faster than ghee.
4. Saponification number decreases with increase in molecular weight of fat.

9

Metabolism of Lipids

DIGESTION AND ABSORPTION OF LIPIDS

Digestion of dietary lipids starts in the small intestine where they are first emulsified by the bile salts. After emulsification, the lipolytic enzymes such as lipase, phospholipase and cholesterol esterase present in the pancreatic juice hydrolyze lipids (Figure 9.1).

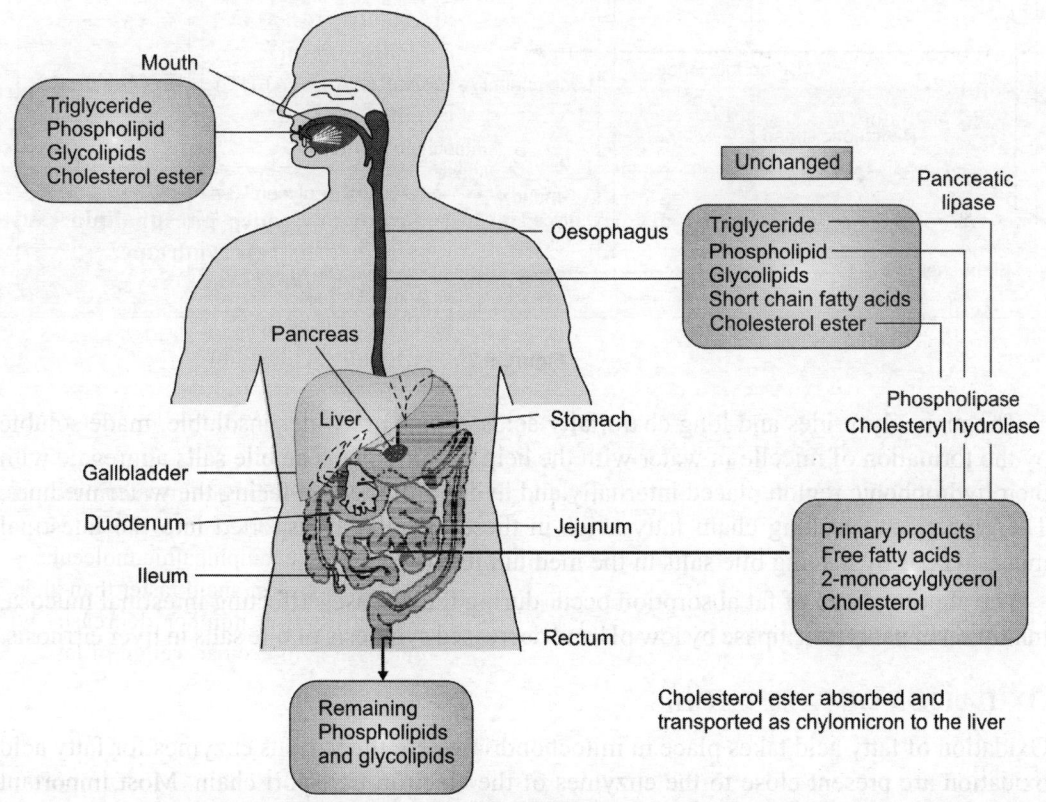

Figure 9.1

After absorption, lipids are either oxidized mainly in the liver or stored in the depots (adipose tissue). For utilization by the body, triglycerides are first hydrolyzed by lipase to release glycerol and free fatty acids. Glycerol is converted into glucose by gluconeogenesis or enters into glycolysis. Fatty acids are oxidized to CO_2 and H_2O with the liberation of large amount of energy.

Inside the mucosal cells, fats are resynthesized and converted to chylomicron and transported to blood via lymphatic vessel.

Fatty acids less than 10 carbon atoms along with glycerol are carried by portal blood to the liver (Figure 9.2).

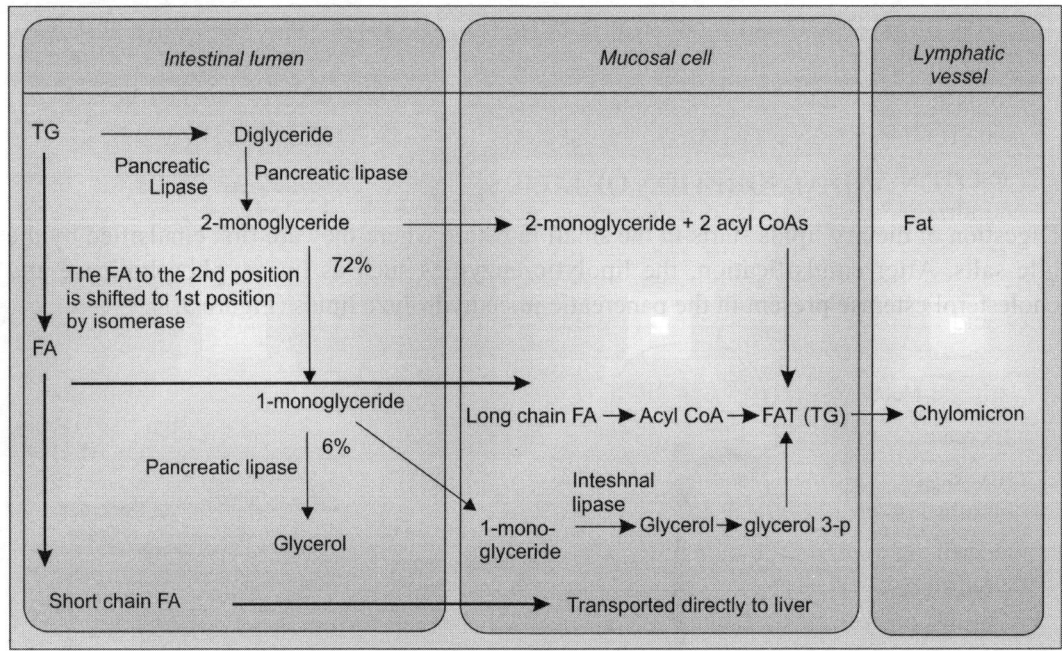

Figure 9.2

The monoglycerides and long chain fatty acids, which are water insoluble, made soluble by the formation of micelle in water with the help of bile salts. The bile salts aggregate with their hydrophobic region placed internally and hydrophilic region facing the water medium. The glycerides and long chain fatty acids in these micelles transported into the intestinal mucosal cells by leaving bile salts in the medium itself.

The abnormalities of fat absorption occur during the diseases affecting intestinal mucosa, inhibition of pancreatic lipase by low pH and decreased synthesis of bile salts in liver cirrhosis.

OXIDATION OF FATTY ACIDS

Oxidation of fatty acid takes place in mitochondria where the various enzymes for fatty acid oxidation are present close to the enzymes of the electron transport chain. Most important theory of the oxidation of fatty acid is the β oxidation of fatty acid.

β-oxidation of fatty acid (Figure 9.4)

➢ Fatty acids are rich sources of energy.

➢ Energy is released when fatty acid undergoes β-oxidation.

➢ The β-carbon atom of fatty acid is oxidized.

➢ It is a cyclic process.

➢ Oxidation of fatty acid occurs at the β-carbon atom resulting in the elimination of two terminal carbon atoms as acetyl CoA leaving fatty acyl CoA, which has 2 carbon atoms less than the original fatty acid.

➢ Active form of fatty acid is called as fatty acyl CoA.

➢ If the starting fatty acid is palmitic acid, which has 16 carbon atoms, at a time 2 carbon atoms are removed as acetyl CoA, then 7 cycles of β-oxidation occurs to convert palmitic acid (16C) into 8 acetyl CoA (2C) molecules.

➢ First step is the activation to its fatty acyl CoA form and this occurs outside the mitochondria.

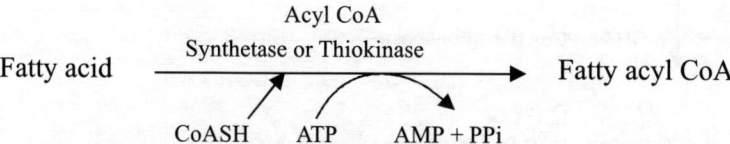

This reaction occurs outside the mitochondria.

Fatty acyl CoA formed, cannot cross the inner mitochondrial membrane."Carnitine", a carrier substance carries the acyl group into the mitochondrial membrane.

1. Once the activated fatty acid enter into the mitochondria, flavoprotein linked acyl CoA dehydrogenase (DH) removes two hydrogen atoms from the α and β position forming α, β-unsaturated fatty acyl CoA. This contains a double bond at α and β positions.

2. Enoyl CoA hydratase enzyme adds a molecule of water at the double bond position of α, β-unsaturated fatty acyl CoA forming β-hydroxyacyl CoA.

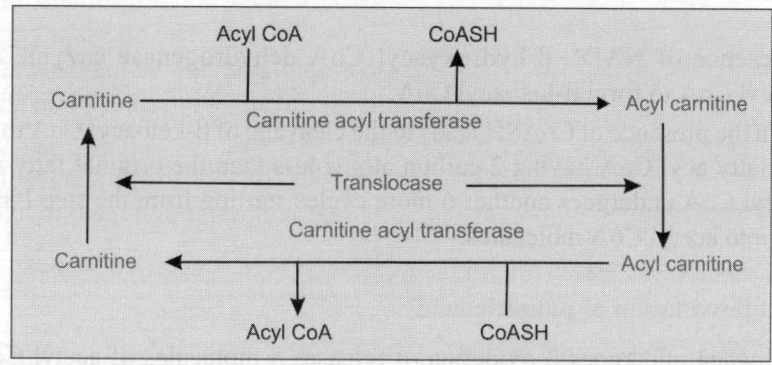

Figure 9.3 *Role of carnitine in β-oxidation*

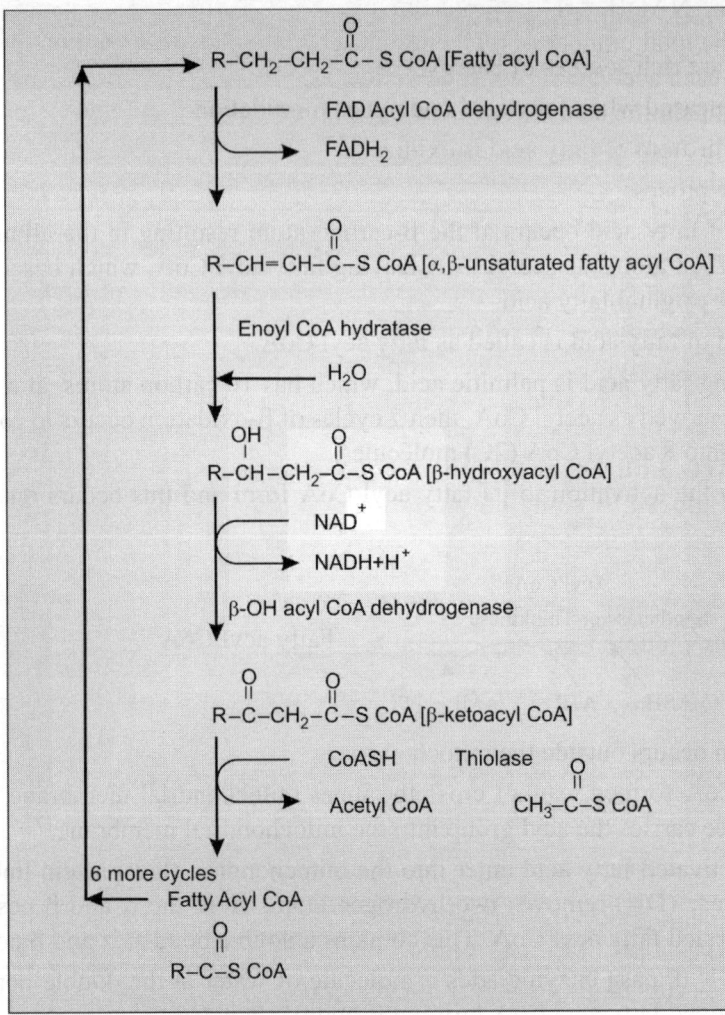

Figure 9.4

3. In the presence of NAD$^+$, β-hydroxyacyl CoA dehydrogenase enzyme oxidizes β-hydroxyacyl CoA to form β-ketoacyl CoA.

4. Thiolase in the presence of CoASH leads to the cleavage of β-ketoacyl CoA to yield acetyl CoA and fatty acyl CoA having 2 carbon atoms less than the original fatty acid. Newly formed acyl CoA undergoes another 6 more cycles starting from the step I and is finally degraded into acetyl CoA molecules.

Energetics of β-oxidation of palmitic acid

Palmitic acid when undergoes β-oxidation, it releases 8 molecules of acetyl CoA in seven cycles of the oxidative process. In each round of β-oxidation, one molecule of FADH$_2$ and one molecule of $NADH + H^+$ is produced. Which generates 2 and 3 molecules of ATP respectively. The total number of ATPs produced in 7 rounds of oxidation process is 35. In addition, when each acetyl CoA molecule oxidized in TCA cycle, 12 ATPs are generated.

Energetics of palmitic acid oxidation:

Per cycle of β-oxidation

Step I ($FADH_2$) ⟶	= 2 ATP
Step III ($NADH + H^+$) ⟶	= 3 ATP
	5 ATP

7 cycles of β-oxidation ⟶ = 35 ATP

Number of ATPs produced in TCA cycle = 12 ATP

Total number of acetyl CoAs formed from palmitic acid = 8

Total number of ATPs produced by complete oxidation of palmitic acid
$$= (8 \times 12) = 96 + 35 \quad = 131 \text{ ATP}$$

Number of ATPs **utilized** for activation of fatty acid = 2 ATP

Net ATPs produced by complete oxidation of palmitic acid = 129 ATP

The standard free energy of palmitate = 2,340 cal
$$129 \times 7.3 \text{ cal} = 940 \text{ cal}$$

The efficiency of energy conservation by FA oxidation = 940 × 100 = 2,340 = 40%

Fatty acids are predominantly oxidized by the process of β-oxidation in mitochondria.

α-oxidation

α-oxidation of fatty acid can also occur in human body mainly in liver and brain by removing one carbon from carboxyl end. There is no activation step.

Hydroxylation occurs at α-carbon atom done by monooxygenase system and then oxidized to keto acid.

Keto acid undergoes decarboxylation.

Liberates a molecule of CO_2 and a fatty acid.

This process occurs in the endoplasmic reticulum.

It is not requiring any CoA and it does not release energy.

Defect in enzyme system leads to Refsum's disease.

ω-oxidation

It is a minor pathway of oxidation of long chain fatty acid in microsomes.

It occurs from both the ends of fatty acid chain.

It needs hydroxylase enzymes with NADPH and cytochrome P-450.

Dicarboxylic acids are produced during this process.

It is important when β-oxidation is defective. The dicarboxylic acids are excreted in urine causing dicarboxylic aciduria.

Unsaturated fatty acid can also be activated and transported across the inner mitochondrial membrane and undergoes β-oxidation.

Oxidation of odd chain fatty acids

It is same as oxidation of even chain fatty acids, but only difference is that in the final β-oxidation cycle, a three-carbon fragment is left behind (in place of 2-carbon unit for saturated fatty acids). This component is propionyl CoA which is converted to succinyl CoA.

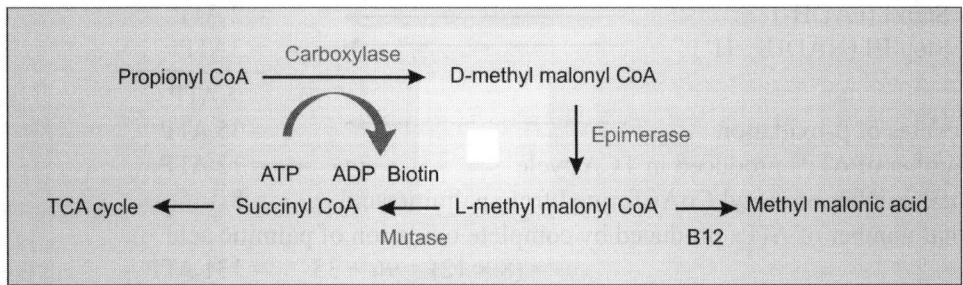

Figure 9.5

Metabolic fate of acetyl CoA

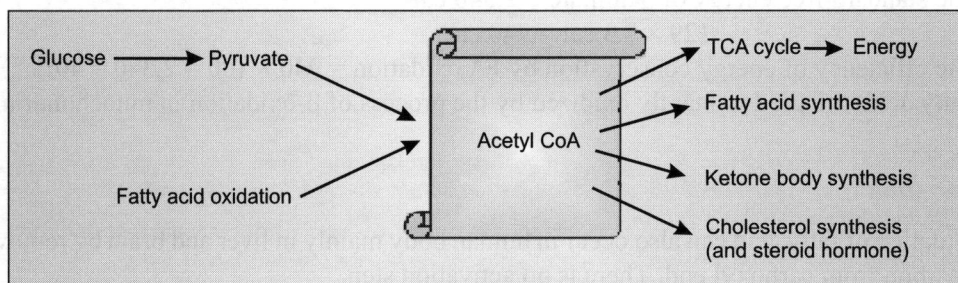

Figure 9.6

BIOSYNTHESIS OR DENOVO SYNTHESIS OF FATTY ACID

➢ Fatty acid synthesis involves the similar steps involved in β-oxidation of fatty acid but in a reverse way.

➢ Mammals can synthesize major portion of the saturated fatty acid as well as monounsaturated fatty acids.

➢ The system for the fresh synthesis of fatty acid is known as denovo synthesis of fatty acid, occurs in liver, adipose tissue, kidney and lactating mammary glands.

➢ The enzyme machinery is located in cytoplasm.

➢ It is referred to as extra mitochondrial or cytoplasmic fatty acid synthase system.

➢ Palmitic acid is the major FA synthesized.

➢ All 16 carbon atoms are from acetyl CoA.

➢ Acetyl CoA and NADPH are the prerequisites for the fatty acid synthesis.

➢ Acetyl CoA produced in the mitochondria cannot enter to cytoplasm through inner mitochondrial membrane. So acetyl CoA condenses with oxaloacetate in mitochondria to form citrate. Citrate is freely transported to cytosol where it is cleaved by citrate lyase to liberate acetyl CoA and oxaloacetate.

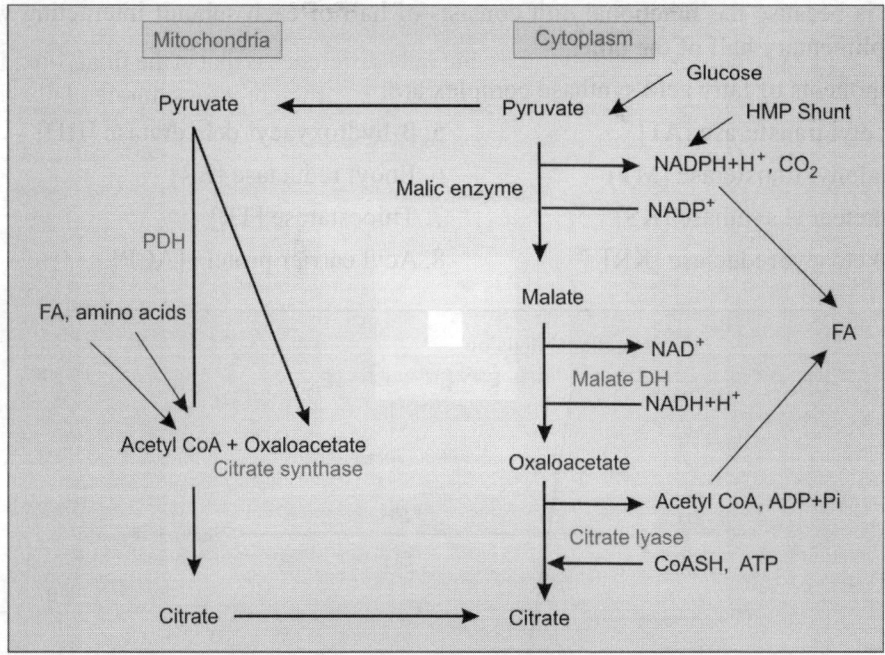

Figure 9.7

For the synthesis of FA, 8 acetyl CoAs are transported from the mitochondria to cytosol, which is linked with the synthesis of 8 NADPHs.

As such 14 NADPHs are needed to synthesize one molecule of palmitate.

The remaining 6 NADPHs supplied from HMP shunt.

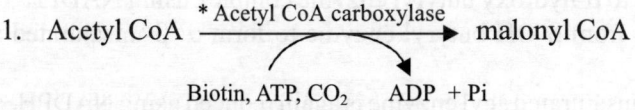

1. Acetyl CoA $\xrightarrow[\text{Biotin, ATP, } CO_2 \quad\quad \text{ADP} + \text{Pi}]{\text{* Acetyl CoA carboxylase}}$ malonyl CoA

* Regulatory enzyme in FA synthesis.

➤ The remaining reactions of FA synthesis are catalyzed by multifunctional enzyme known as *fatty acid synthase complex* (Fig. 9.8).
➤ It is a dimer with two identical subunits.
➤ Each monomer possesses the activities of seven different enzymes and an *acyl carrier protein (ACP)* bound to 4′-phosphopantetheine-SH group.
➤ Two subunits lie in antiparallel (head to tail) orientation.
➤ The –SH group of phosphopantetheine of one subunit is in close proximity to the –SH of cysteine residue of the other subunit.
➤ Each monomer of FAS contains all the enzyme activities of fatty acid synthesis.
➤ But only the dimer is functionally active.

➤ This is because the functional unit consists of half of each subunit interacting with the complimentary half of the other.

➤ Components of fatty acid synthase complex are:

1. Acetyl transferase [AT]

2. Malonyl transferase [MT]

3. β-ketoacyl synthase [KS]

4. β-ketoacyl reductase [KR]

5. β-hydroxyacyl dehydratase [HD]

6. Enoyl reductase [ER]

7. Thioestarase [TE]

8. Acyl carrier protein [ACP].

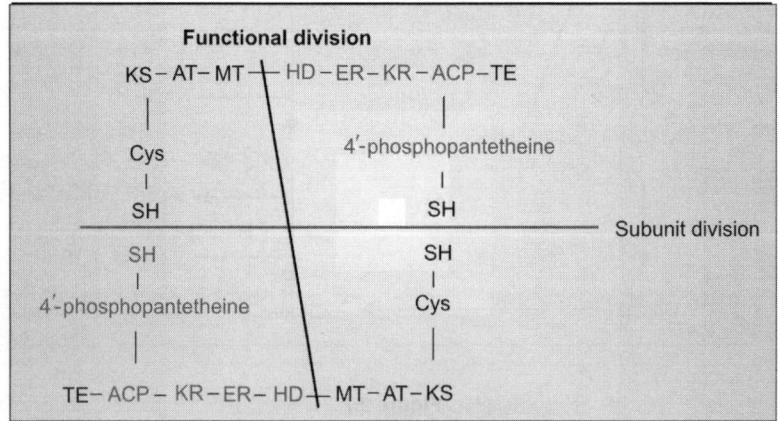

Figure 9.8: *Fatty acid synthase enzyme complex*

1. Fatty acid synthesis starts with the transfer of an acetyl CoA to cysteinyl –SH group of ACP.

2. Malonyl CoA-ACP transferase transfers malonate from malonyl CoA to bind to ACP.

3. The acetyl unit attached to cysteine is transferred to malonyl group attached to ACP. Malonyl moiety loses CO_2, which was added by acetyl CoA carboxylase and form β-ketoacyl enzyme.

4. β-ketoacyl enzyme is reduced to β-hydroxy butyryl enzyme complex using $NADPH + H^+$.

5. Molecule of H_2O is removed from β-OH butyryl enzyme to form α, β-unsaturated acyl enzyme.

6. The unsaturated bond in α, β-unsaturated acyl enzyme is again reduced using $NADPH + H^+$ to form butyryl or acyl enzyme. The carbon chain attached to ACP is transferred to cysteine residue and the reactions 2–6 are repeated 6 more times and finally palmitic acid is synthesized.

7. The completely synthesized fatty acid is released from the enzyme system by the action of thioesterase enzyme.

   Chain elongation of fatty acid occurs in the mitochondria and liver microsomes.

   Of the 16 carbons present in palmitate, only two come from acetyl CoA directly. The remaining 14 are from malonyl CoA which, in turn, is produced by acetyl CoA (Figure 9.9).

   8 acetyl CoA + 7 ATP + 14 NADPH + 14 H^+ → Palmitate + 8 CoA + 7 ADP + 7 Pi + 6 H_2O

Regulation

Acetyl CoA carboxylase enzyme controls a committed step in fatty acid synthesis. This enzyme exists as an inactive protomer (monomer) or an active polymer. Citrate promotes polymer

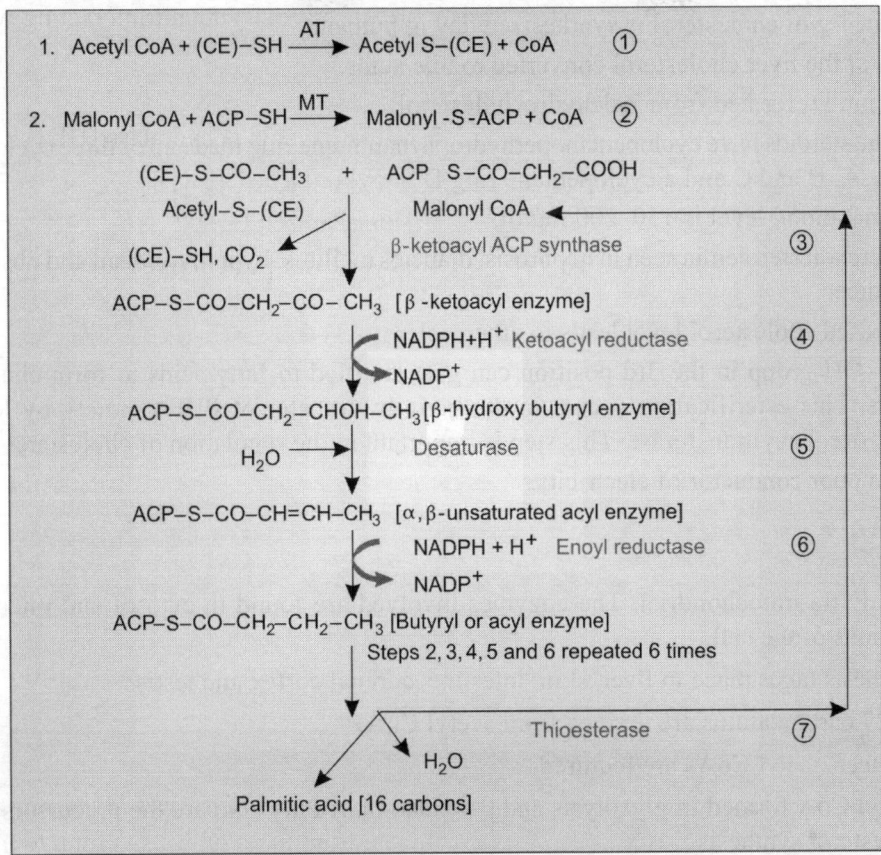

1. Acetyl CoA + (CE)−SH $\xrightarrow{AT}$ Acetyl S−(CE) + CoA   ①

2. Malonyl CoA + ACP−SH $\xrightarrow{MT}$ Malonyl -S -ACP + CoA   ②

(CE)−S−CO−CH$_3$ +   ACP S−CO−CH$_2$−COOH

Acetyl−S−(CE)   Malonyl CoA

(CE)−SH, CO$_2$ β-ketoacyl ACP synthase   ③

ACP−S−CO−CH$_2$−CO− CH$_3$ [β -ketoacyl enzyme]

NADPH+H$^+$ Ketoacyl reductase   ④

NADP$^+$

ACP−S−CO−CH$_2$−CHOH−CH$_3$ [β-hydroxy butyryl enzyme]

H$_2$O   Desaturase   ⑤

ACP−S−CO−CH=CH−CH$_3$ [α, β-unsaturated acyl enzyme]

NADPH + H$^+$ Enoyl reductase   ⑥

NADP$^+$

ACP−S−CO−CH$_2$−CH$_2$−CH$_3$ [Butyryl or acyl enzyme]

Steps 2, 3, 4, 5 and 6 repeated 6 times

Thioesterase   ⑦

H$_2$O

Palmitic acid [16 carbons]

Figure 9.9: *Reactions of fatty acid synthesis*

formation, hence, increases FA synthesis. Palmitoyl CoA and malonyl CoA cause depolymerization of the enzyme and inhibits FA synthesis.

Hormonal influence: Glucagon, epinephrine and norepinephrine inactivate the enzyme by cAMP dependent phosphorylation.

Insulin dephosphorylates and activates the enzyme.

Insulin promotes and glucagon inhibits FA synthesis.

Dietary regulation: High carbohydrate or fat free diet increases the synthesis of acetyl CoA carboxylase and FA synthase, which promote FA synthesis.

Fasting or high fat diet decreases FA production.

NADPH influences FA synthesis.

Cholesterol metabolism

➤ Cholesterol is a sterol, present in cell membrane, brain and lipoprotein.
➤ It is a precursor for all steroids.
➤ It is amphipathic in nature (hydrophilic and hydrophobic).

➤ About 1 g of cholesterol is synthesized/day in humans.

➤ 80% of the liver cholesterol converted to bile acids.

➤ Vitamin D_3 formed from 7-dehydrocholesterol.

➤ All the steroids have cyclopentanoperhydrophenanthrene ring made up of three cyclohexane rings, A, B and C and a cyclopentane ring D.

➤ Normal blood level is 150–200 mg/dl.

➤ Hypercholesterolemia seen in nephrosis, diabetes mellitus, hypothyroidism and obstructive jaundice.

➤ Increased cholesterol level leads to atherosclerosis.

➤ The –OH group in the 3rd position can get esterified to fatty acids to form cholesterol esters. This esterification occurs in the body by transfer of PUFA moiety by lecithin-cholesterol acyltransferase. This step is important in the regulation of cholesterol level.

➤ It is a poor conductor of electricity.

Synthesis

➤ Site: Extra mitochondrial. The enzymes involved are found in cytosol and microsomal fractions of the cell.

➤ Synthesis takes place in liver, skin, intestine, adrenal cortex and testis.

➤ All 27 carbon atoms are derived from acetyl CoA.

➤ Eighteen acetyl CoAs are required.

➤ Acetyl CoA formed in glycolysis and β-oxidation of fatty acid are the precursors for the cholesterol synthesis.

Acetyl CoA $\xrightarrow{\text{Thiolase}}$ Acetoacetyl CoA $\xrightarrow[\text{HMG CoA synthase}]{}$ β-hydroxymethyl glutaryl CoA [HMG CoA](6C)

HMG CoA reductase

Squalene (30C) × 6 ←——— Isoprene unit ←——— Mevalonic acid
                              (5C)   (6C)

Cholesterol (27C)

Regulation of cholesterol synthesis

➤ Cholesterol biosynthesis is controlled by the rate limiting enzyme HMG CoA reductase.

1. *Feedback control*: The end product cholesterol controls its own synthesis of the enzyme by a feedback mechanism. Increase in the cellualar concentration of cholesterol reduces the synthesis of the enzyme by decreasing the transcription of the gene responsible for the production of HMG CoA reductase.

2. *Hormonal regulation*: The HMG CoA reductase exists in two interconvertible forms.

The dephosphorylated form of the enzyme is more active, phosphorylated is less active. Hormones exert their influence through cAMP.

1. *Inhibition by drugs*: The drugs compactin and lovastatin are fungal drugs which inhibits HMG CoA reductase and which is used to decrease the cholesterol level.
2. HMG CoA reductase is inhibited by bile acids.

➤ LDL transports cholesterol from the liver to peripheral tissues.
➤ HDL transports cholesterol from tissues to liver.

Role of LCAT

High density lipoprotein (HDL) and the enzyme lecithin-cholesterol acyltransferase (LCAT) are responsible for the transport and elimination of cholesterol from the body.

LCAT is a plasma enzyme, synthesized by the liver.

LCAT catalyzes the transfer of fatty acid from the second position of phosphatidyl choline (lecithin) to the –OH group of cholesterol.

HDL cholesterol is the real substrate for LCAT and this reaction is freely reversible.

LCAT activity is associated with apo-A1 of HDL.

$$\text{Cholesterol} \xrightarrow[\substack{\text{Lecithin} \quad \text{Lysolecithin}}]{\text{LCAT}} \text{Cholesterol ester}$$

Metabolic fate of cholesterol

Cholesterol is converted into following compounds as shown below.
Cholesterol is mainly excreted in the form of bile salts in stool.

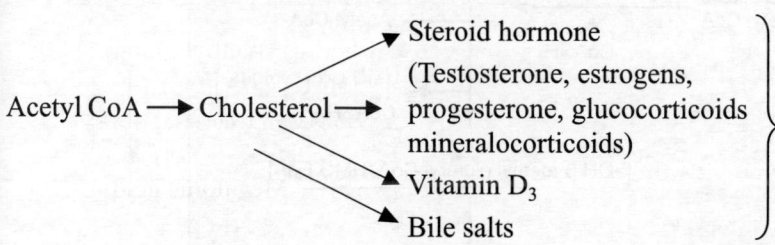

Increased plasma cholesterol results in the accumulation of cholesterol under the tunica intima of the arteries causing atherosclerosis. The progression of the disease process leads to narrowing of the blood vessels. Dietary intake of polyunsaturated fatty acid (PUFA) helps in transport and metabolism of cholesterol and prevents atherosclerosis.

Ketone body formation and utilization

➤ Acetoacetate, β-hydroxy butyrate and acetone are collectively called as ketone bodies.
➤ The process of formation of ketone bodies in the liver is called as ketogenesis.
➤ Ketone body level in the blood is usually less than 2 mg% in well-fed state.

> The ketone body excretion in the urine is 100 mg/24 hours.
> Increased production of ketone bodies is known as ketosis.
> High level of ketone bodies in blood are referred to as ketonemia.
> If the level of ketone bodies is high in the urine, it is called as ketonuria.
> Lungs mainly eliminate acetone.

Conditions in which ketone body formation takes place are:

a. *Prolonged starvation*: During the starvation, the carbohydrate level will be low so the stored fat of the adipose tissue breakdown to free fatty acids. The free fatty acids formed to enter in the liver and undergoes oxidation to release energy.

b. *Uncontrolled diabetes mellitus*: Because of the lack of insulin the carbohydrate is not utilized. The adipose tissue fat becomes the main source of energy and its degradation is generally accelerated. It results in the excessive production of acetyl CoA, which cannot be utilized by the liver through TCA cycle due to lack of oxaloacetate. So it is converted into ketone bodies.

c. *Feeding high fat diet*: Excess breakdown of fatty acids in the liver takes place. This leads to the formation of more acetyl CoA. Once the acetyl CoA formation exceeds more than the requirement of the liver tissues, it is converted to ketone bodies and exported to muscle, heart and kidney to meet the energy requirement. So the peripheral tissues switch over to utilize ketone bodies.

Formation of ketone bodies (Figure 9.10)

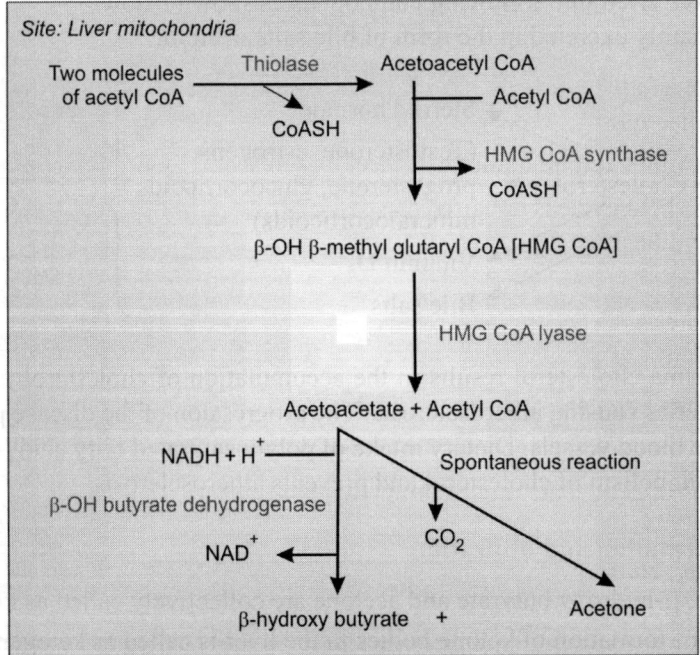

Figure 9.10

Both acetoacetate and β-hydroxy butyrate are week acids, which slowly deplete alkali reserves (bicarbonate) of the body and cause metabolic acidosis. This condition is known as ketoacidosis.

Utilization of ketone bodies (ketolysis) (Figure 9.11)

Acetoacetate and β-hydroxy butyrate can be used as a source of energy in kidney and muscle. During starvation, even brain utilize ketone bodies. Ketone bodies are transported from liver to the extra hepatic tissues and are oxidized in Krebs TCA cycle.

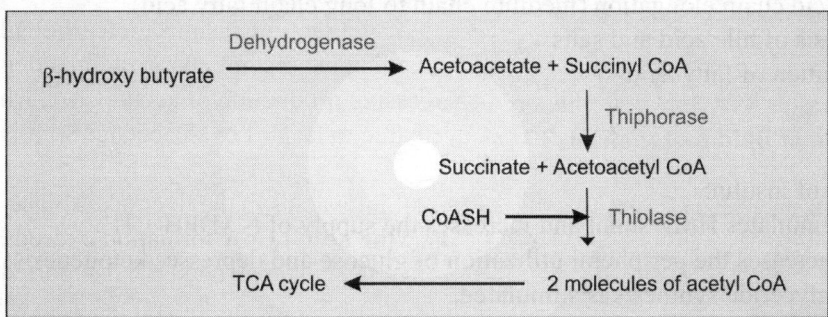

Figure 9.11

Thiophorase is absent in liver. Hence, ketone bodies are not utilized by the liver.

➤ Ketone bodies are water soluble.

➤ They are easily transported from the liver to various tissues.

➤ Acetoacetate and β-hydroxy butyrate serve as an important source of energy for skeletal muscle, cardiac muscle, renal cortex, etc.

➤ During starvation, ketone bodies can meet 50–70% energy needs of brain.

➤ In starvation, TCA cycle is impaired due to the deficiency of oxaloacetate which is diverted to glucose synthesis.

Regulation

➤ Glucagon stimulate ketogenesis.

➤ Insulin inhibits ketogenesis.

➤ The increased ratio of glucagon/insulin in diabetes mellitus promotes ketone body formation.

Ketogenic substances: Fatty acids, amino acids.

Antiketogenic substances: Glucose, glycerol and glucogenic amino acids (Glycine, alanine, serine, glutamate, etc.)

Role of liver in lipid metabolism

Lipids are mainly stored in adipose tissue but liver has a central role in lipid metabolism.

1. Fatty acid synthesis (glucose →   →   acetyl CoA   →   →   fatty acid)
2. Cholesterol synthesis

Glucose
Fatty acid breakdown   →   Acetyl CoA   →   Cholesterol
Ketogenic amino acid

3. Plasma lipoproteins such as VLDL, LDL and HDL are synthesized in liver.
4. Ketone bodies are synthesized in the liver..
5. Fatty acid chain elongation (medium chain to long chain fatty acid).
6. Synthesis of bile acid and salts.
7. β-oxidation of fatty acid.

Regulation of lipid metabolism

1. Actions of insulin:
   a. It stimulates HMP shunt and increases the supply of NADPH + H$^+$.
   b. It increases the peripheral utilization of glucose and depresses ketogenesis.
   c. Triglyceride synthesis is stimulated.
2. Glucocorticoids:
   These hormones increase the rate of release of fatty acid from adipose tissue which in turn leads to ketogenesis and increase cholesterol synthesis.

Self Test

1. Briefly discuss on the digestion and absorption of lipids in the gastrointestinal tract.
2. Add a note on β-oxidation of fatty acids.
3. How many ATPs are produced when one mole of palmitic acid is completely metabolized to acetyl CoA?
4. Explain the denovo synthesis of fatty acid. What is the source of NADPH?
5. Name the compounds formed from cholesterol.
6. Write a short note on atherosclerosis.
7. Name the ketone bodies and mention the conditions in which ketone bodies are formed.
8. Briefly discuss on the formation and utilization of ketone bodies.
9. Write short notes on the following:
   a. Role of liver in lipid metabolism
   b. Metabolic fate of acetyl CoA
   c. Carnitine cycle
   d. Ketoacidosis
10. Explain the terms ketonemia, ketonuria and ketolysis.
11. Outline β-oxidation of fatty acids.
12. How many ATPs are produced when one mole of palmitic acid is completely metabolized to acetyl CoA?
13. Explain the synthesis of fatty acid briefly. What is the source of NADPH?
14. Write short notes on:
   a. Compounds formed from cholesterol
   b. Atherosclerosis
   c. Ketone bodies

Fill in the blanks

1. Net ATPs produced during complete oxidation of palmitic acid is _____.
2. _____ compound is required for the transport of activated fatty acid inside the mitochondria.

3. _____ enzyme digest triglycerides.

4. Lipid absorption requires _____ for emulsification.

Match the following

Enzyme	Action	Match
1. Thiokinase	a. splits HMG CoA	
2. Thiolase	b. β-ketoacyl CoA synthesis	
3. HMG CoA reductase	c. Interconverts β-OH-butyrate and acetoacetate	
4. HMG CoA lyase	d. Required for the activation of fatty acid	
5. β-OH butyrate DH	e. Synthesis of mevalonic acid	
6. β-OH acyl CoA DH	f. β-ketoacyl CoA to acyl CoA and acetyl CoA	

Multiple choice questions

1. **Which of the following is an inaccurate description of cholesterol?**
   a. it is a low water soluble lipid found in blood.
   b. it exists in only one form in plasma.
   c. it is a major structural component of cell surfaces.
   d. it is esterified to some long chain fatty acids, which enhance its hydrophobicity.

2. **Regarding cholesterol determination on serum, the following statements are true EXCEPT**
   a. it is determined by a modified method of Zak's reaction.
   b. The reddish brown color produced is due to the action of $FeCl_3H_2SO_4$.
   c. The color is directly proportional to the concentration of the substance present and quantitated spectrophotometrically at 550 nm.
   d. The color is inversely proportional to the concentration of the substance present and quantitated spectrophotometrically at 550 nm.

3. **If 20 mg standard cholesterol dissolved in 100 ml absolute ethanol then concentration of cholesterol in 1.0 ml solution is**
   a. 0.02 mg   c. 0.2 mg
   b. 0.8 mg   d. 2.0 mg

4. **All of the following are synthesized from cholesterol EXCEPT**
   a. bile acids   c. vitamin D
   b. vitamin C   d. steroid hormones

5. **In all the following clinical conditions, we find high blood cholesterol EXCEPT**
   a. pernicious anemia
   b. nephrosis
   c. obstructive jaundice
   d. diabetes mellitus

6. **Which of the following is an inaccurate statement regarding the structure of cholesterol?**
   a. it has a molecular formula of $C_{27}H_{46}O$.
   b. it has a molecular formula of $C_{25}H_{45}O$.
   c. it has cyclopentanoperhydrophenanthrene ring.
   d. it has three cyclohexane and one cyclopentane rings.

7. **Which of the following is an accurate description of cholesterol?**
   a. low density lipoprotein is responsible for the transport and elimination of cholesterol from the body.
   b. in healthy individuals, the total plasma cholesterol is in the range of 90–150 mg%.

c. cholesterol is not found in animals.

d. high density lipoproteins and lecithin-cholesterol acyl transferase are responsible for the transport and elimination of cholesterol from the body.

8. **Which of the following is an accurate description of ketone bodies?**
   a. their synthesis is stimulated by insulin and inhibited by glucagon.
   b. they are in water-soluble form of acetyl units that are synthesized in the liver and used by many other tissues in the body as a fuel source.
   c. they are the major fuel source for the brain under basal metabolic conditions.
   d. they are not produced during starvation.

9. **Which of the following accurately describes how fatty acids are synthesized in humans?**
   a. fatty acid synthase sequentially adds two-carbon unit from malonyl CoA until palmitate is made.
   b. complex of seven enzymes makes C16 palmitate directly from eight molecules of acetyl CoA.
   c. acetyl CoA is transported out of the mitochondrial matrix as the three-carbon activated molecule malonyl CoA.
   d. Fatty acid synthesis generates large quantities of NADPH, which can be used by the electron transport chain and ATP synthase to generate ATP.

10. **Net amount of ATPs formed when one molecule of palmitic acid undergoes beta-oxidation is**
    a. 29   b. 140
    c. 129   d. 130

11. **The regulatory enzyme of cholesterol synthesis is**
    a. glucosyl transferase
    b. HMG CoA reductase
    c. HMG CoA synthase
    d. mevalonate kinase

12. **One of the following is NOT a biochemical action of prostaglandin**
    a. regulation of blood pressure
    b. reproduction
    c. development of bone
    d. inflammation

13. **Regarding fatty acid synthase complex, all the following statements are true EXCEPT**
    a. is a dimmer with identical subunits
    b. monomer form is functionally active
    c. monomer has seven different enzymes and an acyl carrier protein
    d. two subunits lie in antiparallel orientation

14. **All of the following involve acetyl CoA EXCEPT**
    a. ketone body synthesis
    b. cholesterol synthesis
    c. nucleotide synthesis
    d. fatty acid synthesis

15. **During prolonged starvation, the brain mainly depends on one of the following for energy.**
    a. glucose residues
    b. ketone bodies
    c. amino acids
    d. lactose molecules

16. **For the synthesis of 16-carbon palmitic acid, number of acetyl CoAs transported from mitochondria to cytosol is**
    a. 10   c. 2
    b. 20   d. 8

17. **The substance, which carries acyl CoA into the inner mitochondrial membrane for oxidation is**
    a. β-carotene   c. malate
    b. carnitine   d. creatinine

18. **The main regulatory enzyme of fatty acid synthesis is**
    a. acetyl CoA carboxylase
    b. hexokinase
    c. phosphofructokinase
    d. thioesterase

19. **All of the following are the biochemical actions of prostaglandins EXCEPT**
    a. regulation of blood pressure
    b. reproduction
    c. inhibition of platelet aggregation
    d. destruction of free radical

20. **Regarding starvation, all of the following statements are true EXCEPT**
    a. increased gluconeogenesis
    b. increased glycogen degradation
    c. decreased fatty acid oxidation
    d. increased fatty acid oxidation

21. **All of the following are the ketone bodies EXCEPT**
    a. acetoacetate
    b. beta-hydroxyl butyrate
    c. HMG CoA
    d. acetone

22. **Ketosis occurs in all of the following conditions EXCEPT**
    a. starvation
    b. uncontrolled diabetes mellitus
    c. in the well-fed state
    d. feeding high-fat diet

23. **In humans, most of the prostaglandins are predominantly formed from**
    a. linoleic acid   c. palmitic acid
    b. arachidonic acid   d. stearic acid

24. **All of the following are the components of fatty acid synthase complex EXCEPT**
    a. Acetyl transferase (AT)
    b. Malonyl transferase (MT)
    c. β-ketoacyl synthase (KS)
    d. Succinate dehydrogenase (SD)

25. **Compound required for the transport of activated fatty acid inside the mitochondria is**
    a. Lipoprotein   b. Apoprotein
    c. Carnitine   d. β-carotene

26. **One of the following enzymes mainly digests triglycerides**
    a. Amylase   b. lipase
    c. chymotrypsin   d. pepsin

27. **Micelle formation with bile salts is essential for**
    a. Lipid absorption
    b. Carbohydrate absorption
    c. Lipid digestion
    d. Protein transport

28. **The enzyme which splits HMG CoA is**
    a. Thiokinase
    b. Thiolase
    c. HMG CoA lyase
    d. HMG CoA reductase

29. **One of the following is an example for ketone bodies**
    a. acetoacetic acid   b. lactic acid
    c. pyruvic acid   d. gluconic acid

10

Integration of Metabolism

All organisms possess their variable energy demands; hence, the supply is also equally variable.

The consumed metabolic fuel may be oxidized to CO_2 and H_2O or stored to meet the energy requirements as per the body needs.

ATP serves as the energy currency of the cell.

Glycolysis

Degradation of glucose to pyruvate (Lactate under anaerobic) generates 8 ATPs.

Fatty acid oxidation

Fatty acid (FA) oxidizes to acetyl CoA.
Energy is trapped in the forms of NADH and $FADH_2$.

Amino acid degradation

When amino acids consumed more than the required, are degraded to meet the fuel demands of the body. The glucogenic amino acids can serve as the precursor for the synthesis of glucose via pyruvate or intermediates of TCA cycle. The ketogenic amino acids form the precursor for acetyl CoA.

Citric acid cycle

Acetyl CoA is the common metabolite, produced from different fuel sources. It enters into citric acid cycle and gets oxidized to CO_2. Most of the energy is trapped in the forms of NADH and $FADH_2$.

Oxidative phosphorylation

The NADH and $FADH_2$, produced in different metabolic pathways, are finally oxidized in the electron transport chain, which is coupled with oxidative phosphorylation to generate ATP.

Hexose monophosphate shunt

Concerned with the liberation of NADPH, which is utilized for biosynthesis of several compounds, including fatty acids and ribose sugar, which are essential components of nucleotides.

Gluconeogenesis

Many noncarbohydrate compounds serve as precursor for gluconeogenesis.

Glycogen metabolism: Glycogen is the storage form of glucose in liver and muscle. Glycogen serves as a fuel reserve to meet body needs for a brief period.

The metabolic pathways, in general, are controlled by four different mechanisms:
1. The availability of substrates
2. Covalent modification of enzymes
3. Allosteric regulation
4. Regulation of enzyme synthesis

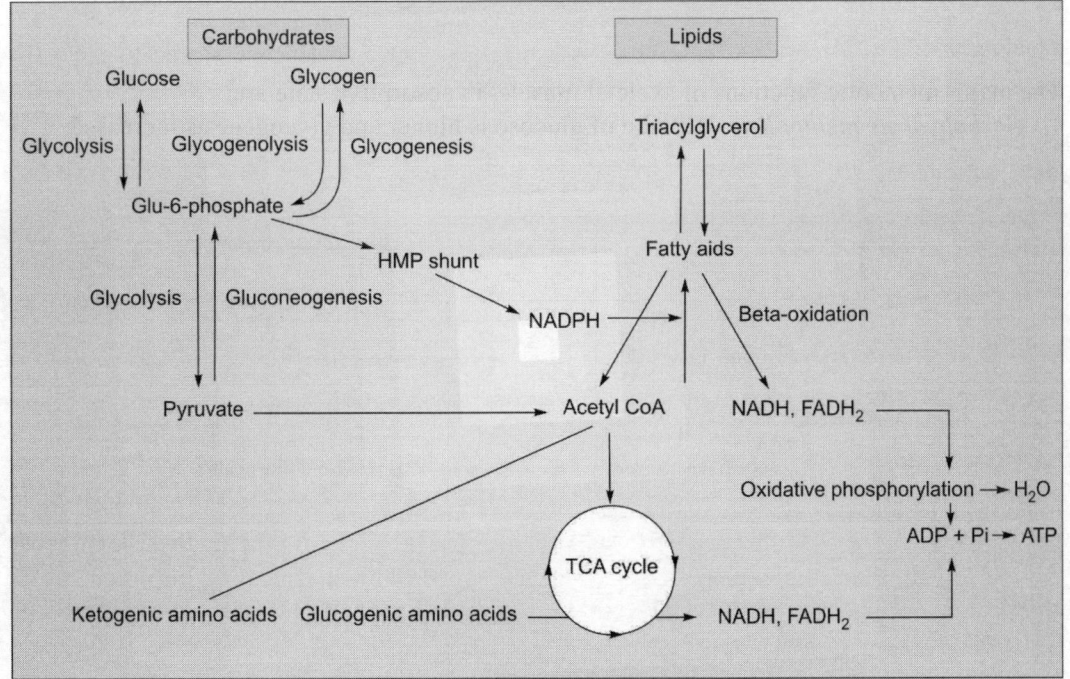

Figure 10.1

1. **Briefly explain the role of different organs and tissues in integrating the metabolism after 2–4 hours of food intake.**

Or

A person went to a marriage party and he had heavy lunch which provided him enough carbohydrates, proteins and fats. How the various tissues and organs of his body work in a well-coordinated manner to meet his metabolic demands?

The various tissues and organs of the body work in a well-coordinated manner to meet its metabolic demands (usually 2–4 hours after food consumption) (Figure 10.2).

Liver

It is specialized to serve as the body's *central metabolic clearing house.* After a meal, the liver takes up the carbohydrates, lipids and amino acids, processes them and routes to other tissues. The major metabolic functions of liver, in absorptive state are:
1. *Carbohydrate metabolism*: Increased glycolysis, glycogenesis, HMP shunt and decreased gluconeogenesis.
2. *Lipid metabolism*: Increased fatty acid and triacylglycerol synthesis.
3. *Protein metabolism*: Increased degradation of amino acids and protein synthesis.

Adipose tissue

It is regarded as the energy storage tissue.
1. *Carbohydrate metabolism*: Increases uptake of glucose, glycolysis and HMP shunt.
2. *Lipid metabolism*: Increases FA and TG synthesis. Degradation of TG is inhibited.

Skeletal muscle

The major metabolic functions of skeletal muscle, in absorptive state are:
1. *Carbohydrate metabolism*: Uptake of glucose is higher and glycogenesis increased.

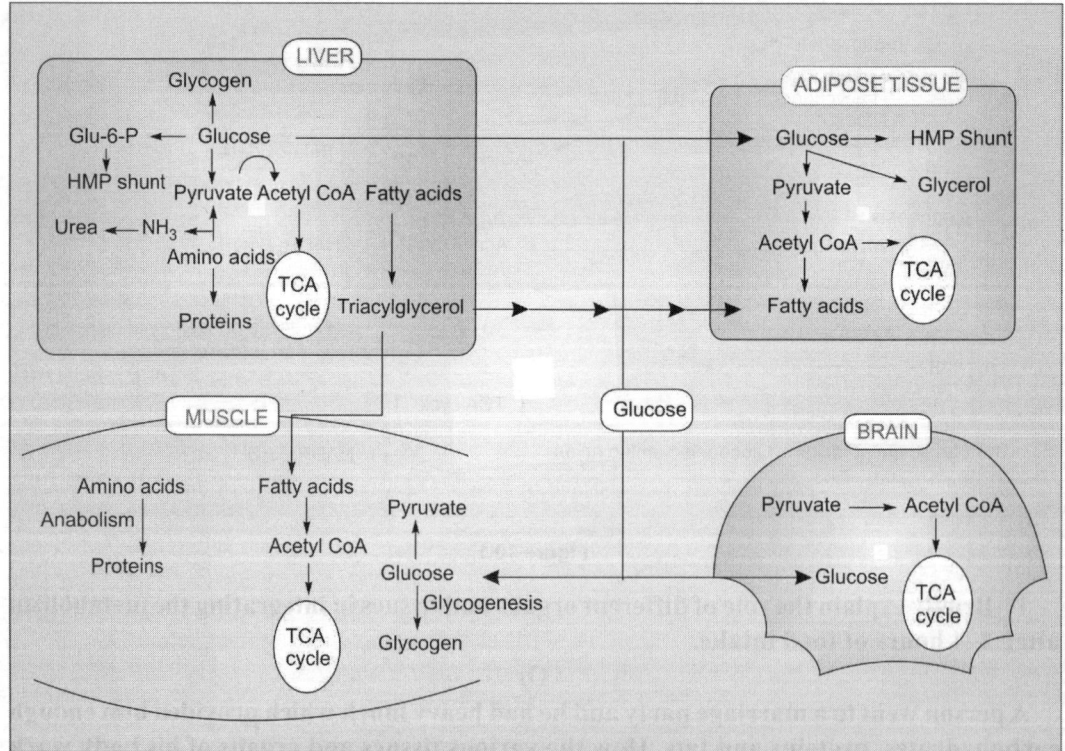

Figure 10.2: *Integration of organs in a well-fed state*

2. *Lipid metabolism*: FA taken up from the circulation.
3. *Protein metabolism*: Incorporation of amino acids into proteins is higher.

Brain

1. *Carbohydrate metabolism*: Glucose is the only source of fuel in an absorptive state. About 120 g of glucose is utilized per day.
2. *Lipid metabolism*: Free fatty acids cannot cross the blood-brain barrier; hence, their contribution for the supply of energy to the brain is insignificant.

2. Briefly discuss the integration of metabolism during starvation.
Or

Steel factory workers went on hunger-strike on demanding the hike in salary. The management did not respond to them still. So they continued their hunger-strike. Discuss the different organs and tissues take part in integrating the metabolism during this condition to meet their energy requirement.

This part explains how all the metabolisms are integrated in different organs and tissues of our body followed by starvation (Figure 10.3).

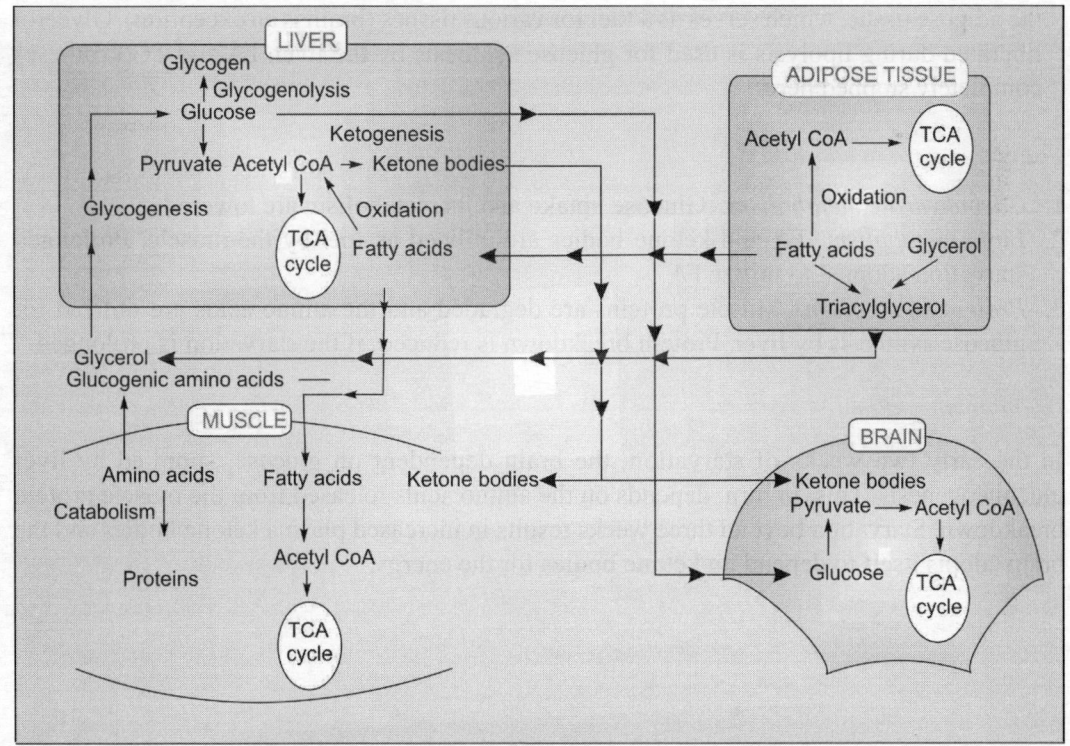

Figure 10.3: *Metabolic interrelationship during starvation*

➢ Starvation may be due to food scarcity or the desire to rapidly lose weight or during surgery and burns.
➢ It is a metabolic stress, which imposes certain metabolic compulsions on the organism.
➢ The metabolism is reorganized to meet the new demands of starvation.
➢ Glucose is the fuel of choice for brain and muscle. Unfortunately, the carbohydrate is not sufficient to meet the requirements.
➢ The triacylglycerol (TG) of adipose tissue is the predominant energy reserve of the body.
➢ Protein can also meet the fuel demands of the body.
➢ Starvation associated with decreased insulin and increased glucagon.

Liver in starvation

1. *Carbohydrate metabolism*: Increased gluconeogenesis and glycogen degradation.
2. *Lipid metabolism*: FA oxidation increased. The TCA cycle cannot cope up with the excess production of acetyl CoA, so it is diverted for ketone body formation. The fuel demands of the brain are met by ketone bodies.

Adipose tissue in starvation

1. *Carbohydrate metabolism*: Glucose uptake and its metabolism are lowered.
2. *Lipid metabolism*: Degradation of TG increased, leading to increased release of FA from the adipose tissue, which serves as a fuel for various tissues (brain is an exception). Glycerol liberated during lipolysis is used for glucose synthesis by the liver. FA and TG syntheses completely stopped here.

Skeletal muscle in starvation

1. *Carbohydrate metabolism*: Glucose uptake and its metabolism are lowered.
2. *Lipid metabolism*: FA and ketone bodies are utilized as fuel by the muscle. Prolonged starvation adopted to utilize FA.
3. *Protein metabolism*: Muscle proteins are degraded and the amino acids are utilized for glucose synthesis by liver. Protein breakdown is reduced, if the starvation is prolonged.

Brain in starvation

In the early two weeks of starvation, the brain dependent on glucose, supplied by liver gluconeogenesis. This, in turn, depends on the amino acids released from the muscle protein breakdown. Starvation beyond three weeks results in increased plasma ketone bodies and the brain adopts itself to depend on ketone bodies for the energy.

11

Hemoglobin Synthesis

Introduction

Hemoglobin is the red pigment present in RBC and transports O_2 to the tissues. It is made up of 2 parts, they are heme, a pigment and a protein part called globin. There are 4 heme molecules and 4 polypeptide chains in one molecule of Hb.

Hemoglobin synthesis takes place in the bone marrow. Its level in blood is 12–16 g/dL. The synthesis of hemoglobin depends on three important factors; they are iron, folic acid, and vitamin B_{12} along with amino acids. Deficiency of any of these factors decreases the ability of the bone marrow to synthesize RBC, thus, causing anemia.

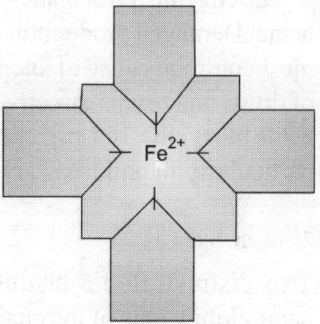

Figure 11.1

Structure of heme

Heme consists of a porphyrin ring with one iron (Ferrous Fe^{2+}) at the centre.

Normal hemoglobin

- Hemoglobin is a conjugated metalloprotein of molecular weight 68,000.
- It is involved in oxygen transport in erythrocytes.
- It consists of 4 heme molecules linked to the protein portion called "globin". Globin part consists of 4 polypeptide chains.
- Each heme molecule is located in a pocket formed by the folding of polypeptide chain.
- Normal adult blood consists of 2 types of Hb, they are HbA_1 and HbA_2.
- HbA_1 comprises 97% of the total Hb and HbA_2 is about 3% of the total Hb.
- The blood of the newborn baby contains another type of Hb called fetal hemoglobin (HbF). The amount of HbF is up to 90% in the neonatal stage and falls gradually by about 4–5 months.

- In normal adults HbF concentration is about 1%.

  The polypeptide chain compositions of various hemoglobins are as follows:

HbA$_1$	$\alpha_2\beta_2$ chains
HbA$_2$	$\alpha_2\delta_2$ chains
HbF	$\alpha_2\gamma_2$ chains

  The numbers of amino acids in the polypeptide chains are as follows:

α-chain	141
β-chain	146
δ-chain	146
γ-chain	146

Heme Synthesis

Heme is synthesized in a complex series of steps involving enzymes in the mitochondrion and in the cytosol of the cell (Figure 11.2). The first step in heme synthesis takes place in the mitochondrion, with the condensation of succinyl CoA and glycine by ALA synthase to form 5-aminolevulinic acid (ALA). This molecule is transported to the cytosol where a series of reactions produce a ring structure called coproporphyrinogen III. This molecule returns to the mitochondrion where an addition reaction produces protoporphyrin IX.

The enzyme ferrochelatase inserts iron into the ring structure of protoporphyrin IX to produce heme. Deranged production of heme produces a variety of anemias. Iron deficiency, the world's most common cause of anemia, impairs heme synthesis thereby producing anemia. A number of drugs and toxins directly inhibit heme production by interfering with enzymes involved in heme biosynthesis. Lead commonly produces substantial anemia by inhibiting heme synthesis, particularly in children.

Globin Synthesis

Two distinct globin chains (each with its individual heme molecule) combine to form hemoglobin. One of the chains is designated as alpha. The second chain is called "non-alpha". With the exception of the very first weeks of embryogenesis, one of the globin chains is always alpha. A number of variables influence the nature of the non-alpha chain in the hemoglobin molecule. The fetus has a distinct non-alpha chain called gamma. After birth, a different non-alpha globin chain called beta, pairs with the alpha chain. The combination of two alpha chains and two non-alpha chains produces a complete hemoglobin molecule (a total of four chains per molecule).

Regulation of heme biosynthesis

➤ Although heme is synthesized in all tissues, the principal sites of synthesis are erythroid cells (~85%) and hepatocytes. The differences in these two tissues and their needs for heme result in quite different mechanisms for regulation of heme biosynthesis.

➤ In hepatocytes, heme is required for incorporation into the cytochromes, in particular, the P_{450} class of cytochromes that are important for detoxification. In addition, numerous cytochromes of the oxidative-phosphorylation pathway contain heme.

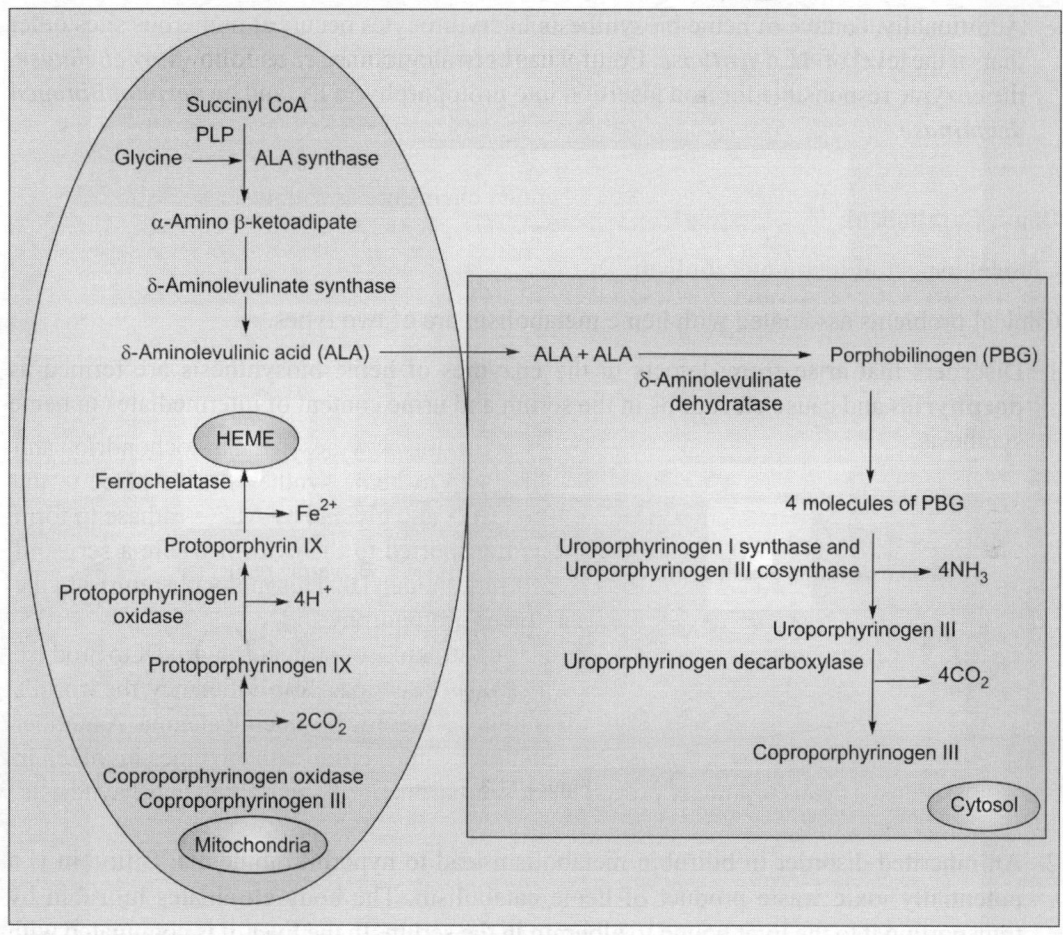

Figure 11.2

➢ The rate-limiting step in hepatic heme biosynthesis occurs at the *ALA synthase* catalyzed step, which is the committed step in heme synthesis.

➢ The Fe^{3+} oxidation product of heme is termed as **hemin**. Hemin acts as a feedback inhibitor on *ALA synthase*.

➢ Hemin also inhibits transport of *ALA synthase* from the cytosol (it's site of synthesis) into the mitochondria (it's site of action) as well as represses synthesis of the enzyme.

➢ In erythroid cells, all of the hemes are synthesized for incorporation into hemoglobin and occur only upon differentiation when synthesis of hemoglobin proceeds.

➢ When red cells mature, both heme and hemoglobin syntheses ceased. The heme (and hemoglobin) must, therefore, survive for the life of the erythrocyte (normally this is 120 days).

➢ In reticulocytes heme stimulates protein synthesis.

➢ Additionally, control of heme biosynthesis in erythrocytes occurs at numerous sites other than at the level of *ALA synthase*. Control has been shown to be exerted on *ferrochelatase*, the enzyme responsible for iron insertion into protoporphyrin IX, and on *porphobilinogen deaminase*.

Heme Catabolism

Clinical aspect of heme metabolism

Clinical problems associated with heme metabolism are of two types.

1. Disorders that arise from defects in the enzymes of heme biosynthesis are termed as **porphyrias** and cause elevations in the serum and urine content of intermediates in heme synthesis.

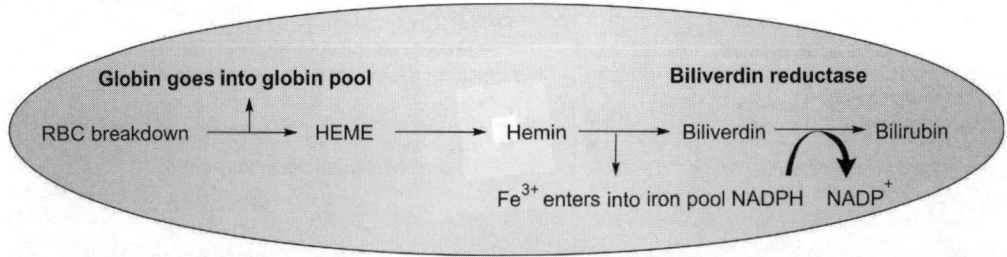

Figure 11.3

2. An inherited disorder in bilirubin metabolism lead to hyperbilirubinemia. Bilirubin is a potentially toxic waste product of heme catabolism. The body eliminates bilirubin by transporting it to the liver bound to albumin in the serum. In the liver, it is conjugated with glucuronide which makes it water soluble. The glucuronide conjugate is then excreted in the bile.

- Persons with extreme elevation in unconjugated bilirubin are susceptible to **bilirubin encephalopathy**, also referred to as **kernicterus**.

- Accumulation of bilirubin in the plasma and tissues results in **jaundice**.

- **Gilbert's syndrome** and **Crigler-Najjar syndrome** result predominantly from unconjugated hyperbilirubinemia.

- **Dubin-Johnson syndrome** and **Rotor's syndrome** result from conjugated hyperbilirubinemia.

- The **porphyrias** are both inherited and acquired disorders in heme synthesis. These disorders are classified as either erythropoietic or hepatic, depending upon the principal site of expression of the enzyme defect (Table 11.1).

Table 11.1

Porphyria erythropoietic class	Enzyme defect	Primary symptom
Congenital erythropoietic porphyria (CEP)	Uroporphyrinogen III cosynthase	Photosensitivity (itching and burning skin of skin when exposed to light.) Excrete more uro and coproporphyrinogen I which then oxidized to uro and coproporphyrin. (red pigments)
Erythropoietic protoporphyria (EPP)	Ferrochelatase	Photosensitivity. Protoporphyrin IX excreted into urine and feces.
Hepatic Class		
ALA dehydratase deficiency porphyria (ADP)	ALA dehydratase	Neurovisceral
Acute intermittent porphyria (AIP)	PBG deaminase or uroporphyrinogen I synthase	Neurovisceral. Increased excretion of porphobilinogen and ALA and urine gets darkened.
Hereditary coproporphyria (HCP)	Coproporphyrinogen oxidase	Neurovisceral, some photosensitivity. Coproporphyrinogen, ALA and PBG are excreted in urine and feces.
Variegate porphyria (VP)	Protoporphyrinogen oxidase	Neurovisceral, some photosensitivity. All the intermediates of heme synthesis accumulate and excreted in urine and feces.
Porphyria cutanea tarda (PCT)	Uroporphyrinogen decarboxylase	Photosensitivity. Increased excretion of uroporphyrins.
Hepatoerythropoietic porphyria (HEP)	Uroporphyrinogen decarboxylase	Photosensitivity, some neurovisceral.

Binding Sites for Oxygen, Hydrogen and Carbon Dioxide

Oxygen binds with ferrous (Fe^{2+}) atoms of the heme to form oxyhemoglobin.

Carbon dioxide binds with alpha amino group of N-terminal end of the polypeptide chains of hemoglobin to form carbaminohemoglobin (Figure 11.4).

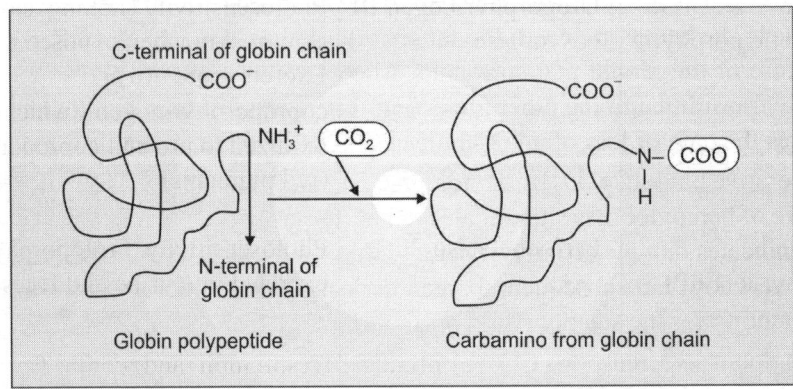

Figure 11.4: *Binding of carbon dioxide to hemoglobin*

Formation of Oxyhemoglobin (Relaxed R structure)

The binding of the first-oxygen molecule to deoxyhemoglobin shifts the heme iron towards the plane of the heme ring, from a position about 0.6 nm beyond it.

This is transmitted to the proximal histidine and other residues lying next.

The salt bridges between the carboxyl terminal residues of all four subunits breaks.

The pair of a and b subunits rotates 15 degrees with respect to the other, compacting the tetramer. The changes in secondary, tertiary and quaternary structures accompany the high-affinity O_2—induced transfer of Hb from the low-affinity, stressed or tense (T) or taut state to the high-affinity relaxed (R) state (Figure 11.5). These changes increase the affinity of the remaining unoxygenated hemes for O_2.

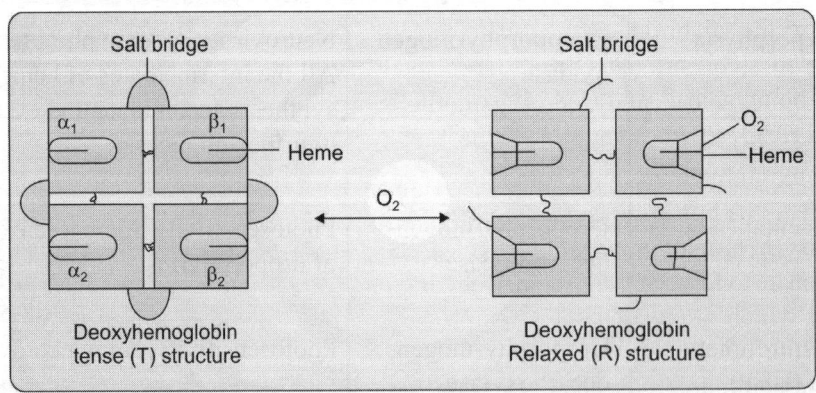

Figure 11.5: *Tense and relaxed structure of hemoglobin*

Cooperative Oxygen Binding of Hemoglobin

The cooperative interaction between different binding sites makes hemoglobin an unusually good oxygen-transport protein because it enables the molecule to pick up as much oxygen as possible once the partial pressure of this gas reaches a particular threshold level, and then give off as much oxygen as possible when the partial pressure of O_2 drops significantly below this threshold level. The hemes are much too far apart to interact directly. But, changes that occur in the structure of the globin that surrounds a heme when it picks up an O_2 molecule, are mechanically transmitted to the other globins in this protein. These changes carry the signal that facilitates the gain or loss of an O_2 molecule by the other hemes (Figure 11.6).

The cooperative binding of O_2 by hemoglobin enhances oxygen transport. The shape of O_2 binding curve of hemoglobin is sigmoidal (S-shaped) because oxygen binding is cooperative. This shape indicates that the affinity of hemoglobin for binding the first molecule of oxygen is relatively very low, but subsequent oxygen molecules are bound with a very much higher affinity accounting for the steeply rising portion of the S-shaped curve.

The hemoglobin also transports CO_2 (by product of respiration) and protons from peripheral tissues to the lungs. Hemoglobin carries CO_2 as carbamates (15%) formed with the amino terminal nitrogen of the polypeptide chains.

$$CO_2 + Hb–NH_2 \leftrightarrow H^+ + Hb–NH–COO^-$$

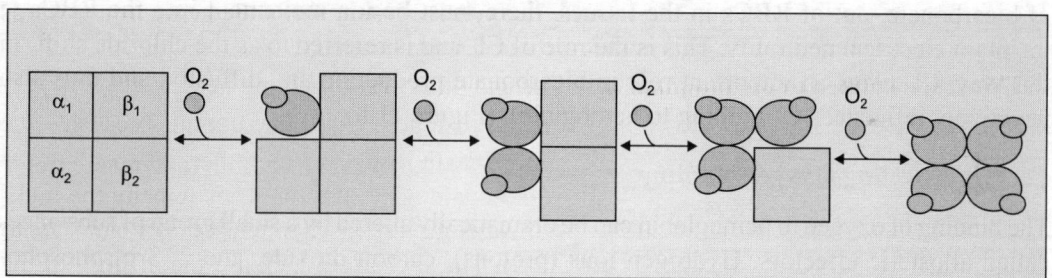

Figure 11.6: *Cooperative binding of oxygen to hemoglobin*

This favors the salt bridge formation between α and β chains of hemoglobin. The remaining CO_2 is carried as bicarbonate, which is formed in erythrocyte by the hydration of CO_2 to H_2CO_3 (carbonic acid), catalyzed by carbonic anhydrase. The venous blood pH dissociates H_2CO_3 into HCO_3^- (bicarbonate) and a proton.

Deoxyhemoglobin binds one proton for every two oxygen molecules released, contributing significantly to the buffering capacity of blood. In the lungs, the process reverses. As oxygen binds to deoxyhemoglobin, protons are released (due to rupture of salt bridges) and combine with bicarbonate to form carbonic acid. Dehydration of H_2CO_3 catalyzed by carbonic anhydrase, forms CO_2, which is exhaled. This reciprocal coupling of protons and oxygen binding is termed as Bohr effect. This effect mainly depends on cooperative interactions between the hemes of the hemoglobin tetramer. Therefore, myoglobin (monomer) does not exhibit Bohr effect (Figure 11.7).

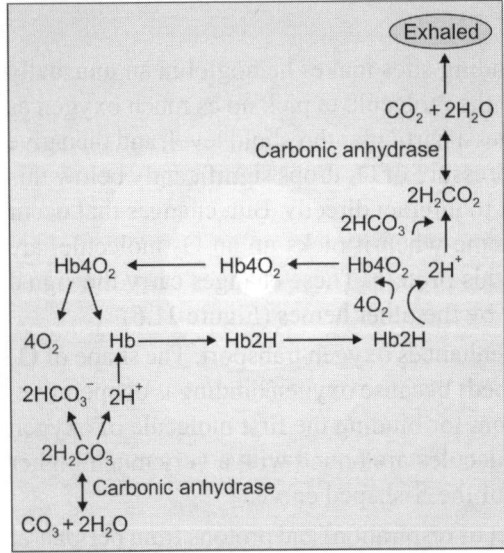

Figure 11.7: *Bohr effect*

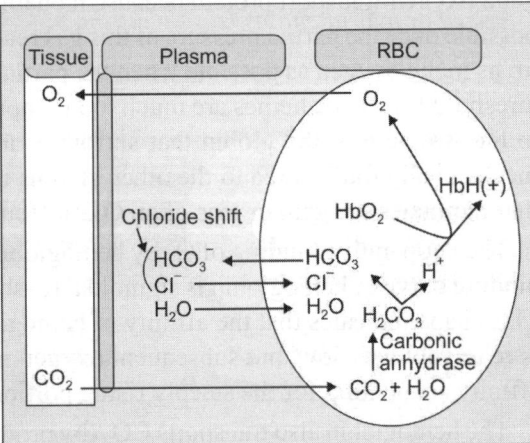

Figure 11.8: *Chloride shift*

Bohr effect increases in hydrogen ion concentration and decreases the amount of oxygen bound by hemoglobin at any oxygen concentration (partial pressure). Coupled to the diffusion of bicarbonate, out of RBCs in the tissues, there must be ion movement into the RBCs to maintain electrical neutrality. This is the role of Cl^- and is referred to as the chloride shift. In this way, Cl^- plays an important role in bicarbonate production and diffusion and thus also negatively influences O_2 binding to hemoglobin (Figure 11.8).

Factors Affecting Oxygen Binding

The binding of oxygen to hemoglobin can be dramatically altered by a small group of substances called allosteric effectors. Hydrogen ions (protons), carbon dioxide, and 2, 3-bisphosphoglycerate are effectors that can promote the release of oxygen by favoring the deoxygenated form of hemoglobin.

Role of 2, 3-Bisphosphoglycerate

Low PO_2 (Partial pressure of oxygen) in peripheral tissues promotes the synthesis of 2, 3-BPG in erythrocytes from 1, 3-BPG. This 2, 3-BPG binds with deoxygenated hemoglobin (T) and stabilizes it. The BPG binds more weakly with HbF than with HbA. Therefore, the HbF has higher affinity for O_2 than HbA.

ABNORMAL HEMOGLOBIN

The abnormal hemoglobin of sickle cell anemia was first demonstrated by Linus Pauling in 1949. Structurally, each globin chain has its own genetic locus. The individual chain of hemoglobin is under genetic control. Based on the genetics of the globin chain production, structural abnormalities can be divided into four groups:

- *Amino acid substitutions*: HbS, HbC, HbD and HbE
- *Amino acid deletion (deletion of three nucleotides in DNA)*: Hb Gun Hill
- Elongated globin chains (resulted from chain termination, shift mutation or other mutations)
- *Fused* or *hybrid chains (resulted from nonhomologous crossing over)*: Hb Lepore.

Most of the hemoglobin variants arised by a single amino acid substitution which is called "point mutations".

Deletion of one or two nucleotide bases can shift the reading frame of all code words which follow. Such an event observed in microorganisms was called as "Frame shift mutation".

Abnormal hemoglobins are inherited as autosomal codominants. Thus, subjects who inherit one normal and one abnormal genes are heterozygous and those who have two identical abnormal genes are homozygous.

Hemoglobinopathy

When biological functions of hemoglobin are altered due to a mutation in hemoglobin, the condition is known as **hemoglobinopathy,** which may be grouped into two types:

Quantitative hemoglobinopathies, characterized by α decreased synthesis of either α or β globin chain, leading to altered combination of normal α, β, γ or Δ chains, e.g. thalassemia.

Qualitative hemoglobinopathies, characterized by an altered sequence of amino acids, usually in one of the constituent chains, e.g. sickle cell disease, hemoglobin C disease, hemoglobin D disease, hemoglobin M disease.

In normal adults, amount of HbF is about 1%. Presence of HbF more than 1% in adults and children above the age of 1 year is abnormal and the condition is known as hemoglobinopathy.

Thalassemia

The name derived from the Greek word, *thalassa*, which means "sea". Greeks inherited this disease present around Mediterranean sea. Absence or diminished synthesis of one of the polypeptide chains of human hemoglobin is characterized as "thalassemia". The reduction in the α-chain synthesis is called α-thalassemia and decreased synthesis of β-chain synthesis is called β-thalassemia. The α-thalassemia is more common.

α-thalassemia: α-globin chain is structurally normal but production of a globin chain is impaired, resulting in the production of excess β-globin and γ-globin chains, which result in the:

Formation of β-globin tetramer, called HbH and tetramer of γ-globin Hb Bart. These two forms cannot deliver oxygen to the tissues, leading to fetal death.

Decreased production of hemoglobins but contains α-chains, i.e. HbA_1, HbA_2 and HbF.

β-thalassemia: In this type, β-globin chain is structurally normal but the production of β-globin chain is decreased. This decreased production of β-globin chain leads to:

A large excess of α-chains and form α-globin tetramer that precipitates immediately within the RBC as Heinz bodies and responsible for damage of the cell membrane and premature breakdown of RBCs.

There are two types of β-thalassemias:
1. β-*thalassemia major*: This is the homozygous state for the β-thalassemia gene. It is a severe disease. Splenomegaly and skin pigmentation are the clinical pictures. Blood picture shows anemia, erythrocyte shows marked anisocytosis. The MCV and MCH decrease and MCHC increases. Both HbA and HbF are present (HbF 10–98%).
2. β-*thalassemia minor*: This is the heterozygous state for the β-thalassemia gene. In this condition, both HbA and HbF are present with less symptoms.

SICKLE CELL HEMOGLOBIN (HbS)

The sickle cell hemoglobinopathies are hereditary disorders in which the red cells contain HbS. They include heterozygous (sickle cell trait, HbA and HbS present) and homozygous (sickle cell anemia, only HbS is present with the complete absence of HbA) for HbS. HbS causes a condition called sickle cell anemia. HbS differs from HbA in the substitution of valine for glutamic acid in the 6th position from the N-terminal end of the β-chain.

HbA—Val-His-Leu-Thr-Pro-Glu-Glu-Lys

HbS—Val-His-Leu-Thr-Pro-Val-Glu-Lys

- The side chain of valine is distinctly nonpolar, whereas that of glutamate is highly polar. This generates hydrophobic contact point called sticky patch, at position six of the β-chain
- This sticky patch is present on the outer surface of the oxygenated and deoxygenated HbSs. This is not found in normal HbA.
- A complementary sticky patch is also present on the surface of the deoxygenated HbS. It is masked in oxygenated HbS.
- This alteration in polarity markedly reduces the solubility of deoxygenated HbS.
- When this HbS is deoxygenated, the sticky patch can bind to the complementary patch on another deoxygenated HbS molecule. This binding causes polymerization of deoxy-HbS forming insoluble long tubular fibrous precipitates (Figure 11.9).

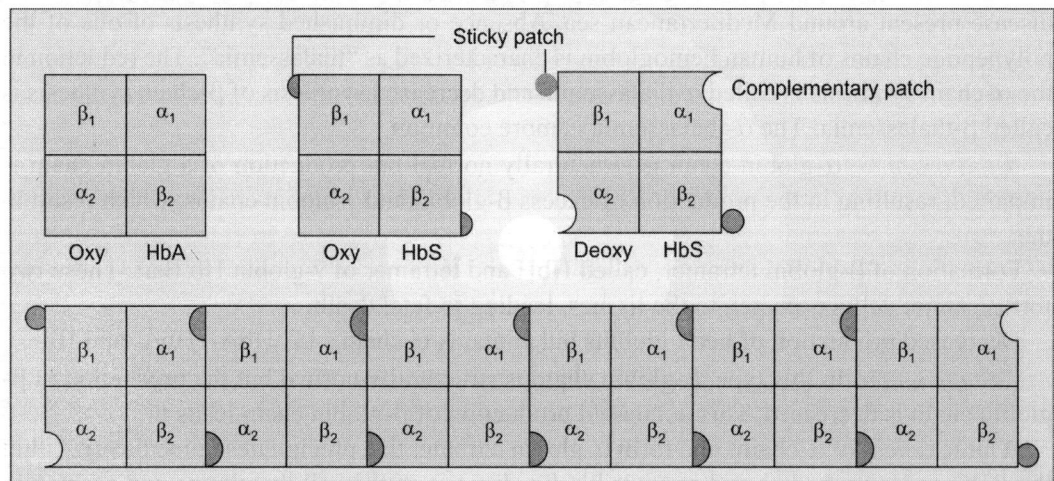

Figure 11.9: *Polymerization of deoxyhemoglobin*

- The insoluble fibers of deoxygenated HbS distort the red cells into sickle-shaped (crescent-shaped) cells (Figure 11.10). Hence, this condition is known as sickle cell anemia. The change in the shape of the cell causes hemolysis leading to anemia.

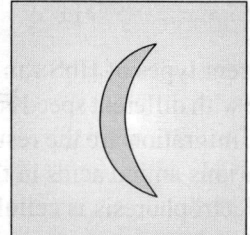

Clinical Symptoms

Figure 11.10: *Sickle red blood cells*

- Chronic hemolytic anemia
- Hypoxia (Breathlessness) due to less blood supply to the tissues and decreased oxygen
- Pain and swelling in the joints
- Persons with sickle cell trait show an increased resistance to malaria specifically for *Plasmodium falciparum*. This parasite spends an obligatory part of its lifecycle in the red blood cell.

Detection of Abnormal Hb (Figure 11.11)

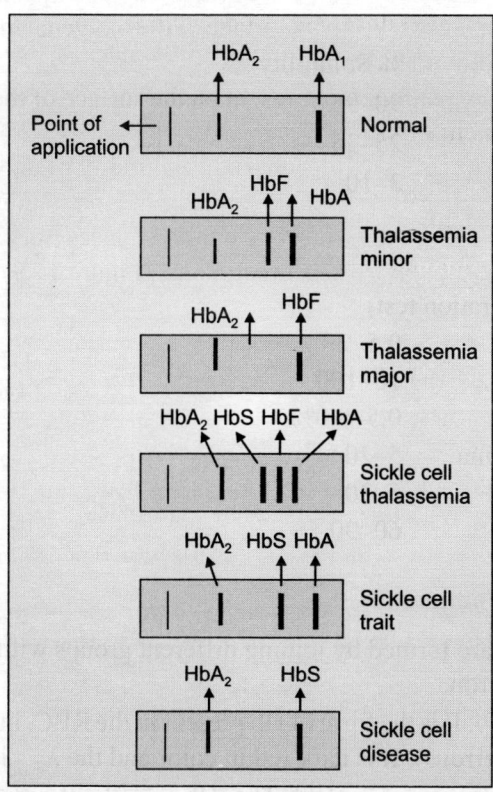

Figure 11.11: *Normal and abnormal hemoglobin patterns on cellulose acetate electrophoresis*

Electrophoresis of HbS

Different types of HbS can be separated from each other by electrophoresis. The Hb variants move with different speeds in an electrical field, and appear as separate bands. These differences in the migration are the result of different electrical charges of each Hb variant brought about by various amino acids in the polypeptide chains of Hb molecules. Support medium used for Hb electrophoresis is cellulose acetate strip.

Detection of HbS

Sickling test: Red cells containing HbS when mixed with a freshly prepared solution of sodium metabisulfite (reducing agent). This can be detected under microscope. This test is simple and will detect both homozygous and heterozygous sickle genes. False results may be obtained, if the patient has had a recent transfusion of normal red cells, or if the blood sample is infected.

Solubility test: HbS is less soluble in concentrated buffer solution at a pH of 6.5 whereas normal Hb is soluble. This principle is used in differentiating HbS from normal Hb. When Hb is added to a solution of sodium hydrosulfite, a reducing agent in phosphate buffer, the solubility decreases and the solution becomes turbid, if HbS is present.

Reference Range

	% Solubility
Normal	90–95
Hb AS	25–35
Hb SS	3–10

Reference Range

Hb F% (Alkali denaturation test)	
Normal	0.5–2
Thalassemia major	10–100
Thalassemia minor	0.5–8.0%
Sickle cell β-thalassemia	5–20
Sickle cell anemia	5–30
Normal newborn	60–90

Derived Hemoglobin Compounds

Hemoglobin derivatives are formed by joining different groups with the heme part or change in the oxidation state of iron.

- *Oxyhemoglobin (Hb-O)*: It is the form of Hb present in the RBC, in the body. O_2 is combined to Hb through Fe^{2+} (Ferrous). It is dark red in color and the λ_{max} is 577 nm.
- *Reduced Hb or deoxyhemoglobin (Hb)*: This Hb is without oxygen. This is purple red in color.

- *CarboxyHb (Hb-CO)*: CarboxyHb is formed by binding of CO with Hb. CO binds with the iron atom in the same way as oxygen binds. CO has more affinity towards Hb than O_2; hence, even small quantity of CO present, will bind to the Hbλ_{max} of Hb-CO is 572 nm.
- Exposure to CO occurs in the following conditions:
  - In the mines (also deep wells)
  - Heavy cigarette smoking
  - Incomplete burning of petrol.
- *Methemoglobin (MetHb)*: A substitution of tyrosine for the histidine at either the proximal or distal histidine residues of either the α- or β-chains locks the heme iron into a trivalent state (Fe^{3+}) or the action of oxidizing agents on ferrous form of Hb converts Fe^{2+} into Fe^{3+} state. Fe^{3+} cannot bind oxygen and, hence, oxygen transport is not possible. Increased Met-Hb in the blood is known as methemoglobinemia.

Causes of Methemoglobinemia

- Congenital MetHb reductase deficiency
- Ingestion of nitrites, nitrates, sulfa drugs, or certain dyes (aniline dyes)
- Household substances like shoe polishes (nitrobenzene), furniture

When MetHb in the blood increases up to 15% of the total pigment cyanosis occurs (Bluish color of the skin). Normally small amount of MetHb is produced in the blood. The enzyme MetHb reductase presents in the RBC converts the Fe^{3+} into Fe^{2+} form thus converting the MetHb to normal Hb.

Thus, under normal conditions MetHb concentration is less than 1% of the total Hb.

$$\lambda_{max} \text{ of MetHb} = 630 \text{ nm}$$

There are again two types of methemoglobinemia:

1. Hereditary methemoglobinemia associated with NADH-methemoglobin reductase deficiency. This is an autosomal recessive trait and affected subjects are persistently cyanotic.

2. Hereditary methemoglobinemia associated with HbM: This is associated with cyanosis. This disorder is transmitted as an autosomal dominant trait.

   - *Sulfhemoglobin (HbS)*: This is an abnormal sulfur containing Hb (attached to the porphyrin ring). It does not act as an oxygen carrier and it is not present in the normal red blood cells. It is formed by the toxic action of drugs and chemical agents that contains sulfur. It results in cyanosis.

   - *Cyanomethemoglobin*: Hb is converted to cyan MetHb by Drabkin's reagent (Potassium ferricyanide + Potassium cyanide). It is a complex formed by MetHb with cyanide and it is a stable compound having λ_{max} at 540 nm. This provides an accurate method for the estimation of Hb in the blood.

   - *Carbonyl Hb (Hb-CO$_2$)*: This is the form of Hb transporting CO_2 from tissues to the lungs.

Muscle Fiber

Skeletal muscle is made up of thousands of cylindrical muscle fibers often running all the way from origin to insertion. The fibers are bound together by connective tissue through which run blood vessels and nerves.

Each muscle fiber contains:

• An array of myofibrils that are stacked lengthwise and run the entire length of the fiber
• Mitochondria
• An extensive smooth endoplasmic reticulum (SER)
• Many nuclei

The multiple nuclei arise from the fact that each muscle fiber develops from the fusion of many cells (myoblasts).

A muscle fiber is not a single cell; its parts are often given special names such as:

• Sarcolemma for plasma membrane
• Sarcoplasmic reticulum for endoplasmic reticulum
• Sarcosome for mitochondrion
• Sarcoplasm for cytoplasm

The striated appearance of the muscle fiber is created by a pattern of alternating dark A bands and light I bands.

• The A bands are bisected by the H zone
• The I bands are bisected by the Z line
• Each fiber is composed of myofibrils and each myofibril is made up of arrays of parallel filaments which is a series of repeating structural units called sarcomeres.
• Sarcomeres are composed of thick (myosin) and thin (actin) filaments.

Thick Filament

• The thick filaments have a diameter of about 15 nm.
• Composed of numerous protein strands which are called myosin filaments.
• Each myosin filament is composed of a two twisted strands called heavy chains and two others, but each different pairs of twisted strands, called light chains. These light chains are found in the myosin heads.
• Myosin filament is flexible at the point of the myosin head, and the stacking of the myosin molecules leaves the myosin heads protruding from the filament at ~60°. This spacing maximizes chances for interaction with actin binding sites.
• Myosin ATPase is found in the myosin heads.
• Another structural element, titin, connects the ends of the myosin filaments to the Z-disks.
• The M-region, centered in the middle of the myosin filaments and crosslinks with other myosin, serves as structural support for the sarcomeres; a part of the M-region contains creatine phosphokinase (CPK).

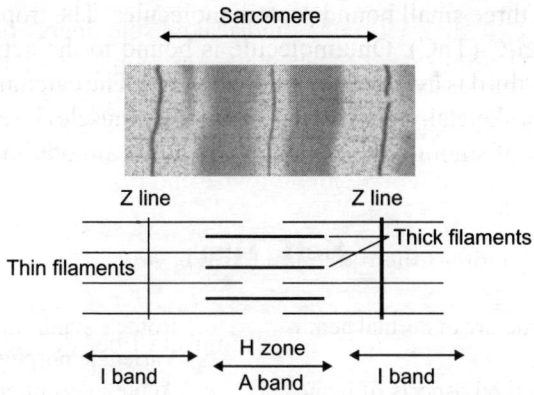

Figure 11.12: *Structure of sarcomere*

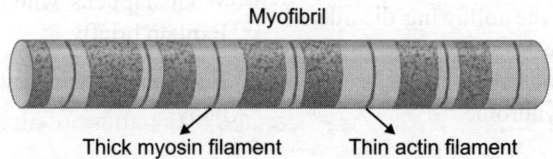

Figure 11.13: *Structure showing thick and thin filaments*

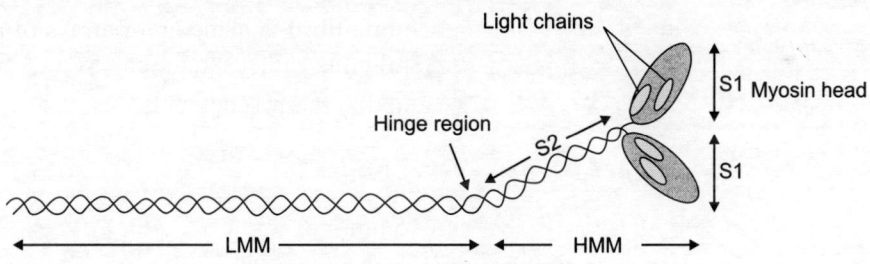

Figure 11.14: *Thick filament*

Thin Filament

- The thin filaments have a diameter of about 5 nm.
- Actin exists as a polymer of repeating globular proteins called G-actin.
- Two actin filaments are twisted into a single stranded filament. These strands are anchored at one end to the Z-disk.
- An ADP molecule on each G-actin molecule is thought to be the active or binding site on the actin filament.
- Lying in the groove formed by the actin filaments are a series of rod-shaped protein molecules called tropomyosin. Each tropomyosin molecule is 6–7 G-actin molecules in length.

- Bound to the end of each tropomyosin is a third protein called *troponin*.
- Troponin consists as three small bound protein molecules. The troponin-I (TnI), troponin-T (TnT) and troponin-C (TnC). One molecule is bound to the actin filament, one to the tropomyosin, and the third is available to bind with Ca^{2+}. The calcium-mediated contraction of striated muscle (fast skeletal, slow skeletal and cardiac muscle) is regulated by the troponin complex; contraction of smooth muscle is regulated by calmodulin.

Self Test

1. Write briefly on the structure of normal hemoglobin.
2. Draw discuss the structural aspects of hemoglobin.
3. Draw the flowchart showing hemoglobin synthesis.
4. Write the causes for the following disorders of hemoglobin synthesis.
   a. Crigler-Najjar syndrome
   b. Dubin-Johnson syndrome
   c. Rotor's syndrome
   d. Variegate porphyria
   e. Acute intermittent porphyria (AIP)
   f. Erythropoietic protoporphyria (EP)
   g. Porphyria cutanea tarda
5. What happens when heme is catabolized? Explain briefly.
6. How hemoglobin synthesis is regulated in our body?

12

Hormones

Hormones are the substances secreted by highly specialized cells and carried by the extra-cellular fluid (mainly blood) and act through the receptor on the target organ to alter the activity of the cells quantitatively to influence:

- Metabolism
- Growth
- Reproduction
- Adaptation to the environment

➤ Hormones carry messages from glands to cells to maintain chemical levels in the bloodstream that achieve homeostasis.

➤ Glands manufacture hormones.

➤ Hormones circulate freely in the bloodstream, waiting to be recognized by a target cell, their intended destination.

➤ The target cell has a receptor that can only be activated by a specific type of hormone. Once activated, the cell knows to start a certain function within its walls.

➤ There are two types of hormones known as steroids and peptides.

➤ In general, steroids are sex hormones related to sexual maturation and fertility. Steroids are made from cholesterol.

➤ Cortisol, an example of a steroid hormone.

➤ Peptides regulate other functions such as sleep and sugar level. They are made from long strings of amino acids, so sometimes they are referred to as "protein" hormones.

➤ Growth hormone helps us to burn fat and build up muscles.

➤ *Insulin*, starts the process to convert sugar into cellular energy.

➤ As special categories, autocrine hormones act on the cells of the secreting gland, while paracrine hormones act on nearby, but unrelated cells.

In classical endocrinology the hormones are:

1. Pituitary hormones
2. Thyroid hormones

3. Parathyroid hormones
4. Pancreatic hormones
5. Suprarenal cortical hormones
6. Suprarenal medullary hormones
7. Ovarian hormones
8. Testicular hormones
9. Hypophyseal hormones

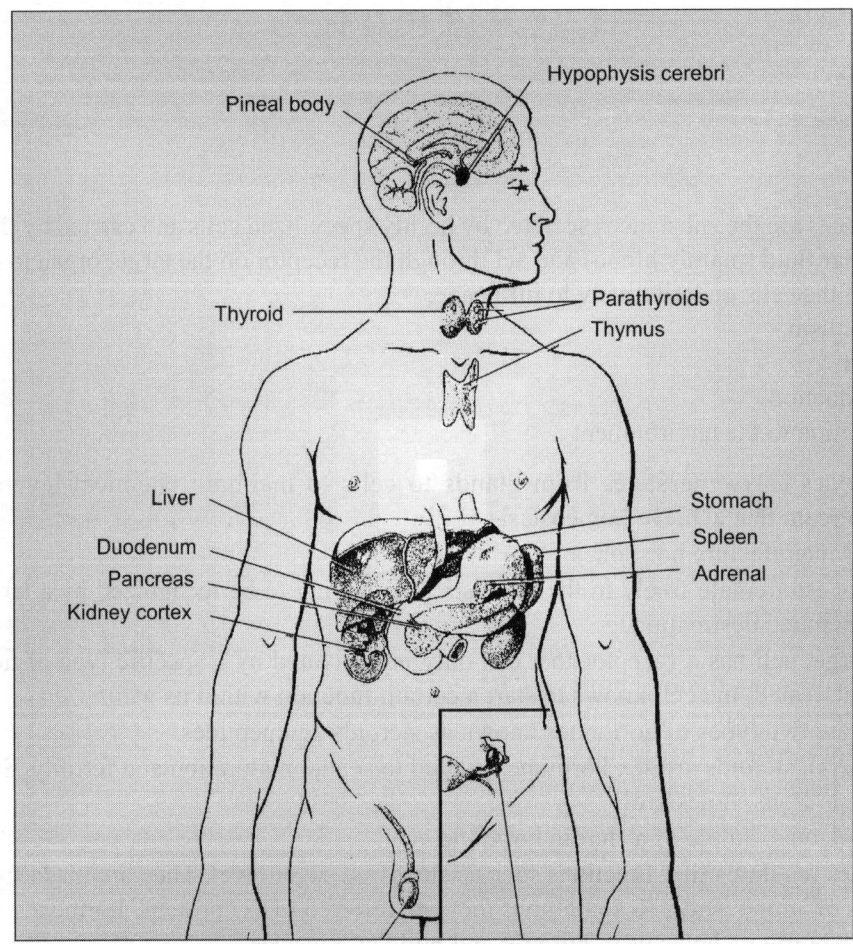

Figure 12.1: *Endocrine glands location in humans*

➤ The hormone binds to a site on the extracellular portion of the receptor.
➤ The receptors are transmembrane proteins that pass through the plasma membrane 7 times, with their *N-terminal* exposed at the exterior of the cell and their *C-terminal* projecting into the cytoplasm.
➤ Binding of the hormone to the receptor activates a **G protein**.

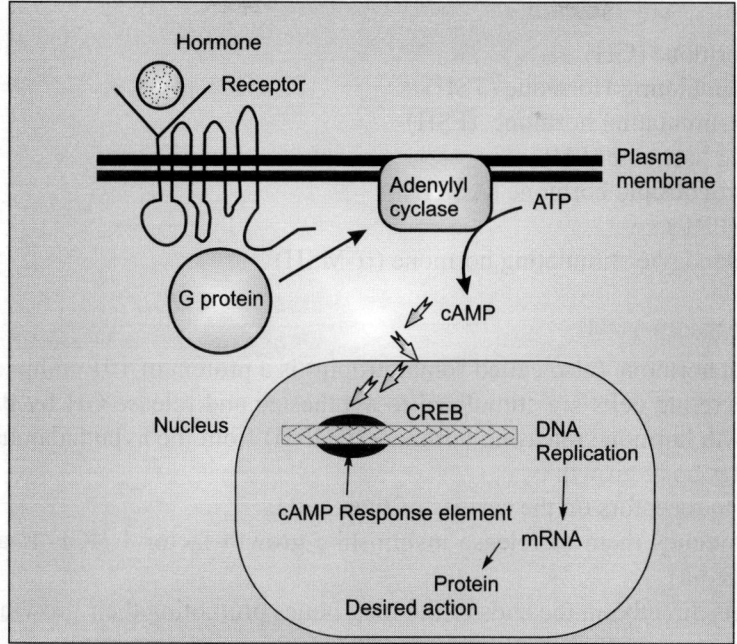

Figure 12.2: *Mechanism of hormonal action*

➢ This initiates the production of a **second messenger** like **cyclic AMP, (cAMP)** which is produced by **adenylyl cyclase** from **ATP, inositol 1, 4, 5-trisphosphate (IP$_3$)**.

➢ The second messenger, in turn, initiates a series of intracellular events such as, phosphorylation and activation of enzymes; release of Ca^{2+} into the cytosol from stores within the endoplasmic reticulum.

➢ In the case of cAMP, these enzymatic changes activate the **transcription factor (cAMP response element binding protein) CREB**.

➢ Bound to its **response element** in the promoters of genes that are able to respond to the hormone, activated CREB turns on gene *transcription*.

➢ Then to translation to produce the desired protein.

➢ Finally biochemical response.

➢ The cell begins to produce the appropriate gene products in response to the hormonal signal it had received at its surface.

Pituitary hormones

The endocrine is a gland, which secretes hormone also called as ductless glands, as the hormone is carried not by the duct, but by the blood.

Pituitary gland comprises:

➢ Anterior pituitary
➢ Posterior pituitary
➢ Intermediate lobe

A. Anterior pituitary hormones

a. Growth hormone (GH)
b. Thyroid stimulating Hormone (TSH)
c. Follicular stimulating hormone (FSH)
d. Luteinizing hormone (LH)
e. Adrenocorticotropic hormone (ACTH)
f. Prolactin (PRL)
g. Alpha-melanocyte stimulating hormone (α-MSH)

a. Growth hormone (GH)

Human growth hormone (also called somatotropin) is a protein of 191 amino acids.

The GH secreting cells are stimulated to synthesize and release GH by the intermittent arrival of growth hormone releasing hormone (GHRH) from the hypothalamus.

GH promotes body growth by:

- Binding to receptors on the surface of liver cells.
- This stimulates them to release insulin-like growth factor 1 (IGF 1; also known as somatomedin).
- IGF 1 acts directly on the ends of the long bones promoting their growth.

Pathophysiology

In childhood, hyposecretion of GH produces the stunted growth of a dwarf.

Dwarfism can also result from an inability to respond to GH.

This can result from inheriting two mutant genes encoding the receptors for

- GHRH or
- GH

Hypersecretion leads to gigantism.

In adults, a hypersecretion of GH leads to acromegaly.

Gigantism   If the growth hormone secretion increases before the epiphysial plate closure take place during the long bone development.

Acromegaly   A condition in which growth hormone secretion increases after the epiphyseal plate closure takes place.

b. Thyroid stimulating hormone (TSH)

TSH (also known as thyrotropin) is a glycoprotein consisting of:

- A β-chain of 112 amino acids and an α-chain of 89 amino acids. The alpha chain is identical to that found in two other pituitary hormones, FSH and LH. Thus, it is its β-chain that gives TSH, its unique properties.

The secretion of TSH is:

- Stimulated by the arrival of thyrotropin releasing hormone (**TRH**) from the hypothalamus.
- Inhibited by the arrival of somatostatin from the hypothalamus.

As its name suggests, TSH stimulates the thyroid gland to secrete its hormone **thyroxine** (T_4).

c. Follicular stimulating hormone (FSH)

➢ In female, it acts on the ovary to stimulate the development of ovarian follicle.
➢ In male, FSH acts on the testes for the maturation of sperm.

d. Luteinizing hormone (LH)

➢ In females, it stimulates the ovarian follicle to mature and also to secrete the estrogen.
➢ In males, it stimulates the secretion of testosterone.

e. Adrenocorticotrophic hormone (ACTH)

➢ ACTH is a peptide of 39 amino acids.
➢ It is cut from a larger precursor proopiomelanocortin (POMC).
➢ ACTH acts on the cells of the adrenal cortex stimulating them to produce their hormone.

Pathophysiology

1. If ACTH secretion is increased by the pituitary or by ectopic production from a tumour results in Cushing's syndrome.
2. The decreased ACTH production leads to Addison's disease.

f. Prolactin (somatomammotropin)

➢ Prolactin is a protein of 198 amino acids.
➢ During pregnancy, it helps in the preparation of the breasts for future milk production. After birth, prolactin promotes the synthesis of milk.
➢ Prolactin secretion is:
  • Stimulated by **TRH**.
  • Repressed by estrogens and dopamine.

Pathophysiology

Hyperprolactinemia is a cause of infertility in females.
  Secretion of prolactin is stimulated by TRH and inhibited by PIF.
  Normal range: Females: 5.4–22.5 ng/ml (mid cycle) 4.5–15 ng/ml (menopausal women).
  Men: 4.2–15 ng/ml.

Posterior pituitary hormone

a. Vasopressin
➢ It was originally named because of its ability to control blood pressure when administered in pharmacological amounts.
➢ But, more appropriately it is called antidiuretic hormone (ADH), because of its important function to promote reabsorption of water from the distal convoluted tubules.
➢ If there is defect in the ADH secretion or the decreased action, it may lead to diabetes insipidus.

➤ Diabetes insipidus is characterized by excretion of large volumes of diluted urine.
  • Primary diabetes insipidus: An insufficient secretion of hormone, which is due to the destruction of the hypothalamic-hypophyseal tract.
  • Arises due to basal skull fractures
  • Tumour or infection
  • It may be hereditary also.

Biochemical findings

• Decreased specific gravity of the urine
• Decreased ADH
• Diluted urine
• Polyurea

b. Oxytocin

➤ Produced in hypothalamus and transported to posterior pituitary gland.
➤ Appropriate stimulation releases the hormones into the blood.
➤ The neural impulses that result from stimulation of the nipples are the primary stimuli for oxytocin release.
➤ Vaginal and uterine distention is the secondary stimuli.
➤ Estrogen also stimulates the production of oxytocin.
➤ Oxytocin causes contraction of uterine smooth muscles and thus is used in pharmacological amount to induce labor in humans.
➤ The most likely physiologic function of oxytocin is stimulation for the contraction of cells surrounding mammary alveoli. This promotes the movement of milk into the system and allows milk ejection.

Thyroid hormones

➤ The thyroid gland synthesizes and secretes: T_4 and T_3.
➤ Thyroxine (T_4) is a derivative of the amino acid tyrosine with four atoms of iodine.
➤ In the liver, one atom of iodine is removed from T_4 converting it into triiodothyronine (T_3).
➤ T_3 is the active hormone.
➤ It has many effects on the body. Among the most prominent of these are:
  • An increase in metabolic rate (seen by a rise in the uptake of oxygen).
  • An increase in the rate and strength of the heart beat.
➤ The thyroid cells responsible for the synthesis of T_4 and take up circulating iodine from the blood.

Pathophysiology

1. Hypothyroid diseases; caused by inadequate production of T_3.
   Cretinism: Hypothyroidism in infancy and childhood leads to stunted growth and intelligence. It can be corrected by giving thyroxine, if started in the early stage.

Myxedema: Hypothyroidism in adult's leads to lowered metabolic rate and vigor. It can be reversed by giving thyroxine.

Goiter: Enlargement of the thyroid gland. Can be caused by:

- Inadequate iodine in the diet resulting in low levels of T_4 and T_3.
- An autoimmune attack against components of the thyroid gland (called Hashimoto's thyroiditis).
- The region for hypothyroid disease produces an enlarged gland is:
  - The activity of the thyroid is under negative feedback control.
  - The synthesis and release of TRH and TSH are normally inhibited as the levels of T_4 and T_3 rise in the blood.
  - When the iodine supply is inadequate, T_4 and T_3 levels fall.
  - This stimulates the hypothalamus and pituitary to increased TRH and TSH activities respectively. This stimulates the thyroid gland to enlarge (fruitlessly).

Symptoms

- Reduced basal metabolic rate (BMR)
- Slow heart rate
- Diastolic hypertension
- Sluggish behavior
- Sleepiness
- Constipation
- Sensitivity to cold
- Dry skin and hair

Biochemical findings

- Dcreased T_3, T_4 and increased TSH especially in primary hypothyroidism.
- Decreased T_3, T_4 and decreased TSH in secondary hypothyroidism.
2. Hyperthyroid diseases; caused by excessive secretion of thyroid hormones.
   Graves' disease.
   Osteoporosis: High levels of thyroid hormones suppress the production of TSH through the negative-feedback mechanism mentioned above. The resulting low level of TSH causes an increase in the numbers of bone-reabsorbing osteoclasts resulting in osteoporosis.

Symptoms

- Rapid heart rate
- Nervousness
- Inability to sleep
- Weight loss in spite of hyperthyroidism, weakness
- Excessive sweating
- Sensitivity to heat

Biochemical findings

Increased T_3 and T_4 and TSH is decreased.

Normal levels

T_3 = 0.8–2.0 ng/ml

T_4 = 4.5–12.0 µg/dL

Parathyroid hormones (PTH)

Functions

1. Calcium homeostasis (regulation)

PTH restores normal ECE calcium concentration by acting directly on bone and kidney and acting indirectly on intestinal mucosa.

Bone: It increases the resorption in both organic and inorganic phases, which lose Ca^{2+} into ECF.

Kidney: It reduces renal clearance or excretion of calcium and hence increases ECF concentration of calcium.

GIT: It increases efficiency of calcium absorption from the intestine by promoting the synthesis of calcitriol. It acts upon the intestine to increase Ca^{2+} absorption and plays a permissive role of PTH on bone and kidney.

PTH increases renal phosphate clearance also. Thus, the net effect of PTH on bone and kidney is to increase ECF-Ca^{++} concentration and decrease ECF-PO_4 concentration.

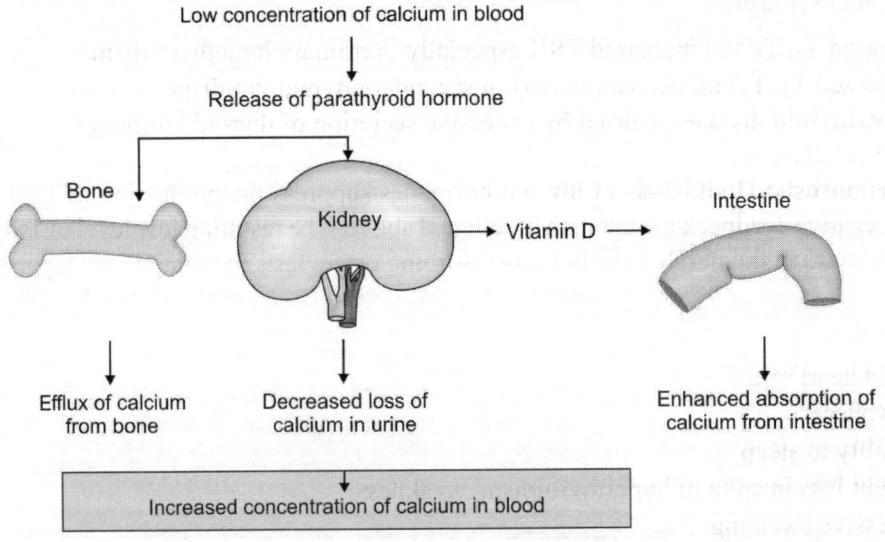

Figure 12.3: *Regulation of calcium*

Adrenal gland

The adrenal gland comprises cortex and medulla.

Cortex has again three zones:

Zona glomerulosa	→	produces mineralocorticoids.
Zona fasciculata	→	produces glucocorticoids.
Zona reticularis	→	secretes sex steroids like androgens and estrogens.

Glucocorticoids

It is a steroid hormone; it is mainly derived from cholesterol.

The functions of glucocorticoid in the human body are:

- The glucocorticoids get their name from their effect of raising the level of blood sugar. They do this by stimulating gluconeogenesis in the liver.
- The conversion of fat and protein into intermediate metabolites that are ultimately converted into glucose.
- The most abundant glucocorticoid is **Cortisol** (also called hydrocortisone).
- Cortisol and the other glucocorticoid also have a potent antiinflammatory effect on the body.
- They depress the immune response, especially cell mediated immune response.
- They are widely used in therapy: To reduce the inflammatory destruction of rheumatoid arthritis and other autoimmune diseases.
  - To prevent the rejection of transplanted organs.
  - To control asthma.

Pathophysiology

Addison's disease (Adrenal insufficiency)

Addison's disease has many causes, such as:

- Destruction of the adrenal glands by infection
- Their destruction by an autoimmune attack
- An inherited mutation in the ACTH receptor on adrenal cells.

Symptoms

- Hypoglycemia
- Extreme sensitivity of insulin
- Intolerance to stress
- Weight loss
- Nausea
- Severe weakness
- Patients have low blood pressure.

The essential role of the adrenal hormones means that a deficiency can be life threatening. Fortunately, replacement therapy with glucocorticoid and mineralocorticoids can permit a normal life.

Cushing's syndrome: Excessive levels of glucocorticoids.

In Cushing's syndrome, the level of adrenal hormones, especially of the glucocorticoids, is too high.

Causes:

- Excessive production of ACTH by the anterior lobe of the pituitary.
- Excessive production of adrenal hormones themselves (e.g. because of a tumour).
- As a result of glucocorticoid therapy for some other disorder such as rheumatoid arthritis or decreased glucocorticoid hormone synthesis.

Symptoms

- Hyperglycemia
- Severe protein catabolism results in thinning of skin, muscle wasting, osteoporosis and negative nitrogen balance.
- There is a peculiar redistribution of fat in trunks.
- Obesity and typical buffalo hump.
- Resistant to infection and inflammatory response is impaired.

Mineralocorticoids

- ➢ It is a steroid hormone and mainly derived from the cholesterol.
- ➢ The mineralocorticoids get their name from their effect on mineral metabolism. The most important of them is the steroid **aldosterone**.
- ➢ Aldosterone acts on the kidney promoting the reabsorption of sodium ions (Na^+) into the blood.
- ➢ Water follows the salt and this helps to maintain normal blood pressure.
- ➢ Aldosterone also acts on sweat glands to reduce the loss of sodium in perspiration.
- ➢ Acts on taste cells to increase the sensitivity of the taste buds to sources of sodium.
- ➢ The secretion of aldosterone is stimulated by:
  - A drop in the level of sodium ions in the blood.
  - A rise in the level of potassium ions in the blood.
  - Angiotensin II.
  - ACTH.

Primary aldosteronism or Conn's syndrome

- ➢ Results from an aldosterone-secreting tumour which leads to elevated levels of plasma aldosterone.
- ➢ The plasma pH in this condition increases because of hypokalemic alkalosis and the plasma osmolality also increases.

Adrenal medulla

Secretes
- Dopamine
- Adrenaline (epinephrine)
- Noradrenaline (norepinephrine).

Functions

- The adrenal medulla consists of masses of neurons that are part of the sympathetic branch of the autonomic nervous system.
- Instead of releasing their neurotransmitters at a synapse, these neurons release them into the blood. Thus, although part of the nervous system, the adrenal medulla functions as an endocrine gland.
- The adrenal medulla releases:
  o **Adrenaline** (also called epinephrine) and
  o **Noradrenaline** (also called norepinephrine).
- Both are derived from the amino acid tyrosine.
- Release of adrenaline and noradrenaline is triggered by nervous stimulation in response to physical or mental stress.
Some of the effects are:
- Increase in the rate and strength of the heartbeat resulting in increased blood pressure.
- Blood shunted from the skin and viscera to the skeletal muscles, coronary arteries, liver, and brain.
- Rise in blood sugar
- Increased metabolic rate
- Bronchi dilate
- Pupils dilate
- Hair stands on end
- Reduced clotting time
- Increased ACTH secretion from the anterior lobe of the pituitary

Pathophysiology

The tumour of the adrenal medulla results in over secretion of its hormones and leads to a condition called pheochromocytoma.

Pancreas

Alpha-cells of pancreas secrete glucagon and β-cells of islets of langerhan's of pancreas secrete insulin.

Insulin

Insulin is a polypeptide hormone synthesized from the β-cells of islets of langerhans of pancreas.

It is synthesized as a larger precursor called pre-pro-insulin. Pre-pro-insulin has 109 amino acids. It is immediately converted into pro-insulin in the endoplasmic reticulum by the removal of 23 amino acids. So the pro-insulin formed contains 86 amino acids. The pro-insulin is transported to Golgi apparatus. There the pro-insulin is cleaved to form insulin and C-peptide.

The C-peptide contains 33 amino acids. Insulin formed from pro-insulin contains 53 amino acids from which 2 amino acids are cleaved to from insulin with 51 amino acids.

Insulin mainly controls blood glucose by the following mechanisms:
1. Increases the uptake of glucose by the peripheral cells.
2. Increases the utilization of glucose by stimulating the glycolysis.
3. Stimulates glycogenesis and inhibits glycogenolysis.
4. Inhibits lipolysis.
5. Inhibits gluconeogenesis.

Glucagon

It is a polypeptide secreted by the α-cells of islets of langerhans of pancreas. It is called as anti-insulin hormone since its actions are entirely opposite to that of insulin. Glucagon stimulates the production of glucose in the liver by promoting glycogenolysis and gluconeogenesis. (Also refer blood sugar regulatiuon).

Ovary

The ovarian follicles secrete the following hormones:
- Estrogen is secreted from the follicular tissue.
- Progesterone is secreted from the corpus luteum.
- Androgens

Estrogen

- Primarily responsible for the conversion of girls into sexually mature women.
  o Development of breasts.
  o Further development of the uterus and vagina.
  o Broadening of the pelvis.
  o Growth of pubic and axillary hair.
  o Increase in adipose (fat) tissue.
- Participate in the monthly preparation of the body for a possible pregnancy.
- Participate in pregnancy, if it occurs.

Progesterone

- It is a steroid hormone synthesized from a parent compound cholesterol.
  1. Causes the development of endometrium and prepares it for the implantation of fertilized ovum for conception.
  2. Stimulates the mammary glands.

Normal range:

0.175 – 0.7 ng/ml—follicular and mid cycle

4.7 – 20 ng/ml—luteal cycle

Testes

- Secretes testosterone
  - ➤ Promotes the growth and function of epididymis, vas deferens, prostate and seminal vesicles.
  - ➤ It enhances and maintains the mobility and fertilizing power of the sperms.
  - ➤ Promotes protein synthesis in the body.

Self Test

1. What are hormones?
2. Name the hormones secreted from anterior and posterior pituitary glands.
3. Describe the mechanism of hormonal action.
4. Explain the pathophysiology of growth hormone.
5. Mention the hormones secreted from thyroid gland and which hormones stimulate the thyroid hormone release?
6. Write short notes on the following:
   a. Cretinism
   b. Goiter
   c. Myxedema
7. How the parathyroid hormones act to maintain the calcium homeostasis?

8. Mention the hormones secreted from three zones of adrenal cortex.
9. List the functions of glucocorticoid and mineralocorticoid hormones.
10. Write the cause, signs and symptoms of:
    a. Addison's disease
    b. Cushing's syndrome
11. List the adrenal medullary hormones and their functions.
12. Mention few functions of female sex hormones and mention on what influence they enter into the circulation to act finally?
13. What are the hormones secreted from pancreas?

13

Acid-Base Balance

Introduction

The human body can be described as a complex system, which consists of several levels and subsystems. At the chemical level, acids and bases are one of the essential compounds upon which all biochemical processes depend. The biochemical reactions, which are taking place in our body, are extremely sensitive to small changes in the acidity or alkalinity of the environment. The acid-base homeostasis should be maintained for cellular viability, enzymatic reactions, protein conformation and CNS functions, etc. These functions are modified when there is change in the cellular and extracellular acid-base status. For these reactions, the acids and bases that are formed constantly should be in balance.

To understand acid-base homeostasis, a definition of some of the terms needed, are explained below.

Acids: Bronsted defined an acid as a chemical entity that donates protons in solution.

$$HCl \rightleftharpoons H^+ + Cl^-$$
$$H_2CO_3 \rightleftharpoons H^+ + HCO_3^-$$
$$NH_4 \rightleftharpoons H^+ + NH_3$$
$$H_2PO_4 \rightleftharpoons H^+ + HPO_4$$

Bases: Are those, which accept protons.

pH: Sorensen expressed pH as the negative log of H^+ concentration, i.e. log $[H^+]$.

Buffers

Buffer is a solution that resists changes in pH when acid or base is added. The effectiveness depends on its pK or (pK_a). pK is the pH at which the buffer is 50% ionized, means, the acid concentration is exactly equal to that of the base conjugate. The buffer is very efficient at a pH of ± 1 around its pK.

For example, phosphate buffer pK = 6.8.

This buffer will have maximum buffer capacity between pH levels 5.8 and 7.8.

A buffer solution is a mixture of a weak acid and its Na or K salt (base).

Henderson-Hasselbalch equation

$$pH = pK_a + \log_{10} \frac{[Base]}{[Acid]}$$

This indicates the relationship between the pH, pK of the buffer and the ratio of conjugate base to the undissociated acid. It enables to relate quantitatively the changes in pH, [acid] and [base].

H^+ balance

In a healthy individual, the normal pH of arterial blood is 7.4 ± 0.05 and that of venous blood is 7.4 ± 0.02. When the arterial pH raises above 7.45 then the individual is considered to have alkalosis, if the pH is below 7.35, is considered to have acidosis. In a healthy subject, the pH of blood is always between 7.35 and 7.45. The change in pH leads serious effects, therefore, the control of pH is necessary.

There are two types of metabolic acids:
1. Fixed acids
2. Volatile acids

CO_2 is the volatile acid.

Lactic acid (–CHO), acetoacetic acid, β-hydroxy butyric acid, H_2SO_4 and H_3PO_4 are non-volatile or fixed acids.

CO_2 is the major end product in the oxidation of carbohydrates, fats and amino acids. It has the ability to react with H_2O to form H_2CO_3 and again they dissociate to H^+ and HCO_3^-. The CO_2 can be regarded as an acid by virtue of its ability to react with H_2O to form H_2CO_3, which in turn can dissociate to form $H^+ + HCO_3^-$. In vivo, it is the carbonic anhydrase in tissues of liver and kidney which catalyzes the following reaction either the way of depending on the blood pH.

$$CO_2 + H_2O \underset{}{\overset{\text{Carbonic anhydrase}}{\rightleftharpoons}} H_2CO_3$$

$$H_2CO_3 \longrightarrow H^+ + HCO_3^-$$

The fixed acids H_2SO_4 and H_3PO_4 are the end products of the sulfur containing amino acids, phospholipids, nucleic acids, phosphoproteins and phosphoglycerides.

Organic acids like lactic acid and β-hydroxy butyric acids are formed during the metabolism of carbohydrates and lipids.

Accumulation of lactic acid is called lactic acidosis. Normally, lactic acid produced by the anaerobic glycolysis is taken up by the liver and converted to glucose through a Cori's cycle.

Pyruvate and lactate accumulate in conditions like arsenic or mercury poisoning and also in thiamine deficiency. Inherited enzyme *pyruvate dehydrogenase* deficiency also leads to lactic acidosis.

Regulation of acid-base balance

The pH of the plasma is 7.4 and is normally maintained within a narrow range of 7.35 to 7.45. Blood buffer system regulates small changes in acids or bases.

Next one is the respiratory system by increasing the expulsion of the CO_2 (hyperventilation) or by conservation of CO_2 (hypoventilation) regulates the blood pH. These two compensatory mechanisms cannot go longer. It is only a temporary balance.

The renal system maintains acid-base balance of blood by adjusting the rate of reabsorption and excretion of H^+ or HCO_3^- or HPO_3^-, in addition to the formation and excretion of NH_3 and NH_4^+.

Blood buffer system

ECF Buffers

1. Carbonate-bicarbonate—H_2CO_3/HCO_3^- (20:1)
2. Phosphate buffer—$HPO_4/H_2PO_4^-$ (4:1)
3. Basic proteins/acidic proteins
4. Organic base/organic acid

Bicarbonate buffer system

The most important buffer system in the plasma is the bicarbonate-carbonate system. It accounts for 60% of buffering action in plasma and 40% in the whole body. The bicarbonate (HCO_3^-) level is regulated by the kidney; the acid part of carbonic acid (H_2CO_3) is under respiratory control. The buffer is most active when the ratio of salt and acid is equal according to the Henderson-Hasselbalch equation. The normal plasma bicarbonate level is 24 mmol/l. The normal pCO_2 of arterial blood is 40 mm of Hg. The normal carbonic acid is 1.2 mmol/l. The pKa of carbonic acid is 6.1. Substituting these values in Henderson-Hasselbalch equation.

$$pH = pK + \log_{10} \frac{[Base]}{[Acid]}$$

$$pH \text{ of blood} = 7.4 = 6.1 + \log \frac{(HCO_3^-)}{(H_2CO_3)}$$

$$7.4 = 6.1 + \log \frac{24}{1.2}$$

$$= 6.1 + \log 20 \text{ (antilog of } 20 = 1.3)$$
$$= 6.1 + 1.3$$

So, the ratio between (HCO_3^-) and (H_2CO_2) = 20:1
(HCO_3^-): (H_2CO_3) = 20:1

So the ratio of HCO_3^- to H_2CO_3 at pH 7.4 is 20 in normal conditions. The bicarbonate represents the alkali reserve and it is sufficient to meet the acid load. During the compensation, if (HCO_3^-) is 24, then (H_2CO_3) is adjusted to 1.2. This is how compensatory mechanism operates to bring the ratio back to 20:1.

Whenever metabolic acid is added to the blood, it reacts with the basic component of the buffer system, producing salt and water and helps to prevent the fall in blood pH. Reversal of this mechanism takes place in the event of addition of base by metabolic processes.

Phosphate buffer system

It is the main intracellular buffer. The pK_a value, 6.8 is nearer to the physiological pH 7.4. When equation is applied

$$pH = pK_a + \log \frac{[Base]}{[Acid]}$$

$$7.4 = 6.8 + \log \frac{[Base]}{[Acid]}$$

$$0.6 = \log \frac{[Base]}{[Acid]}$$

Antilog of 0.6 is 4.

Therefore, the ratio is 4.

The phosphate buffer system is effective at wide range of pH; because of the more ionizable groups, it has different pK_a values.

$$H_3PO_4 \xrightarrow{pK_a = 1.96} H^+ + H_2PO_4^-$$

$$H_2PO_4^- \xrightarrow{pK_a = 6.8} H^+ + HPO_4^-$$

$$HPO_4^- \xrightarrow{pK_a = 12.4} H^+ + PO_4^{2-}$$

The $Na_2HPO_4/NaH_2PO_4^-$ is an effective buffer system in the human body because of its pK_a value nearer to the physiological pH.

Protein buffer system

The buffering action of protein mainly depends on the pK_a value of its ionizable side chains. The effective group is histidine with a pK_a value of 6.1. Therefore, the albumin and hemoglobin with more histidine residues play an important role in buffering action in the body.

Respiratory regulation of acid-base balance

The second line of defense against acid-base disturbance is the control of CO_2 by the lungs by increasing or decreasing the rate of respiration.

The rate of respiration is known to be controlled by the receptors in the respiratory center, which are sensitive to changes in pH and pCO_2 of blood. When there is a fall in pH of plasma, the respiratory center is stimulated, resulting in hyperventilation, which eliminate more CO_2 thus lowering H_2CO_3 concentration in blood. If the blood pH increases, the respiratory center is inhibited so that elimination of CO_2 is decreased by hypoventilation till the blood pH comes to normal.

The hemoglobin transports CO_2 formed in the tissues and also it serves to generate bicarbonate or alkali reserve by the activity of carbonic anhydrase system.

Renal Regulation of pH (Figure 13.1)

An important function of kidney is to regulate the function by excreting either acidic or basic urine. The pH of urine ranges from 4.5 to 9.5 because the renal system plays a significant role in long-term pH maintenance of the blood at 7.4 ± 0.05. This is possible by its capacity of reabsorption, secretion and excretion of the nonvolatile acids like lactic acid; lungs cannot excrete pyruvic acid, inorganic acid, HCl, phosphoric acid and H_2SO_4, which are produced in the body. The first mechanism for removal of acids from the body is by renal excretion. The major mechanism by which the kidney regulate the level of HCO_3^- in plasma are reabsorption of filtered HCO_3^-, generation of new HCO_3^- and by secreting HCO_3^- under condition of chronic alkalosis.

The filtered HCO_3^- combined with H^+ forming H_2CO_3, carbonic anhydrase present in the brush border of the cell wall dissociates H_2CO_3 into H_2O and CO_2. CO_2 diffuses into the cell; in the cell carbonic anhydrase again ionizes H_2CO_3 into HCO_3^- and H^+. It is secreted into the lumen in exchange for Na^+ and HCO_3^- and is reabsorbed into plasma along with Na^+, there is no net excretion of H^+ or generation of new HCO_3^- so that this mechanism helps to maintain a steady state of acid-base balance.

Another function of the kidney is to buffer acids and thus to conserve fixed base is through the production of NH_3 from amino acids with the help of an enzyme glutaminase. Whenever there is excess acid production, the NH_3 production is also increased which combines with H^+ to form NH_4^+ which is excreted as NH_4Cl. This occurs in the event of acidosis. When alkali is in excess of H^+ is reabsorbed into the cell in exchange to Na^+/K^+.

Acid-base Disorders (Figures 13.2 and 13.3)

Acid-base disorder results from a variety of pathological conditions. The normal pH of blood is referred as euphamia. If the pH is more than the normal range, it is termed as alkalemia and pH lesser than the normal range, it is called acidemia and the conditions are called alkalosis and acidosis respectively.

There are two reasons for the pH abnormalities in blood, which are metabolic and respiratory causes. Metabolic causes are responsible for metabolic acidosis and metabolic alkalosis. The respiratory causes are responsible for respiratory acidosis and respiratory alkalosis.

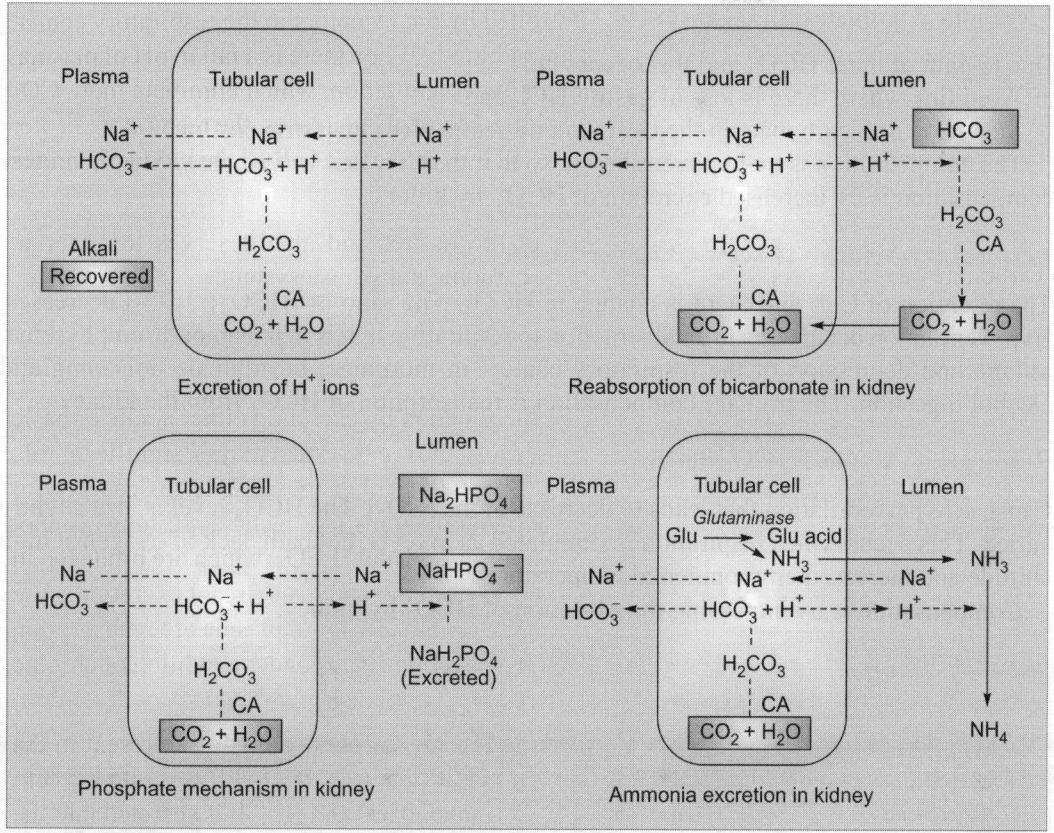

Figure 13.1

Metabolic Acidosis (HCO_3^- deficit or fall in pH)

The most common acid-base disturbance is decreased HCO_3^- concentration. This is due to the increased production of acids. These acids dissociate to give H^+ ions, which are buffered by HCO_3^-. This occurs in:

a. Uncontrolled diabetes mellitus,
b. Starvation, and
c. Severe exercise.

In first two conditions, the acidosis is due to the formation of ketone body. During severe exercise, the lactic acid produced by anaerobic glycolysis leads to acidosis that is called lactic acidosis.

The metabolic acidosis is also due to ingestion of acids like ammonium chloride, the ammonia part after detoxified leaves behind the H^+. It also occurs in diarrhea, which leads to the loss of HCO_3^- from the intestinal fluid.

The primary compensation in metabolic acidosis is by hyperventilation that removes CO_2, and also through the elimination of acids in the urine and the urinary ammonia is also increased.

Metabolic Alkalosis (HCO_3^- excess or rise in pH)

Due to gain of more HCO_3^- and this occurs in:
a. Vomiting where there is loss of gastric HCl, and
b. Ingestion of bicarbonate in the treatment of peptic ulcer in gastric suction.

The compensation is by hypoventilation, so that the CO_2 loss will be slow. The secondary compensation is by increased excretion of HCO_3^- by kidney.

Respiratory Acidosis (Excess CO_2)

The retention of CO_2 and there is change in HCO_3^-. The ratio of $[HCO_3^-]$: $[CO_2]$ decreases. Hypoventilation occurs due to an obstruction to respiration that is in pneumonia, emphysema, asthma and depression of the respiratory centers in morphine, bicarbonate poisoning and alcohol ingestion. The primary compensation is reabsorption of HCO_3^- from the kidney.

Respiratory Alkalosis (CO_2 deficit)

Cause is hyperventilation that leads to decrease in the $[CO_2]$. The HCO_3^- level is also slightly varied. This occurs when respiration is stimulated as in fever, hot bath, lack of oxygen at high altitude and increased environmental temperature.

Compensation is by increasing the excretion of HCO_3^- by kidney.

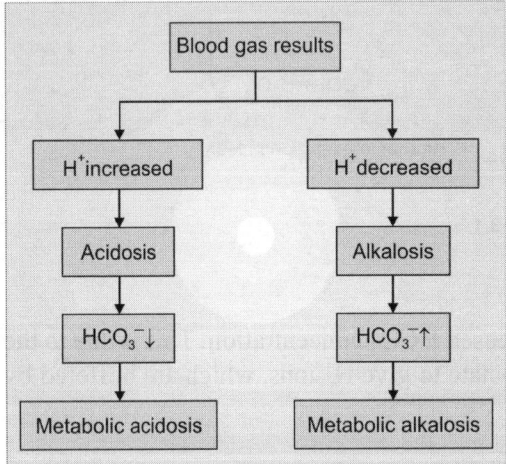

Figure 13.2: *Metabolic acidosis and alkalosis*

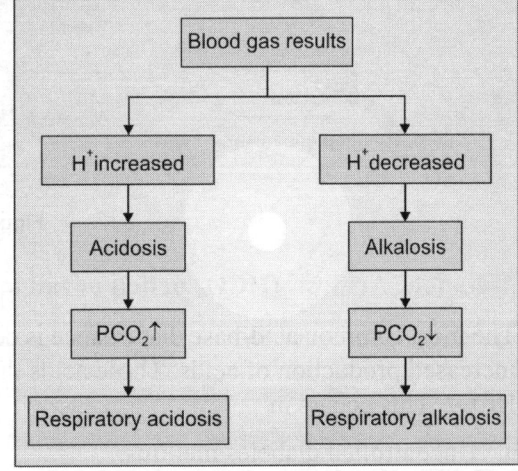

Figure 13.3: *Respiratory acidosis and alkalosis*

Table 13.1: *Laboratory findings in acid-base disturbances*

	pH	*pCO$_2$*	*HCO$_3^-$*	*HCO$_3^-$/H$_2$CO$_3$*
Normal	7.4 ± 0.05	40 mm Hg	20 mm Hg	20
Metabolic acidosis	Decreased	Normal	Decreased	Decreased
Metabolic alkalosis	Increased	Normal	Increased	Increased
Respiratory acidosis	Decreased	Increased	Normal	Decreased
Respiratory alkalosis	Increased	Decreased	Decreased	Increased

Anion Gap

The sum of cations and anions in extracellular fluid is always equal so as to maintain the electrical neutrality. Cations (95%) were maintained by Na^+ and K^+, whereas, chloride and, HCO_3^- account for 86% of anions. These are the commonly measured electrolytes and, hence, there is a difference between cations and anions. The difference of cations and anions or the unmeasured anions constitute the anion gap, which is due to the presence of phosphorous, SO_4^-, PO_4^{3-} and organic acid salts.

The difference between $Na^+ + K^+$ and $Cl^- + HCO_3^-$ is normally about 12 ± 5 mEq/L (mmol/L). Alteration in anion gap is extremely useful in the clinical assessment with acid-base disorders.

Self Test

1. Name the blood buffer systems.

2. Briefly discuss the bicarbonate buffer system to show how it helps to regulate the blood pH.

3. Explain the regulation of blood pH through renal mechanism.

4. Discuss the various acid-base disorders. Mention the causes and findings of each disorder.

5. Mention the laboratory findings for metabolic acidosis and respiratory alkalosis.

6. What is metabolic alkalosis and respiratory acidosis?

14

Biological Oxidation

- Oxidation/reduction reactions are coupled chemical reactions in which one atom or molecule loses one or more electrons (oxidation) while another atom or molecule gains those electrons (reduction).
- The compound that loses electrons becomes oxidized.
  The compound that gains those electrons becomes reduced.
- In covalent compounds, however, it is usually easier to lose a whole hydrogen (H) atom, a proton and an electron—rather than just an electron.
- An oxidation reaction during which both a proton and an electron are lost is called dehydrogenation.
- A reduction reaction during which both a proton and an electron are gained is called hydrogenation.
- The large quantity of NADH resulting from TCA cycle activity can be used for reductive biosynthesis.
- The reducing potential of mitochondrial NADH is most often used to supply the energy for ATP synthesis via **oxidative phosphorylation**.
- The oxidation of NADH with phosphorylation of ADP to form ATP is a process supported by the mitochondrial electron transport assembly and ATP synthase, which are integral protein complexes of the inner mitochondrial membrane.
- The electron transport assembly is comprised a series of protein complexes that catalyze sequential oxidation/reduction reactions; some of these reactions are thermodynamically competent to support ATP production via ATP synthase provided a coupling mechanism, such as a common intermediate, is available. Proton translocation and the development of a transmembrane proton gradient provide the required coupling mechanism.

Principles of reduction/oxidation (redox) reactions

- Redox reactions involve the transfer of electrons from one chemical species to another.
- An example of a coupled redox reaction is the oxidation of NADH by the electron transport chain:

$$NADH + (1/2)\ O_2 + H^+ \longrightarrow NAD^+ + H_2O$$

- The description of ATP synthesis through oxidation of reduced electron carriers indicated 3 moles of ATP could be generated for every mole of NADH and 2 moles for every mole of $FADH_2$. However, direct chemical analysis has shown that for every 2 electrons transferred from NADH to oxygen, 2.5 equivalents of ATPs are synthesized and 1.5 for $FADH_2$.

Complexes of the electron transport chain

➤ The system of mitochondrial enzymes and redox carrier molecules which ferry the reducing equivalents from substrates to oxygen are collectively known as the electron transport system, or the respiratory chain.

➤ This system captures the free energy available from substrate oxidation so that it may later be applied to the synthesis of ATP.

➤ The main components participate in the approximate order of their redox potentials, and the bulky complexes are linked by low molecular weight mobile carriers which ferry the reducing equivalents from one complex to the next.

➤ Except for succinate dehydrogenase (complex 2), all these complexes pump protons from the matrix space into the cytosol as they transfer reducing equivalents (either hydrogen atoms or electrons) from one carrier to the next.

➤ NADH is oxidized by a series of catalytic redox carriers that are integral proteins of the inner mitochondrial membrane.

➤ The free energy change in several of these steps is very exergonic. Coupled to these oxidation/ reduction steps is a transport process in which protons (H^+) from the mitochondrial matrix are translocated to the space between the inner and outer mitochondrial membranes.

➤ The redistribution of protons leads to formation of a proton gradient across the mitochondrial membrane.

➤ The size of the gradient is proportional to the free energy change of the electron transfer reactions.

➤ The result of these reactions is that the redox energy of NADH is converted to the energy of the proton gradient.

➤ In the presence of ADP, protons flow down their thermodynamic gradient from outside the mitochondrion back into the mitochondrial matrix.

➤ This process is facilitated by a proton carrier in the inner mitochondrial membrane known as ATP synthase. As its name implies, this carrier is coupled to ATP synthesis.

➤ Electron flow through the mitochondrial electron transport assembly is carried out through several enzyme complexes.

➤ Electrons enter to the transport chain primarily from cytosolic NADH to mitochondrial NADH but can also be supplied by succinate (to mitochondrial $FADH_2$) or by the glycerol phosphate shuttle via mitochondrial $FADH_2$.

➤ Diagram shows the flow of electrons from either NADH or succinate to oxygen (O_2) in the electron transport chain of oxidative phosphorylation.

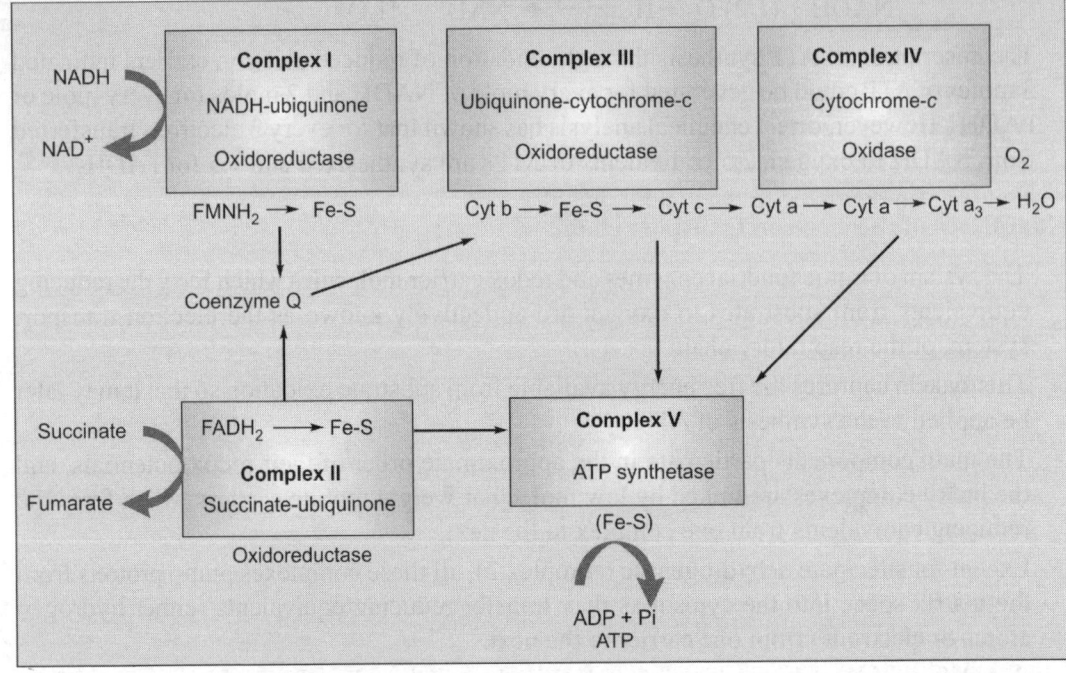

Figure 14.1

➢ Mitochondrial electron transport proteins are clustered into complexes (as shown above) known as **Complexes I, II, III**, and **IV**.

➢ Complex I, also known as **NADH: CoQ oxidoreductase**, is composed of NADH dehydrogenase with FMN as cofactor and 22–24 iron-sulfur (Fe-S) proteins in 5–7 clusters.

➢ Complex II contains $FADH_2$ and 7–8 Fe-S proteins in 3 clusters and cytochrome b_{560}.

➢ Complex III contains cytochrome b, cytochrome c_1 and one Fe-S protein.

  Associated with complex III by electrostatic interaction is cytochrome c, the ultimate electron acceptor in complex III.

➢ Complex IV contains cytochrome a, cytochrome a_3 and 2 copper ions. As the two electrons pass through the proteins of complex I, four protons (H^+) are pumped into the intramembrane space of the mitochondrion. Similarly, four protons are pumped into the intramembrane space as each electron pair flows through complexes III and as four electrons are used to reduce O_2 to H_2O in complex IV.

➢ The free energy released as electrons, flow through complex II is insufficient to be coupled to proton pumping.

➢ These protons are returned to the matrix of the mitochondrion, down their concentration gradient, bypassing through ATP synthase coupling electron flow and proton pumping to ATP synthesis.

➤ With the exception of NADH, succinate, and CoQ, all of the components of the pathway are integral proteins of the inner mitochondrial membrane whose cofactors undergo redox reactions.

➤ NADH and succinate are soluble in the mitochondrial matrix, while CoQ is a small, mobile carrier that transfers electrons between the primary dehydrogenases and cytochrome b.

➤ CoQ is also restricted to the membrane phase because of its hydrophobic character.

Oxidative Phosphorylation

• The NADH and $FADH_2$ formed in glycolysis, fatty acid oxidation, and the citric acid cycle are energy-rich molecules because each contains a pair of electrons having a high transfer potential. When these electrons are used to reduce molecular oxygen to water, a large amount of free energy is liberated, which can be used to generate ATP.

• Oxidative phosphorylation is the process in which ATP is formed as a result of the transfer of electrons from NADH or $FADH_2$ to O_2 by a series of electron carriers and occurs by chemiosmosis.

• The energy of the proton gradient is known as the **chemiosmotic potential**, or **proton motive force (PMF)**.

• This potential is the sum of the concentration difference of protons across the membrane and the difference in electrical charge across the membrane.

• The 2 electrons from NADH generate a 6-proton gradient. Thus, oxidation of 1 mole of NADH leads to the availability of a PMF with a free energy of about -31.2 kcal (6×-5.2 kcal). The energy of the gradient is used to drive ATP synthesis as the protons are transported back down their thermodynamic gradient into the mitochondrion.

Inhibitors of oxidative phosphorylation

➤ The pathways of electron flow through the electron transport assembly, and the unique properties of the PMF, have been determined through the uses of a number of important antimetabolites.

➤ Some of these agents are inhibitors of electron transport at specific sites in the electron transport assembly, while others stimulate electron transport by discharging the proton gradient.

➤ For example, antimycin A is a specific inhibitor of cytochrome b. In the presence of antimycin A, cytochrome b can be reduced but not oxidized.

➤ The cytochrome c remains oxidized in the presence of antimycin A.

➤ An important class of antimetabolites are the uncoupling agents exemplified by 2,4-dinitrophenol (DNP).

➤ Uncoupling agents act as lipophilic weak acids, associating with protons on the exterior of mitochondria, passing through the membrane with the bound proton, and dissociating the proton on the interior of the mitochondrion.

➤ These agents cause maximum respiratory rates but the electron transport generates no ATP, since the translocated protons do not return to the interior through ATP synthase.

Table 14.1: *Inhibitors of oxidative phosphorylation*

Name	Function	Site of action
Rotenone	e⁻ transport inhibitor	Complex I
Amytal	e⁻ transport inhibitor	Complex I
Antimycin A	e⁻ transport inhibitor	Complex III
Cyanide	e⁻ transport inhibitor	Complex IV
Carbon monoxide	e⁻ transport inhibitor	Complex IV
Azide	e⁻ transport inhibitor	Complex IV
2, 4-dinitrophenol	Uncoupling agent	Transmembrane H^+ carrier
Pentachlorophenol	Uncoupling agent	Transmembrane H^+ carrier
Oligomycin	Inhibits ATP synthase	OSCP fraction of ATP synthase

Self Test

1. What is oxidative phosphorylation?
2. Mention the sites of ETC where ATP synthesis takes place.
3. Define the term antimetabolites.
4. Give any two examples of inhibitors of oxidative phosphorylation with the site of action.

15

Vitamins

Vitamins are naturally occurring organic substances. Their coenzyme forms are essential in metabolic processes. They serve nearly the same roles in all forms of life. The daily requirement of any vitamin depends on a number of factors and may increase during growth, pregnancy and lactation. They are essential nutrients and required in small amounts for various roles in the human body.

The vitamins are divided into two groups:

1. Fat-soluble vitamins (A, D, E and K), foods that contain these vitamins will not lose them when cooked.
2. Water-soluble vitamin (B complex).

FAT-SOLUBLE VITAMINS

VITAMIN A

Sources

- Cod liver oil
- Fish liver oil
- Animal liver
- Milk and milk products
- Eggs
- The carotenoid pigments present in carrots, sweet potato, and green leafy vegetables like spinach and amaranth.
- The yellow pigment, beta-carotene present in vegetables is a precursor of vitamin A.
- It has two ionone rings connected by a polyprenoid chain.
- One molecule of beta-carotene can theoretically give rise to two molecules of vitamin A; but it may produce only one in biological systems.

Requirements

- Adult: 800–1000 μg/day (5000 IU/day)

- Pregnancy and lactation: 1000–1200 µg/day (4000 IU/day)
- Infants and children: 400–600 µg/day (3000 IU/day)

Physiological role

There are three active forms of vitamin A.

1. Retinal
2. Retinoic acid
3. Retinol

1. The retinal form of vitamin is required for visual function. Retina of the eye contains two types of cells. *Rod cells* (vision in dim light), *cone cells* (vision in bright light).

   Rod cells have a photosensitive pigment called rhodopsin, is a conjugated protein made up of opsin and 11-*cis* retinal.

   Rhodopsin once exposed to light, it dissociates into all

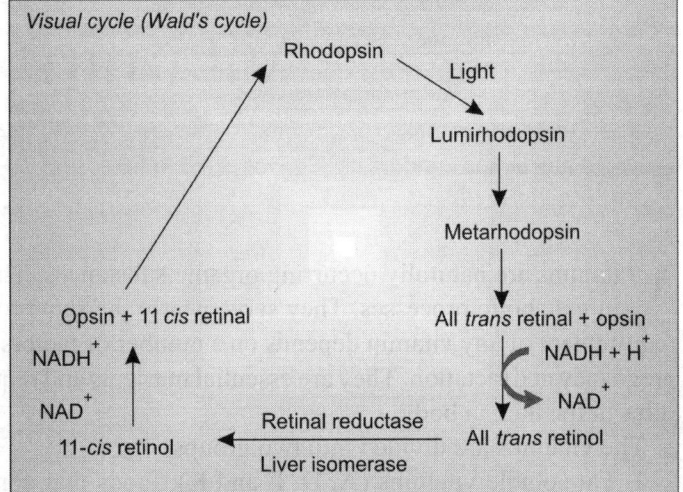

Figure 15.1

trans retinal and opsin. All *trans* retinal reduced to All *trans* retinol in the retina and transported to liver where it is isomerized to 11-*cis* retinol, this is transported back to retina then oxidized to 11-*cis* retinal, which combines with opsin to form rhodopsin.

2. Retinoic acid form of vitamin A maintains structural and functional integrity of epithelium.
3. Retinol form of vitamin A is required for growth and reproductive function.
4. Retinol is also known to require for the formation of bone and teeth.

Deficiency

➢ Night blindness
➢ Keratinization of lacriymal glands
➢ *Keratomalacia:* Dryness of the cornea, corneal epithelium becomes keratinized and opaque and may become softened and ulcerated.
➢ *Follicular keratosis*: Deficiency will affect hair follicles and causes scaly skin.

Hypervitaminosis

It is rare, if occurs, it leads to headache, nausea, vomiting, loss of appetite and pain in bones.

VITAMIN D

Ergocalciferol [D$_2$]
Cholecalciferol [D$_3$]

Sources

- D_2 in plants
- D_3 in fish, egg and liver

- Ergosterol $\xrightarrow{\text{UV light}}$ Vitamin D_2 (Ergocalciferol)

- 7-dehydrocholesterol $\xrightarrow[\text{(Derivative of cholesterol)}]{\text{Sunlight}}$ Vitamin D_3 (Cholecalciferol)

- The 7-dehydrocholesterol, an intermediate of a minor pathway of cholesterol synthesis, is available in the epidermis. The skin on exposure to sunlight, the 7-dehydrocholesterol converted to cholecalciferol.

Requirement

- Children: 10 µg/day (400 IU/day)
- Adults: 5–10 µg/day (400 IU/day)
- Pregnancy and lactation: 10 µg/day (400 IU/day)

Vitamin D_2 and D_3 are not active biologically but converted to active form by hydroxylation.

Vitamin D_3 $\xrightarrow[\text{in liver}]{\text{25-hydroxylase}}$ 25-OH vitamin D_3 $\xrightarrow[\text{in kidney}]{\text{1-hydroxylase}}$ 1, 25-dihydroxy vitamin D_3 [Calcitriol]

Regulation of formation of 1, 25-$(OH)_2$ vitamin D_3

➢ Low calcium level stimulates parathyroid hormone (PTH) secretion; this in turn acts on kidney to secrete 1-hydroxylase.
➢ High level of 1, 25-$(OH)_2$ D_3 inhibits the secretion of 1-hydroxylase.
➢ When calcium level is normal, the production of 1, 25-$(OH)_2$ vitamin D_3 suppressed which results in the stimulation of 24-hydroxylase which converts 25-hydroxy vitamin D_3 to 24, 25-$(OH)_2$ vitamin D_3.

Functions

It maintains an adequate calcium level by the following mechanisms:
a. Increases the absorption of calcium from the intestine: Vitamin D_3 enters to the intestinal cell then binds to cytoplasmic receptor. This complex interacts with DNA in the nucleus results in the synthesis of mRNA. This in turn forms a calcium binding protein (CBP). This calcium binding protein increases the absorption of calcium.
b. Causing removal of calcium from bone (resorption of bone calcium).

Deficiency

➢ The deficiency of vitamin D leads to **rickets** in children.
➢ Signs and symptoms are bowlegs, knock knees, pigeon chest, hypocalcemia and hypophosphatemia.
➢ **Osteomalacia** in adults.
➢ Signs and symptoms are soft and pliable bones.

VITAMIN E (Tocopherol)

Sources

Vegetable oils like wheat germ oil, corn oil, cottonseed oil and safflower oil.

Requirements

• Adult male: 10 mg/day (30 IU/day)
• Female: 12 mg/day (25 IU/day)
• Children: 9 mg/day (10–20 IU/day)

Functions

1. Potent physiological antioxidant: Protects membranes with lipids from oxidative damage.
2. Vitamin E, which is present in cell membranes, prevents the destructive nonenzymatic oxidation of polyunsaturated fatty acids (PUFA) by molecular oxygen, and it maintains the membrane integrity.
3. Protects erythrocytes from hemolysis by oxidizing agents (H_2O_2).
4. Required for normal reproduction in animals.
5. Prevents liver necrosis and muscular dystrophy.
6. It protects cellular and subcellular membranes.

Deficiency

➢ Reproductive failure in animals.
➢ Hemolysis of erythrocytes.
➢ Muscular weakness and fragile RBCs.

VITAMIN K

Phylloquinone [K_1]
Menaquinone [K_2]
Menadione [K_3]
1. Vitamin K_1 (Phylloquinone)
2. Vitamin K_2 (Menaquinone)
   Naturally occurring
3. Vitamin K_3 (Menadione) ⟶ Synthetic form

Sources

- Green leafy vegetables (Spinach, alfalfa grass, cauliflower, cabbage)
- Tomato
- Putrid fish meal

Functions

Required for the maintenance of normal levels of following blood clotting factors.

a. Prothrombin
b. Stable factor
c. Plasma thromboplastin component
d. Stuart Prower factor

Each of these is synthesized in the liver in an inactive form.

Conversion of inactive to active form involves gamma-carboxylation of glutamic acid residues from the N-termini. This process creates negative charges.

This process depends on vitamin K.

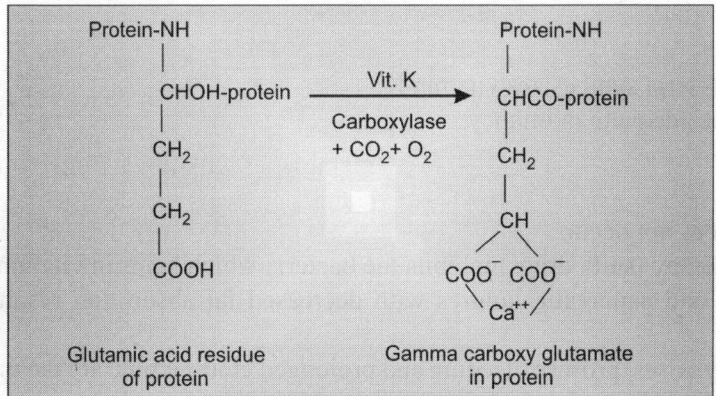

Figure 15.2

The Ca^{++} and phospholipids bind with negative charges and activate prothrombin to thrombin.

$$\text{Fibrinogen} \xrightarrow{\text{Thrombin}} \text{Fibrin}$$

In the absence of gamma-carboxylation, chelation with Ca^{++} is impaired.

The vitamin dependent gamma-carboxylation is also necessary for the functional activity of C-reactive protein and osteocalcin. The osteocalcin binds to hydroxyapatite crystals of bone; this binding mainly dependent on the level of gamma-carboxylation. The vitamin K helps to retain calcium by this mechanism.

The vitamin K-dependent carboxylase enzyme requires oxygen, CO_2, NADPH and reduced vitamin K. In this process the vitamin passes through a cycle. For reconversion of vitamin K, reduced lipoamide is necessary. This process is inhibited by a vitamin K antagonist, warfarin and dicoumarol.

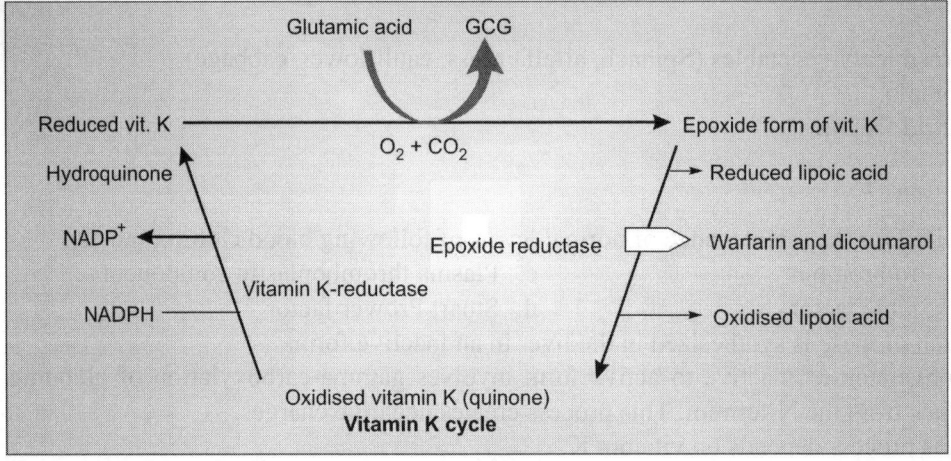

Figure 15.3

Requirements

- Intestinal bacteria synthesizes vitamin K.
- 40–140 µg is adequate in infancy.

Deficiency

➢ Normally does not occur.
➢ The drug therapy (sulfa drugs) inhibits the bacteria which helps in vitamin K synthesis.
➢ Steatorrhea and pancreatic failures with decreased fat absorption result in vitamin K deficiency.
➢ If deficiency arises, profuse bleeding and prolonged clotting time are the main symptoms.

Antagonists

- Dicoumarol
- Warfarin

WATER-SOLUBLE VITAMINS

VITAMIN C (Ascorbic Acid)

Sources

- The rich sources are citrus fruits (orange, lemon)
- Tomatoes
- Strawberries
- Green leafy vegetables
- Guava fruit
- Green pepper

Requirements

- Adults: 60 mg/day
- Children: 40 mg/day

Table 15.1: *Summary of Vitamins A, D E and K.*

Vitamin	Source	Physiological functions	Deficiency	Overconsumption
A (retinol) provitamin A, such as beta-carotene	Liver, fortified milk and dairy products, butter, whole milk, cheese, egg yolk. Provitamin A: Carrots, green leafy vegetables, sweet potatoes, pumpkins, apricots	1. Skin and mucous membranes formation 2. Night vision; 3. Bones and teeth development. 4. Beta-carotene is an antioxidant and may protect against cancer.	Night blindness, diarrhea, intestinal infections, impaired vision. Inflammation of eyes, keratinization of skin and eyes. Blindness in children.	*Mild:* Nausea, irritability, blurred vision. Growth retardation, enlargement of liver and spleen, loss of hair, bone pain, increased pressure in skull, skin changes.
D	Fortified dairy products, fortified margarine, fish oils, egg yolk. Synthesized by sunlight action on skin.	Promotes hardening of bones and teeth, increases the absorption of calcium.	*Severe:* Rickets in children; osteomalacia in adults.	Nausea, weight loss, irritability. Mental and physical growth retardations, kidney damage, movement of calcium from bones into soft tissues.
E	Vegetable oil, margarine, butter, shortening, green and leafy vegetables, wheat germ, whole grain products, nuts, egg yolk, liver	Protects vitamins A and C and fatty acids; prevents damage to cell membranes. Antioxidant.	Almost impossible to produce without starvation; possible anemia in low birth-weight infants.	Nontoxic under normal conditions. *Severe:* Nausea, digestive tract disorders.
K	Dark green leafy vegetables, liver; also made by bacteria in the intestine.	Helps blood to clot.	Excessive bleeding.	None reported.

Functions

1. *Collagen synthesis*. Vitamin C is very important for the hydroxylation of proline and lysine residues, which are the collagen precursors.
2. It helps in the absorption of iron by reducing Fe^{3+} to Fe^{2+} in the stomach.
3. Reaction between amino groups of protein and nitrites formed in the intestine produces nitrosamines that may cause cancer. So vitamin C acts as an antioxidant, scavenging the free radicals and reduces the nitrosamine formation.

4. The conversion of dopa to dopamine and dopamine to noradrenaline requires vitamin C as an activator.

$$\text{Tyrosine} \longrightarrow \text{Dopa} \xrightarrow[\substack{\text{Dopamine oxidase} \\ \text{vitamin C}}]{} \text{Dopamine}$$

$$\text{Dopamine} \longrightarrow \text{Noradrenaline}$$

5. The vitamin C in high dose (1 g/day) decreases the severity of cold.

Deficiency

➢ The vitamin C deficiency leads to **scurvy**.
➢ Signs and symptoms are:
   o Spongy gums
   o Loose teeth
   o Fragile blood vessels
   o Aching swollen joints
   o Anemia
   o Delay in wound healing.

B COMPLEX VITAMINS

THIAMINE (B$_1$)

• It is a sulfur containing vitamin.
• It has thiazole and pyrimidine rings.

Sources

• Whole grains (rice, wheat)
• Legumes (beans, peas)
• Meat

Requirements

• Children: 1.2 mg/day
• Adults: 1.5 mg/day
• Pregnancy and lactation: 2.0 mg/day

Functions

The coenzyme form of thiamine is **thiamine pyrophosphate (TPP)**.

TPP is required as coenzyme for several reactions, which are taking place in the human body.

1. Pyruvate $\xrightarrow[\text{complex TPP}]{\text{Pyruvate dehydrogenase}}$ Acetyl CoA

2. α-KG $\xrightarrow[\substack{\text{Dehydrogenase complex} \\ \text{TPP, FAD}}]{\alpha\text{-ketoglutarate}}$ Succinyl CoA

3. Xylulose-5-P + Erythrose-4-P $\xrightarrow[\text{TPP}]{\text{Transketolase}}$ Fructose-6-P + Glyceraldehyde-3-P

Deficiency

➢ Beriberi: It is of two types and they are **dry and wet beriberi.**
➢ *Dry beriberi:*
  Symptoms
  o Loss of appetite
  o Weight loss
  o Muscle wasting
  o Peripheral neuritis with numbness
  o Tingling sensations in the lower legs and feet
  o Ataxic gait.
➢ *Wet beriberi*
  o With the symptoms of dry beriberi
  o Edema
  o Foot drop and wrist drop
  o Enlargement of heart are the additional symptoms.
➢ Mainly in the alcoholics, the B_1 deficiency occurs, step into peripheral and neurological defects known as **Wernicke-Korsakoff** syndrome.

RIBOFLAVIN (Vitamin B₂)

Chemistry: Riboflavin has a dimethyl isoalloxazine ring attached to ribitol vitamin B_2 is stable to heat but is sensitive to light.

Sources

The sources of vitamin B_2 are:
• Animal liver
• Yeast
• Green leafy vegetables
• Milk
• Eggs

Requirements

- Adults: 2.0 mg/day
- Children: 1.2 mg/day
- Pregnancy and lactation: 2.0 mg/day

The riboflavin has two coenzyme forms, and they are **flavin mononucleotide (FMN) and flavin adenine dinucleotide (FAD)** and both are nucleotides.

Some enzymes have FMN and FAD as their integral part. Such enzymes are called flavoproteins.

Functions of FMN and FAD

They take part in oxidation reactions.
   FMN is required for:
   1. L-amino acid oxidase
   2. Cytochrome C reductase
   FAD is required as coenzyme for:
   1. Succinate dehydrogenase
   2. Pyruvate dehydrogenase complex
   3. α-ketoglutarate dehydrogenase complex
   4. Xanthine oxidase

Deficiency symptoms

- Glossitis (Magenta colored tongue)
- Cheilosis (Fissuring of the lips)
- Fissuring at the corners of mouth
- Seborrheic dermatitis, corneal vascularization are the symptoms of riboflavin deficiency.

NIACIN (nicotinic acid)

Chemistry: Nicotinic acid and its amide, nicotinamide have equal biological activities. Nicotinic acid is also called as niacin. The compounds have pyridine ring. The niacin is stable in nature.

Sources

The major sources are:
- Lean meats (liver)
- Legumes, peanuts (ground nuts)
- Green leafy vegetables
- Whole grains
   Amino acid tryptophan can be converted to the coenzyme NAD.
   About 60 mg of tryptophan yields 1 mg of niacin.
   Milk and eggs are low in niacin but are rich in tryptophan.

Requirements

- Adults: 16–20 mg/day
- Children: 9–16 mg/day
- Infants: 5–8 mg/day

Coenzyme forms

It has two coenzyme forms.
   i. **Nicotinamide Adenine Dinucleotide (NAD)**
   ii. **Nicotinamide Adenine Dinucleotide Phosphate (NADP)**
They take part mainly in oxidation reactions of our body.

NAD is required as a coenzyme for *pyruvate dehydrogenase complex, α-ketoglutarate dehydrogenase complex* to mediate the reactions.

NADP is required for *glucose-6-phosphate dehydrogenase* and *6-phosphate gluconate dehydrogenase* mediated reactions.

Deficiency

➤ The deficiency of niacin leads to a condition called **pellagra.**
   Involves skin, gastrointestinal tract and central nervous system.
   Its symptoms are called 3d symptoms, diarrhea, dermatitis and dementia (disturbances of CNS) and if untreated, is followed by death.
➤ Fate of these vitamins when given in large doses: Nicotinic acid and nicotinamide are converted to their corresponding N-methyl derivatives before they are excreted in urine. This is an example of detoxication by transmethylation.

PYRIDOXINE (B₆)

Chemistry

Pyridoxine, pyridoxal and pyridoxamine, as a group, are designated as vitamin B_6.
   All are equally active.
   They have a pyridine ring.
   Pyridoxine is heat-stable, but decomposes in the light or in alkaline solutions.

Sources

The sources are:
- Whole grains
- Organ meats
- Eggs
- Legumes

Requirements

- Adults: 2.2 mg/day
- Children: 1.2 mg/day
- Infants: 3.0 mg/day

The coenzyme form of pyridoxine is **pyridoxal phosphate (PLP).**

PLP is required as a coenzyme in the reactions involved in amino acid metabolism for the enzymes like:

- Transaminases
- Decarboxylases
- Kynureninase
- Cystathionine β-synthase
- Cystathionine gamma-lyase and ALA synthase.

Enzymes like serine hydroxymethyl transferase and phosphorylase contain PLP, but role of PLP in their action is not known.

Deficiency symptoms

The deficiency leads to:

- Hypochromic microcytic anemia
- Glossitis
- Pigmented scaly dermatitis similar to pellagra
- Numbness and tingling sensations in the extremities
- Irritability, depression and convulsive seizures.

  Tuberculous patients who are on long-term therapy with antituberculosis drug, isonicotinic acid hydrazide (INH) suffer from B_6 deficiency. This drug has a structure similar to B_6 and antagonizes the action of B_6. Hence, along with INH, they have to be given large doses of B_6. The deficiency occurs also in women taking oral contraceptives.

Antagonists

Deoxypyridoxine and methoxypyridoxine.

BIOTIN

Sulfur containing vitamin, consists of two fused rings, one is imidazole and the other is thiophane and an attached valeric acid side chain.

Sources

- Egg yolk
- Organ meats (liver, kidney)
- Milk
- Legumes
- Nuts

Requirements

- Adults: 0.3 mg/day.
- The intestinal bacteria can also synthesize biotin to some extent.
  The coenzyme form: Biotin itself acts as coenzyme.
  It functions as a coenzyme in the reactions involving fixation of CO_2.

1. $\text{Pyruvate} \xrightarrow[\text{H}_2\text{O} + \text{CO}_2 \text{ biotin}]{\text{Pyruvate carboxylase}} \text{Oxaloacetate}$

2. $\text{Propionyl CoA} \xrightarrow[\text{CO}_2 \text{ biotin}]{\text{Propionyl CoA carboxylase}} \text{D-methyl malonyl CoA}$

3. $\text{Acetyl CoA} + \text{CO}_2 + \text{ATP} \xrightarrow[\text{Biotin}]{\text{Acetyl CoA carboxylase}} \text{Malonyl CoA} + \text{ADP} + \text{Pi}$

Antivitamin

Avidin, a glycoprotein present in raw egg white when fed to animals can produce biotin deficiency. Since avidin causes egg-white injury, biotin is called anti-egg white injury factor. Avidin being protein, on heating, it will be denatured and looses its biotin-binding activity.

Deficiency symptoms

➢ It is rare, experimental animals shows the symptoms like anorexia, depression, insomnia, muscle pain and dermatitis.

Antagonists

Desthiobiotin
Oxybiotin

PANTOTHENIC ACID

Consists of a dihydroxy dimethyl butyric acid joined to β-alanine by a peptide bond.

Sources

The good sources are:
- Eggs
- Animal liver
- Meat
- Milk
- Vegetables
- Grains

Requirement

- Adults: 5–10 mg/day
- Children: 4–5 mg/day
- Infants: 1–2 mg/day

The coenzyme form: **Coenzyme A (CoASH).**
Its reactive group is sulfydryl group (–SH)
CoASH is required for:

1. Pyruvate $\xrightarrow{\text{Pyruvate dehydrogenase complex}}$ Acetyl CoA
   +
   CoASH

2. α-ketoglutarate $\xrightarrow[\text{CoASH}]{\text{α-ketoglutarate DH complex}}$ Succinyl CoA

3. Fatty acid $\xrightarrow{\text{Thiokinase}}$ Acyl CoA
   +
   CoASH

4. α-ketoacyl CoA $\xrightarrow[\text{CoASH Acyl CoA}]{\text{Thiolase}}$ Acyl CoA

5. Detoxication of benzoic acid
6. For the synthesis of bile salts

Deficiency

➤ It is rare. When it is produced experimentally have the symptoms like fatigue, sleep disorders, weakness, abdominal cramp and a burning sensation of the feet.

FOLIC ACID

Composed pteridine ring attached to para amino benzoic acid (PABA) and conjugated with glutamic acid residues.

Sources

- Fresh green vegetables
- Liver
- Whole grains
- Meat
- Legumes

Requirements

- Children: 300 µg/day
- Adults: 400 µg/day
- Pregnancy and lactation: 800 µg/day.

The coenzyme form of folic acid is **tetrahydrofolic acid (FH_4)**.
The FH_4 is a carrier of single carbon and it is involved in single carbon transfer reactions. The single carbon may be in the form of:

a. Formyl (–CHO)
   Tryptophan
   $\downarrow$
   Formate $\xrightarrow{FH_4}$ N_{10} formyl FH_4 $\longrightarrow$ C-2 Purine ring

b. Methenyl (=CH)
   Histidine
   $\downarrow$
   FIGLU $\xrightarrow{FH_4}$ N_5, N_{10}-methenyl FH_4 $\longrightarrow$ C-8 Purine ring

c. Glycine N_5 $\xrightarrow{FH_4}$ N_{10} methylene FH_4 $\longrightarrow$ Tymidine monophosphate (TMP)

Deficiency

➢ Megaloblastic anemia
➢ Growth failure
   FH_4 required for purine ring synthesis that again required for the synthesis of DNA and RNA.
   Causes: Low dietary intake, malabsorption syndrome and during pregnancy.
   FIGLU excretion test: In the deficiency of folic acid the availability of FH_4 is less or totally absent. So the intermediate of histidine metabolism, formiminoglutamate accumulates in the blood and excreted in the urine. This is one of the tests to detect the megaloblastic anemia whether it is due to folic acid or vitamin B_{12} deficiency.

VITAMIN B_{12} (Cobalamin)

It has a corrin ring.

Sources

The sources are:
- Liver
- Meat

- Fish
- Eggs
- Milk

Requirements

- Children: 2 μg/day
- Adults: 3 μg/day
- Pregnancy and lactation: 4 μg/day

Absorption

- A glycoprotein is the **Castle's intrinsic factor**.
- **Vitamin B$_{12}$ is called extrinsic factor**.
- Vitamin B$_{12}$ of food binds to intrinsic factor in the stomach, this complex moves to ileum, there it bind to specific receptors.
- Then the B$_{12}$ is transported to mucosal cell and then to blood and carried by B$_{12}$ binding proteins.
- The coenzyme form of vitamin B$_{12}$ is **5'-deoxyadenosylcobalamin**.
- Vitamin B$_{12}$ along with folic acid is required for the development of red blood cells beyond megaloblastic stage.
- It acts as coenzyme for the mutase enzyme which converts methyl malonyl CoA into succinyl CoA.
- It is involved in the conversion of ribonucleotides to deoxyribonucleotide.

Deficiency

- Megaloblastic anemia
- Glossitis and inflammation of mouth
- Methyl malonic aciduria.
  Cause: Intestinal malabsorption and poor dietary intake.

Self Test

Long essay questions

1. Write a note on the sources and requirement of vitamin A.
2. Discuss the functions and deficiency manifestations of vitamin A.
3. What are the functions of vitamin D?
4. What are the deficiency symptoms of vitamin D?
5. Discuss the sources and functions of vitamins E and K.
6. Add a note on the requirement, sources, functions and deficiency manifestations of vitamin C.
7. Name the B complex vitamins.
8. What is the coenzyme or active form of thiamine?

9. Discuss the sources and functions of thiamine.
10. What is beriberi, explain briefly?
11. Name the enzymes, which are dependent on PLP as coenzyme.
12. Mention the symptoms of pyridoxine deficiency.
13. Discuss briefly the sources, requirement, functions and deficiency manifestations of niacin.
14. What is the function of biotin in the body?
15. Mention the coenzyme form for pantothenic acid.
16. What are the enzymes, which need FMN and FAD as coenzymes?
17. Write the deficiency diseases of riboflavin.
18. Discuss the sources, functions and deficiency manifestations of vitamin B_{12}.
19. Write a note on the requirement and deficiency diseases of folic acid.
20. What is FIGLU excretion test?

Short essay questions

1. Which form of vitamin A has a role in vision?
2. Cod liver oil is a rich source for which vitamin?
3. Which vitamin deficiency leads to night blindness?
4. Name the two forms of vitamin.
5. In adults and children, deficiency of vitamin D leads to what?
6. The antioxidant property is observed in which vitamin?
7. Name the naturally occurring form of vitamin K.
8. Which vitamin involved in gamma carboxylation of the glutamic acid residues of the inactive clotting factor?
9. Name the important source for vitamin.
10. Which vitamin is responsible for the hydroxylation of prolyl residues?
11. The vitamin C deficiency leads to what?
12. Name the coenzyme form of thiamine.
13. Which vitamin deficiency leads to beriberi?
14. The pellagra arises due to the deficiency of which vitamin?
15. Mention the coenzyme form of pyridoxine.
16. Name the two coenzyme forms of niacin.
17. Which vitamin deficiency leads to magenta colored tongue?
18. Write the requirement of niacin for adults and children.
19. Name the two coenzyme forms of riboflavin.
20. Which vitamin is called as anti-egg white injury factor?
21. CoASH is the coenzyme form of which vitamin?
22. Give the requirement of folic acid for pregnant and lactating women.
23. What is the other name for vitamin B_{12}.
24. The folic acid deficiency leads to what?
25. Mention the importance of FIGLU excretion test.

Fill in the blanks

1. ———— form of vitamin A has a role in vision.
2. Cod liver oil is a rich source for vitamin ————.
3. Night blindness is due to the deficiency of ————.
4. The two forms of vitamin D are ———— and ————.
5. The deficiency of vitamin D leads to ———— in adults and ———— in children.
6. The antioxidant property is observed in vitamin ————.
7. Phylloquinone is the naturally occurring form of vitamin ————.
8. The vitamin K is involved in ———— of the glutamic acid residues of the inactive clotting factor.

9. The requirement of vitamin C for children is ——————— .
10. The hydroxylation of prolyl residues is brought about by vitamin ——————— .
11. The vitamin C deficiency leads to ——————— .
12. The coenzyme form of thiamine is called ——————— .
13. The beriberi is due to the deficiency of ——————— .
14. The pellagra is due to the deficiency of ——————— .
15. The coenzyme form of pyridoxine is ——————— .
16. The coenzyme forms of niacin are ——————— and ——————— .
17. The magenta colored tongue is due to the deficiency of ——————— .
18. The requirement of niacin for adults is ——————— .
19. The coenzyme forms of riboflavin are ——————— and ——————— .
20. Anti-egg white injury factor is called for ——————— .
21. CoASH is the coenzyme form of ——————— .
22. The requirement of folic acid for pregnants and lactating women is ——————— .
23. The vitamin B_{12} is also called as ——————— .
24. The folic acid deficiency leads to ——————— .
25. The coenzyme form of vitamin B_{12} is ——————— .

Multiple choice questions

1. **The following are the symptoms of vitamin A deficiency EXCEPT**
   a. Night blindness
   b. Fragile RBCs
   c. Keratinization of lacrimal glands
   d. Keratomalacia

2. **Regarding the vitamin D, one of the following statements is INCORRECT.**
   a. Low calcium stimulates the 1- hydroxylase.
   b. Vitamin D_3 increases the absorption of calcium from the intestine.
   c. Deficiency leads to scurvy.
   d. Deficiency leads to rickets.

3. **One of the following is NOT the form of vitamin K.**
   a. Phylloquinone
   b. Menaquinone
   c. Menadione
   d. Ubiquinone

4. **All of the following statements are correct with respect to the function of vitamin E EXCEPT**
   a. Antioxidant
   b. Normal reproduction in animals
   c. Helps in vision
   d. Protects cellular membrane

5. **Scurvy is the result of:**
   a. Deficiency of vitamin A
   b. Deficiency of vitamin C
   c. Deficiency of vitamin D
   d. Deficiency of vitamin E

6. **The INCORRECT statement regarding vitamin B_{12} is**
   a. Called as extrinsic factor.
   b. Vitamin B_{12} of food binds to intrinsic factor in the stomach.
   c. The coenzyme form of vitamin B_{12} is **5'-deoxyadenosyl cobalamine**.
   d. Vitamin B_{12} along with vitamin C is required for the development of red blood cells beyond megaloblastic stage.

7. **The tetrahydrofolic acid (FH$_4$) does the following EXCEPT**
   a. Carrier of single carbon and it is involved in single carbon transfer reactions.
   b. Contributes to C-2 purine ring
   c. Contributes to C-8 purine ring
   d. Synthesis of UMP

8. **One of the following enzymes DOES NOT require coenzyme A (CoASH).**
   a. Pyruvate dehydrogenase complex
   b. α-ketoglutarate DH complex
   c. Hexokinase
   d. Thiokinase

9. **Deficiency of vitamin B$_6$ leads to the following EXCEPT**
   a. Hypochromic microcytic anemia
   b. Glossitis
   c. Pigmented scaly dermatitis similar to pellagra
   d. Megaloblastic anemia

10. **All of the following statements are correct regarding the riboflavin EXCEPT**
    a. Has a dimethyl isoalloxazine ring attached to ribitol.
    b. RDA for adults is 2.0 mg/day.

    c. Flavin mononucleotide (FMN) is its coenzyme form.
    d. Flavin adenine dinucleotide (FAD) is its coenzyme form.

11. **One of the following is NOT dependent on the coenzyme pyridoxal phosphate (PLP) for its activity.**
    a. Transaminases
    b. Decarboxylases
    c. Pyruvate dehydrogenase
    d. ALA synthase

12. **All of the following statements are correct regarding niacin EXCEPT**
    a. Nicotinamide adenine dinucleotide (NAD) is its coenzyme.
    b. Flavin adenine dinucleotide (FAD) is its coenzyme form.
    c. Nicotinamide adenine dinucleotide Phosphate (NADP).
    d. The deficiency of niacin leads to a condition called pellagra.

13. **Thiamine is essential for all of the following EXCEPT**
    a. Pyruvate dehydrogenase complex
    b. α-ketoglutarate dehydrogenase complex
    c. Protect against night blindness
    d. Protect against beriberi

16

Minerals and Electrolyte Metabolism

1. **What are the two types of minerals present in the human body?**
   The minerals present in the human body may be classified as:
   a. Bulk elements (macronutrients) and
   b. Trace elements (micronutrients).
2. **Name the bulk elements.**
   Bulk elements are 7 in number and they are calcium, magnesium, sodium, potassium, phosphorus, sulfur, and chloride. They constitute 60–80% of all inorganic material in the body.
3. **What are trace elements and name them?**
   Trace elements are those, which are required in very small amounts. They are 9 in number and they are iron, iodine, cobalt, manganese, molybdenum, zinc, lead, selenium, and fluoride.

CALCIUM

4. Discuss the calcium under the following headings.
   a. Sources
   b. Requirement
   c. Functions

Sources

Rich sources:
- Milk and its products.

Good sources:
- Meat, fish,
- Green leafy vegetables,
- Cereals,
- Pulses.

Requirements

- Children: 1.2 gm/day
- Adults: 0.8 gm /day
- Pregnancy and lactation: 1.2 gm/day.

Absorption

Factors favoring absorption are:
- 1, 25-dihydroxy vitamin D_3
- Gastric acidity
- Lactose
- Amino acids and citrate
- Calcium: Phosphate ratio of the diet
- Low level of phosphate increases absorption

The substances decrease absorption are:
- Oxalate and phytates of food
- Fatty acids
- All forms of insoluble salts with calcium

Calcium content of body and blood

Calcium is the major inorganic element comprising nearly 2% of the body weight.

Human body contains 1200 gm. Major amount (99% of this) present in bone and teeth as hydroxy appetite. Remaining 1% is present in blood and soft tissues.

Calcium level of serum in adult is 9–11 mg/100 ml.

Blood calcium present in 3 different forms:
  a. Ionized calcium (Ca^{++}) is the physiological active form. It constitutes 50% of the total calcium (4.5–5.5 mg%).
  b. Protein (albumin) bound form. This is 45% of total level.
  c. Calcium complexes with citrate, phosphate and bicarbonate. This fraction is only 5%.

Functions

➢ Calcium is required for the formation of bone and teeth.
➢ Gives hardness and strength to bone and teeth.
➢ Required for blood coagulation process.
➢ Required for contraction of heart and muscle.
➢ Controls the permeability of cell membranes.
➢ Activates pancreatic lipase in the digestion of fats.
➢ Activates phosphorylase during the breakdown of glycogen.
➢ Regulates the excitability of nerve fibers.
➢ Releases hormones like insulin from storage granules.
➢ Serves as a second messenger in the action of hormones like adrenaline.

➢ Responses of calcium are mediated by interaction with a receptor protein called *calmodulin*. This cytosol protein has calcium-binding sites. Calmodulin-calcium complex activates protein kinases, which in turn activates other enzymes and through these, bring about metabolic effects. In this mechanism cAMP is also involved.

Regulation of serum calcium level

The ionic calcium level is maintained by vitamin D and hormones like parathyroid hormone (PTH) and calcitonin.

Actions of vitamin D

a. Increasing the absorption of calcium (and phosphate) from the small intestine.
b. Causing removal of calcium from bone (bone resorption).

The mechanism by which 1,25-dihydroxy vitamin D_3 increases calcium absorption from intestine is as follows:

The 1,25-dihydroxy vitamin D_3 enters to the intestinal cell and binds to a cytoplasmic receptor. The vitamin D_3 receptor complex then moves to the nucleus where it interacts with DNA. This results in the synthesis of mRNA and this in turn forms a calcium binding protein. The calcium binding protein increases the absorption of calcium from intestine.

Actions of PTH on kidney and bone

1. PTH increases the activity of 1-hydroxylase in kidney, which increases the synthesis of 1,25-dihydroxy vitamin D_3 and this in turn enhance the absorption of calcium from intestine.
2. It increases the reabsorption of calcium from glomerular filtrate in kidneys.
3. It causes the resorption of calcium from bone.
   These 3 actions correct the hypocalcemia and bring it to normal level.
4. PTH also causes excretion of phosphate in urine by inhibiting phosphate reabsorption in kidney.

Action of calcitonin

This is a hormone from C cells of thyroid glands.

Hypercalcemia stimulates its secretion.

Calcitonin inhibits calcium reabsorption from kidneys and resorption from bone. Thus, it corrects hypercalcemia.

Hypocalcemia

1. This provokes a characteristic hyperexcitable state of the nerves and muscles called tetany.

Symptoms are:

• Numbness of extremities
• Emotional irritability
• Tightness and spasm of muscles.

2. Hypocalcemia also occurs in hypoparathyroidism, rickets, osteomalacia, pancreatitis, etc. Total calcium level is less than 4.0 mg% in this condition.

Hypercalcemia

This occurs in hyperparathyroidism and hypervitaminosis D.
Total calcium level is more than 12 mg% in this condition.

PHOSPHORUS

1. Mention the sources and functions of phosphorus.

Sources

Good sources:
- Milk
- Meat
- Cereals
- In general, a diet supplying sufficient calcium will supply an adequate amount of phosphorus also.

Requirements

- Adults: 800 mg/day.
- Extra allowance is required during growth and pregnancy.

Phosphorus content of body and blood

Phosphorus forms 1% of the body weight.

Whole body contains 700 gm of phosphorus, 80% of this is present in bones and teeth as hydroxyapatite.

Functions

- Helps in the formation of bone and teeth.
- Act as a buffer in blood.
- Helps in the formation of compounds like nucleic acids, nucleotides like ATP, GTP, ADP, etc, as organic phosphate esters in glycolysis and other metabolic reactions.
- It is also required in energy metabolism, synthesis of phospholipids, cAMP, phospho-proteins, and coenzymes like TPP.

Normal serum inorganic phosphate level:

Adults: 2.5–4.5 mg%

Children: 4–6 mg%

Hypophosphatemia (decreased level of phosphorus)
- Rickets
- Hyperparathyroidism
- Condition associated with decrease in the reabsorption of phosphate from the glomerular filtrate (Fanconi syndrome).

Hyperphosphatemia (Increased phosphorus level)
- Seen in hypoparathyroidism
- Hypervitaminosis D
- Renal failure

MAGNESIUM

Magnesium (Mg^{2+}) is the major intracellular cation (15 mEq/L) next to potassium (155 mEq/L). About 70% of total magnesium is in skeletal tissues, the remainder is in muscle, brain and other tissues.

Source

- Abundant in chlorophyll pigment of vegetables
- Good sources are whole grains
- Nuts
- Milk
- Meat

Requirements

- Adults: 300 mg/day
- Children: 250 mg/day

Functions

- It is an essential activator of many enzymes especially those involving transfer of phosphate groups from ATP.
- Examples are hexokinase and phosphofructokinase.
- It also activates a number of enzymes like:
  - enolase
  - glucose-6-P dehydrogenase
  - pyruvate carboxylase
  - thiokinase
  - G-6-P dehydrogenase

Deficiency

- Deficiency symptoms bear some resemblance to those seen in hypocalcemia, with muscle twitching, spasms and tetany.

IRON

Iron (Fe) is a trace element. Trace elements are present in the body in much smaller amounts. Total body iron is about 5 gm.

Sources

- Liver
- Meat
- Egg yolk
- Vegetables
- Whole wheat
- Legumes
- Cashew nuts
- Dates

Functions

- Iron is necessary for the synthesis of certain proteins.
- Iron containing proteins in the body are of two types: Heme proteins and non-heme proteins.

Examples of heme proteins

1. *Hemoglobin:* This accounts for 70% of total body iron.
2. *Myoglobin:* This is the muscle O_2-binding protein, 5% of total Fe is in this form. Both proteins function in the transport of O_2.
3. *Catalase and peroxidase:* Function of these are in the decomposition of H_2O_2, a toxic compound.
4. Cytochrome b, c_1, c, aa_3. These take part in respiratory chain.

Examples of non-heme proteins

1. *Ferritin and hemosiderin:* These are iron storage proteins in liver, spleen and bone marrow. These comprise 15% of body iron.
2. *Transferrin:* This is the iron transport protein in blood.
3. Aconitase of Krebs TCA cycle.
4. *Iron-sulfur proteins:* Succinate dehydrogenase is an example.
   Some iron-sulfur proteins function in respiratory chain.

Requirement

The amount of iron required for each day to compensate for the losses depends on age and sex; it is highest in pregnancy and menstruating females.

Requirements (RDA)

- Adult males: 12 mg/day
- Females: 20 mg/day
- Pregnancy and lactation: 40 mg/day

Dietary source

Content and the amount of iron absorbed differ from food to food; shell fish, meat, liver is better than vegetables, eggs or milk foods.

Iron absorption

Absorption takes place mainly in the duodenum.

Factors favoring absorption	Factors reducing absorption
Ferrous form	Ferric form
Inorganic iron	Organic iron
Acids—HCl, vitamin C	Alkalis, antacids, pancreatic secretions
Iron deficiency	Iron excess
Increased erythropoiesis	Decreased erythropoiesis
Pregnancy	Infection

HCl of stomach liberate Fe^{3+} from non-heme iron compounds of food.
Iron is absorbed as Fe^{2+}.

Mechanism of Fe absorption

- ✓ After absorption of Fe^{2+} into the intestinal mucosal cell, it is oxidized to Fe^{3+}.
- ✓ This combines with intracellular carrier protein.
- ✓ This complex either delivers a fixed amount of Fe to mitochondria, or transfers some iron to another protein called apoferritin, which binds Fe^{3+} to form ferritin.
- ✓ The ferritin is a storage form of iron.
- ✓ Some iron binds with plasma α1-globulin called apotransferrin to form transferrin. The transferrin is a transport form of iron. Proportions of iron transferred to apoferritin and apotransferrin depend upon the iron status of the person.
- ✓ In the iron deficient state, more iron is delivered to apotransferrin and much less to apoferritin.
- ✓ In the case of iron overload, more iron is transferred to apoferritin and much less to apotransferrin. Thus entry of iron into the body is regulated at the intestine level.

Transport in blood

Fe^{3+} is reduced to Fe^{2+} in the mucosal cell. Fe^{2+} then enters to the plasma where it is reoxidized to Fe^{3+} by a copper-carrying protein called ceruloplasmin (or serum ferroxidase).

Serum content

Hundred milliliter blood contains about 300 mg of transferrin which is capable of carrying 360 µg of Fe, but normally, it carries an average of only 100 µg of Fe. In deficiency, this level is much less.

Deficiency

- Hypochromic microcytic anemia (microcytic RBC of reduced size)
  - o Hemorrhage,
  - o Malabsorption
  - o Hookworm infestation depletes the body iron even if the diet is adequate.

The pronounced and repeated "Fe" losses resulting from menstruation, pregnancy and lactation render women of childbearing age especially vulnerable to depletion of iron stores.

Anemic patients are found to be pale, tired, and restless and have palpitation, lesions of oral cavity and spoon-shaped nails.

Hemochromatosis

- ➢ It is an excessive hemosiderin accumulation in tissues like liver, spleen, skin, etc. caused by an excessive intestinal absorption of iron due to a genetic disorder.
- ➢ This results in bronze colored skin, cirrhosis of liver and damage to pancreas leading to diabetes. This is called bronze diabetes.
- ➢ Hemosiderosis is an excessive accumulation of iron. This may be seen in the Bantu people of Africa who consume large amount of Fe obtained from their cooking pots made of iron.

COPPER (Cu)

Sources

- Fish, liver
- Nuts
- Green leafy vegetables
- Milk and cereals are poor sources.

Requirement

- Adults: 3 mg/day.

Functions

A need for copper is linked to its functional role in several Cu-containing enzymes.
1. Ceruloplasmin (also called serum ferroxidase). This copper containing protein catalyzes the oxidation of Fe^{2+} to Fe^{3+}
2. Cytochrome oxidase of the respiratory chain contains Fe^{3+} and Cu^{2+}
3. Dopamine oxidase of catecholamine synthetic pathway
4. Monoamine oxidase and diamine oxidase

5. Cytoplasmic superoxide dismutase contains Cu^{2+} and Zn^{2+}.
6. P-hydroxyphenyl pyruvate hydroxylase of tyrosine catabolism.
7. Lysyl oxidase involved in cross-linking process in the conversion of tropocollagen to collagen.
8. Tyrosinase of melanin synthetic pathway is a Cu-dependent enzyme.

Transport in blood

The copper absorbed in the intestine enters to the blood, first binds to albumin and later transferred to α-globulin fraction of plasma protein to form ceruloplasmin.

Deficiency

➤ Hypochromic microcytic anemia due to copper deficiency in milk-fed infants has been observed. It responds to copper but not to iron therapy.

➤ Wilson's disease or also called hepatolenticular degeneration: It is a fatal inherited disease. Blood copper level decreases.

There is an excessive storage of copper in the liver, probably owing to defective synthesis of ceruloplasmin by the liver cells. Besides deposition in liver, copper is also deposited in kidney, brain and cornea (brown ring called Kayser-Fleischer ring at the margin of cornea). Cirrhosis of liver, neurologic disorders, tubular damage and high urinary copper are also seen.

Pencillamine, a copper-chelating agent, is used in its treatment. Excess copper is thus excreted.

ZINC (Zn)

Sources

- Meat
- Egg
- Marine fish
- Unmilled cereals
- Legumes, corn
- Spinach and lettuce

Requirements

- Adults: 10–15 mg/day.
- Children: 3–15 mg/day.
- Pregnancy and lactation: 20–25 mg/day.

Functions

The Zn is required as an activator ion for following enzymes.

- Carbonic anhydrase

- Alkaline phosphatase
- Liver alcohol dehydrogenase
- Carboxyl peptidase A
- DNA polymerase
- Cytosolic superoxide dismutase (both Cu^{2+} and Zn^{2+})

Zinc deficiency may cause dwarfism. Other deficiency manifestations are hypogonadism, and loss of taste sensation and impaired wound healing.

- *Acrodermatitis enteropathica:* Is an autosomal recessive disorder and its clinical manifestations appear to be related to zinc deficiency. The clinical manifestations of this are chronic diarrhea, alopecia, wasting and thickened ulcerated skin around the body orifices and extremities.

MANGANESE (Mn)

Sources

- Wheat germ seeds
- Nuts
- Leafy vegetables
- Meat

Requirements

- Adults: 3.5 mg/day.
- Children: 0.2 mg/day.

Functions

Manganese acts as a cofactor or an activator for several enzymes.
The manganese containing enzymes are:

- Acetyl CoA carboxylase
- Mitochondrial superoxide dismutase
- Arginase
- 6-P-gluconate dehydrogenase
- Squalene synthetase
- Isocitrate dehydrogenase

In both birds and mammals, the manganese deficiency is characterized by defective growth, bone abnormalities, reproductive dysfunction and CNS manifestations.

The toxicity has been seen in miners as a result of absorption of manganese through respiratory tract after prolonged exposure to manganese dust.

MOLYBDENUM (Mo)

Sources

- Legumes
- Whole grains
- Milk
- Leafy vegetables
- Organ meat

Requirement

- Adults: 0.5 mg/day

Metabolic functions

It is required as a catalytic component of the metalloenzymes like
- Xanthine oxidase
- Aldehyde oxidase
- Sulfite oxidase.

COBALT (Co)

Sources

- Liver
- Kidney
- Muscle meats
- Oysters
- Clams

Functions

- This occurs in vitamin B_{12} and its coenzymes.
- Cofactor for glycyl-glycine dipeptidase of intestinal juice.

SELENIUM (Se)

Sources

- Fish
- Whole grain
- Meat

Requirement

- Adults: 0.2 mg/day.

Selenium is an integral component of glutathione peroxidase. This enzyme scavenging the free radicals and protect the cells and membranes against oxidative damage.

So, this mineral complements the action of vitamin E. Thus, it acts as an antioxidant.

IODINE

Iodine is a chemical element with symbol **I** and atomic number 53.

Iodine and its compounds are primarily used in nutrition.

Sources

Iodine is found on Earth mainly as the highly water-soluble iodide ion I^- which concentrates it in oceans and brine pools.

Deficiency

Iodine deficiency affects about two billion people and is the leading preventable cause of intellectual disabilities.

Functions

Iodine is required by higher animals, those use it to synthesize thyroid hormones, which contain the element. Because of this function, radioisotopes of iodine are concentrated in the thyroid gland along with non-radioactive iodine. If inhaled, the radioisotope iodine-131, which has a high fission product yield, concentrates in the thyroid, but is easily remedied with non-radioactive potassium iodide treatment.

FLUORIDE (F)

Sources

- Fish
- Tea
- Drinking water

Requirements

- 1–2 mg/day.
- Drinking water provides fluoride (1 part per million (1ppm) fluoride. Two-liter water consumed by an individual provides 2 mg F).

Functions

- It is a component of a hydroxyapettite.
- Fluoride is needed for bone and teeth formation. The surface layer of enamel contains a higher content of fluoride than deeper layers of enamel or dentine. It strengthens the enamel surface of teeth and renders it resistant to dental carries (decay).

Excess fluoride causes fluorosis. In this condition there is mottling of enamel. The mottled enamel is discolored, corroded and pitted. High concentrations of fluoride inhibit magnesium-requiring enzymes enolase.

SODIUM (Na$^+$)

Sodium (Na$^+$) is the major cation of the extracellular fluid.

Sources

The major sources are:
- Milk
- Cereals
- Legumes
- Egg
- Carrot
- Tomato
- Table salt.

Average intake from table salt is 5–10 gm/day.

Requirement

- 5 gm/day.
- **The normal range:** 130–145 mEq/L (intracellular Na$^+$ is 10 mEq/L).

Functions

➤ Maintains the osmotic pressure, thus to maintain the volume of blood (i.e. protection against fluid loss).
➤ Regulate the electrolyte and pH balance of the extracellular compartment.
➤ Control the electronic potentials of excitable tissues such as nerve and muscle.
➤ Helps in the active transport of glucose, galactose and amino acids across intestinal mucosa and for Na$^+$/ K$^+$-ATPase.

Deficiency

- A nutritional deficiency is highly important.
- On a low sodium diet the kidney decreases the excretion of sodium in urine.
- Low blood sodium triggers the kidney to release angiotensin.
- Angiotensin causes the adrenal cortex to secrete aldosterone.
- The aldosterone induces the renal tubules to reabsorb sodium from the glomerular filtrate.

Hyponatremia (decrease in plasma sodium)

Cause

- Defect in kidneys or adrenal cortex.
- Sweating, vomiting or diarrhea can cause loss of sodium containing fluids.
- In adrenocortical insufficiency (Addison's disease), decrease in serum sodium and increase in sodium excretion occur.

Hypernatremia (increased plasma sodium concentration)

- Due to the hyperactivity of adrenal cortex (Cushing's disease).
- Administration of cortisone also leads to increase in serum sodium.

- May also be due to decreased loss of sodium through body fluids, especially in prolonged hyperpnea.
- Hypertensive patients are advised to take less salt, about 1 gm/day.

POTASSIUM (K$^+$)

- It is the most important cation of intracellular fluid.
- Average concentration is 155 mEq/L of intracellular fluid.

Sources

- Orange
- Banana
- Fresh vegetables
  An average diet provides 4 gm K$^+$/day.
  Normal value of serum: 3–5.0 mEq/L

Functions

- The extracellular potassium is important for its controlling influence upon neuromuscular irritability, cardiac muscle (a proper balance between K$^+$ and Ca^{++} is essential for the contraction of heart muscle) and the operation of Na$^+$/ K$^+$-ATPase (the Na pump). In cells, there is a significant concentration gradient of Na$^+$ and K$^+$ across cell membranes.
- The high intracellular (K$^+$) is maintained by an energy requiring extrusion of 3 Na$^+$ out of the cell with replacement by 2 K$^+$.
- Intracellular K$^+$ is essential for a number of enzyme-mediated reactions such as pyruvate kinase, glycogen synthesis and protein synthesis, for maintaining osmotic and acid-base balance.

Hypokalemia (decreased plasma K$^+$ concentration)

- A low serum K$^+$ decreases the heartbeat and interferes with vital muscles such as those involved in respiration.
- Occurs in any illness, wasting disease, malnutrition and in diarrhea.
- Certain diuretics increase the excretion of potassium. It is, therefore, important to supplement enough potassium when these drugs are used.

Hyperkalemia (increased plasma K$^+$ concentration)

- The capacity of kidney to excrete potassium is more, so that hyperkalemia not normally occur.
- It may occur in Addison's disease and in intravenous infusion of potassium at a excess rate of 25 mmol/hour.
- Other causes may be in renal failure, advanced dehydration or shock.
- Tissue trauma (in burns, traumatic injury and intestinal bleeding) causes the cells to release K$^+$ into the ECF.

CHLORIDE (Cl⁻)

➤ Chloride (Cl^-) is the major extracellular anion.
➤ Serum concentration is 105 mEq/L.

Functions

➤ It is involved in maintaining osmotic pressure, proper body hydration and electric neutrality.
➤ Dietary chloride is almost completely absorbed by the intestinal tract. It is filtered out by the glomerulus and passively reabsorbed in conjunction with Na^+ by the proximal tubules. Excess chloride is excreted in urine and through sweating. Excessive sweating stimulates aldosterone secretion, which acts on the sweat glands to conserve Na^+ and chloride.

Hypochloremia (A low serum chloride)

It is associated with loss of gastric HCl due to prolonged vomiting.

Salt-losing during renal disease.

In metabolic acidosis, etc.

Hyperchloremia (high serum chloride)

Seen in dehydration and decreased renal blood flow, etc.

Self Test

Short essay questions

1. Write a note on the requirement and functions of calcium.
2. What are the factors that favor iron absorption?
3. Add a note on the absorption and transport of iron.
4. Name the heme and non-heme proteins, which contain iron.
5. Mention the functions of phosphorus.
6. Name any four enzymes, which need magnesium as an activator ion.
7. Which trace element deficiency leads to Wilson's disease?
8. Mention the important source of fluoride. What is fluorosis?
9. What are the sources for copper?
10. What are trace elements and name any four of them?
11. What are the importances of sodium and potassium in the human body?
12. Give the normal values of Na^+ and K^+.

Short answer questions

1. Whether copper is an example for trace or bulk element?
2. Give the normal serum value of calcium.
3. Name the non-heme protein, which contains iron.
4. Which form of iron is absorbed from GI tract?
5. The deficiency of iron leads to what?
6. Name the storage form of iron.
7. Antioxidant property is observed in which trace element?
8. Give an example for copper containing enzyme.
9. The fluoride deficiency leads to what?
10. Name the major cation of the extracellular fluid.
11. What is hyponatremia?
12. Mention the names of the major extracellular anion.

Fill in the blanks

1. Copper is a ———————— element.
2. The normal serum value of calcium is ——————— .
3. The example for non-heme protein which contains iron is ——————— .
4. The form of iron which absorbed from GI tract is ——————— .
5. The deficiency of iron leads to ——————— .
6. Storage form of iron is called ——————— .
7. Antioxidant property is observed in the trace element is ——————— .
8. Cytochrome oxidase is a ——————— containing enzyme.
9. The fluoride deficiency leads to ——————— .
10. The major cation of the extracellular fluid is ——————— .
11. Hyponatremia means ——————— .
12. The major extracellular anion is ——————— .

17

Nutrition

Calorie

- It is a measurement of energy measured in a bomb calorimeter. "The amount of heat it takes to raise the temperature of 1 gram of water by 1 degree celsius".
- Food is measured in kilocalories (kcal), "Calories" with a large "C" on nutrition label are in kcal.

Caloric values of carbohydrates, fat and protein

Caloric value: It is the amount of heat obtained when 1 gm of substance is completely oxidized. Energy = Calories in nutrition

➤ When 1 gm of carbohydrate is oxidized in the body, 4 calories are formed.
➤ When 1 gm of protein is oxidized in the body, 4 calories are formed.
➤ When 1 gm of fat is oxidized in the body, 9 calories are formed.

Respiratory quotient (RQ) of food stuffs

The **respiratory quotient is** the volume of CO_2 produced, divided by the volume of O_2 consumed at the whole body. Because of inherent chemical differences in the composition of carbohydrates, fats, and proteins, different amounts of oxygen are required to completely oxidize the carbon and hydrogen atoms in carbohydrates, fats, and proteins into carbon dioxide and water. Thus, the quantity of carbon dioxide produced relative to the oxygen consumed will vary depending on the proportional mix of energy nutrients (carbohydrate, fat, protein) metabolized.

$$RQ = \frac{\text{Volume of } CO_2 \text{ produced}}{\text{Volume of } O_2 \text{ utilized}}$$

$$RQ = VCO_2/VO_2$$

Carbohydrates

When carbohydrates are completely oxidized, their RQ is

$$C_6H_{12}O_6 \text{ (glucose)} + 6O_2 \longrightarrow 6CO_2 + 6H_2O$$

$$\frac{VCO_2 \text{ produced}}{VO_2 \text{ utilized}} = \frac{6}{6} = 1$$

Fats

When palmitic acid completely oxidized, their RQ is

$$C_{15}H_{32}COOH \text{ (palmitic acid)} + 23O_2 \longrightarrow 16CO_2 + 16H_2O$$

$$\frac{VCO_2 \text{ produced}}{VO_2 \text{ utilized}} = \frac{16}{23} = 0.7$$

This reaction shows that fats have relatively low RQ, since they have low oxygen content.

Proteins

The protein is not completely oxidized to CO_2 and cannot be represented by formula.

For example, the protein, albumin, is oxidized as follows:

$$C_{72}H_{112}N_2O_{22}S + 77 O_2 \longrightarrow 63CO_2 + 38H_2O + SO_3 + 9CO(NH_2)_2$$

$$\frac{VCO_2 \text{ produced}}{VO_2 \text{ utilized}} = \frac{63}{77} = 0.818$$

The RER for protein is **0.82** (indirect measurements).

The RQ of a mixed diet is 0.8.

The RQ value is important not only in determining the body's rate of energy expenditure, but it also enables the investigator to determine the nutrient mixture being metabolized during rest or exercise.

The RQ is very helpful in understanding the kind of food which is predominantly oxidized at any time.

Importance of carbohydrates, proteins and fats

Carbohydrates

- To some extent every body cell depends on glucose. The cells of the nervous system and the brain almost exclusively use glucose for energy.
- Simple carbohydrates are monosaccharides (glucose, fructose, galactose) and disaccharides (maltose, sucrose, lactose).
- Complex carbohydrates (glycogen, starch and fiber): Foods rich in complex carbohydrates tend to be low in fat and sugar and can, therefore, add bulk to meals.

- Glycogen is not a significant food source of carbohydrate. However, the body stores much of its glucose as glycogen.
- Glycogen is released when the body needs glucose for energy.
- Starch—plants store starch like human bodies store glycogen and when we eat the plant, our body hydrolyzes the starch to glucose.
- Grains are the richest food source of starch and provide much of the food energy.
- Some examples of starches are rice, corn, rye, barley, and oats.
- Fibers are different than starches in that they cannot be broken down by the digestive system, and, therefore, they provide little or no energy for the body.
- Fiber has been shown to **protect against heart disease and diabetes by lowering cholesterol and glucose levels**.
- Fiber has also been shown to provide a **feeling of fullness, and promote proper bowel function**.
- Examples of good sources of fibers are bran cereals, okra, butter beans, kidney beans, navy beans, sweet potatoes and pears.

Protein

The roles of proteins in the body are:
- Whenever our body is growing, repairing or replacing tissue, proteins are involved.
- Proteins form the building blocks of bones, teeth, muscles, skin and blood.
- In addition, proteins help to regulate fluid balance; act as enzymes, act as transporters and some hormones are proteins as well.
- As antibodies, proteins also help with the body's defense against disease.
- Proteins can also be used as a source of energy, if needed.

Complete and Incomplete Proteins

- **Complete proteins:** These contain all of the essential amino acids needed for growth.
- **Sources:** Milk, fish, poultry, cheese, eggs, yogurt
- **Incomplete proteins:** These are missing one or more essential amino acids needed for growth. Incomplete proteins are found in the plant form.
- **Sources:** Vegetables, seeds, nuts, grains and legumes.

Complementary proteins: Two or more dietary proteins whose amino acids composition complement each other in such a way that the essential amino acids missing from one are supplied by the other. By combining two or more plant proteins, we can consume all of the essential amino acids needed to support growth.

Protein and weight gain

- Ideally, protein should contribute to 10–35% of energy intake.
- Protein-rich foods are often higher in fat, which can contribute to weight gain.
- To prevent weight gain, choose lean cuts of meat and trim away visible fat from meats and poultry before cooking.
- Broil or grill meat instead of frying.

Protein and weight loss

- It is generally not advisable to use a high protein diet to lose weight.
- High protein diets can be effective in weight loss. However, the reason that high protein diets work is because, they increase the feeling of satiety and are lower in calories.
- Eating excess protein may trouble the kidney with extra work. As the kidneys work to eliminate the excess protein, they also excrete a lot of water out of our system.
- While the scale may show a dramatic weight loss, this is may not be a real weight loss.
- It is generally wise to consume extra amounts of water, if eating extra protein.

Recommended Daily Allowance for Protein

- The RDA for adults is 0.8 grams of protein per/kg/body weight/per day.

Fats

- Fat provides us with 60% of our energy needs at rest, it spares protein, insulates our bodies against extreme temperatures, and protects us against shock by providing a cushion for bones and vital organs.
- Fat also helps to maintain cell membranes and aids in the absorption of vitamins A, D, E, and K.
- As a food ingredient, fat provides flavor, consistency, stability and satiety.

  Unsaturated fats: The most effective dietary strategy in preventing heart disease may be replacing saturated fats in the diet with monounsaturated and polyunsaturated fats.
- *Sources of monounsaturated fats:* Olive oil, canola oil, peanut oil and avocados
- *Sources of polyunsaturated fats:* Vegetable oils (safflower, sesame, soya, corn and sunflower), nuts and seeds

  Essential fatty acids: The body can make all except two linoleic and linolenic acids. These two acids must be supplied by our diet.
- *Linoleic acid sources:* Sunflower, safflower, corn and soyabean oils
- *Linolenic acid sources:* Soyabean and canola oils, walnuts and salmon

Saturated Fats and their Risks

Main sources come from animal sources such as: whole milk, cream, butter, cheese and fatty cuts of beef and pork. Coconut, palm and palm kernel oils and products containing them (pastries, pies, doughnuts and cookies and the like) are also sources of saturated fat.

- Saturated fat is implicated in raising LDL cholesterol.
- LDL cholesterol raises risk of heart disease.

DIETARY FIBER

- Dietary fiber is a complex mixture of plant materials that are resistant to breakdown (digestion) by the human digestive enzymes.

- There are two major kinds of dietary fiber—insoluble (cellulose, hemicelluloses, and lignin) found in wholegrain products such as wholewheat bread; soluble (gums, mucilages, pectins) fibers found in fruits, vegetables, dry beans and peas.
- Insoluble fiber promotes normal elimination by providing bulk for stool formation and thus hastening the passage of the stool through the colon. Insoluble fiber also helps to satisfy appetite by creating a full feeling. Some studies indicate that soluble fibers may play a role in reducing the level of cholesterol in the blood.
- Eating a variety of foods that contain dietary fiber is the best way to get an adequate amount.
- Breads, cereals, other grain products, fruits, vegetables, meat, poultry, fish and alternates are the sources.

IMPORTANCE

The use of fiber in the irritable bowel

Irritable bowel syndrome (IBS) is one of the most common disorders of the lower digestive tract.

- It creates bothersome symptoms such as altered bowel habits, constipation, diarrhea, or both alternately.
- There may also be bloating, abdominal pain, cramping, and spasm. An attack of IBS can be triggered by emotional tension and anxiety, poor dietary habits, and certain medications.
- Increased amounts of fiber in the diet can help to relieve the symptoms of irritable bowel syndrome by producing soft, bulky stools.
- This helps to normalize the time it takes for the stool to pass through the colon.
- Liquids help to soften the stool.
- Irritable bowel syndrome, if left untreated, may lead to diverticulosis of the colon.

Fiber and Colon Polyps/Cancer

Colon cancer is a major health problem and is most common in Western cultures.
- Most colon cancer starts out as a colon polyp, a benign mushroom-shaped growth.
- In time, it grows, and in some people, it becomes cancerous.
- Colon cancer is usually always curable, if polyps are removed when found or, if surgery is performed at an early stage.
- There is a very low rate of colon cancer in residents of countries where grains are unprocessed and retain their fiber.
- The theory is that in the Western world, cancer-containing agents (carcinogens) remain in contact with the colon wall for a longer time and in higher concentrations. So, a large bulky stool may act to dilute these carcinogens by moving them through the bowel more quickly.
- Less carcinogenic exposure to the colon may mean fewer colon polyps and less cancer.

Fiber and Diverticulosis

Prolonged, vigorous contraction of the colon, usually in the left lower side, may result in diverticulosis.

- This increases pressure causing small and eventually larger ballooning pockets to form. These pockets usually cause no problems.
- However, sometimes they can become infected (diverticulitis) or even break open (perforate) causing pockets of infection or inflammation of the sac lining the abdomen (peritonitis).
- A high-fiber diet may increase the bulk in the stool and thereby reduce the pressure within the colon.
- The formation of pockets is reduced or possibly, even stopped.

Fiber, Cholesterol and Gas

- Insoluble fiber is found in wheat, rye, bran, and other grains.
- Insoluble fiber means it does not dissolve in water.
- It also cannot be used by intestinal-colon bacteria as a food source, so these beneficial bacteria generally do not grow and produce intestinal gas.
- Soluble fiber, on the other hand, does dissolve in water forming a gelatinous substance in the bowel.
- Soluble fiber is found in oatmeal, oat bran, fruit, barley, and legumes.
- Soluble fiber, among its other benefits, seems to bind up cholesterol allowing it to be eliminated with the stool (10–15%).
- The down side of soluble fiber is that it can be metabolized by gas forming bacteria in the colon.
- These bacteria are harmless but for those who have an intestinal gas or flatus problem are probably best to avoid or carefully test soluble fibers to see, if they are contributing to intestinal gas.
- Whenever possible, both soluble and insoluble fibers should be eaten on a daily basis.

Basal metabolic rate (BMR)

➢ Defined as the minimum amount of energy required by the body to maintain life at complete physical and mental rests in the post-absorptive period (12 hours after the intake of last meal).
➢ BMR is expressed as Cal/square metre body surface/hour.

Resting metabolic rate (RMR) is the energy expended while an individual is resting quietly in a supine position.

RMR and BMR are sometimes used interchangeably but there are some small differences.

RMR includes the thermal effect of substrate metabolism and heightened metabolic activity due to prior physical or mental activity. These factors, collectively known as facultative thermogenesis, may be thought of as components of a person's **resting metabolic rate** (RMR), and are not part of the BMR.

Measurement of metabolic rate or energy expenditure

- Energy expenditure can be measured in two different ways.
- The determination of energy expenditure by measuring the amount of *heat* produced over a period of time is called **direct calorimetry**.

- The determination of energy expenditure by measuring the amount of *carbon dioxide* consumed over a period of time is called **indirect calorimetry**.
- Two procedures of indirect calorimetry are closed-circuit and open-circuit spirometry (Douglas bag).
- During metabolic energy transformations, oxygen is consumed and heat is produced. Either of these variables can, therefore, be used to estimate energy expenditure.
- Using the fact that one liter of oxygen liberates 4.82 kcal of heat energy when a mixture of carbohydrate, fat and protein is burned in a bomb calorimeter; a highly accurate indirect measure of energy production is possible.

Factors which affect basal metabolic rate (BMR)

1. **Body surface area**
   - This is a reflection of height and weight.
   - The greater the body surface area factor, the higher the BMR.
2. **Sex:** Males average a higher BMR because of a greater proportion of lean body mass.
3. **Body temperature:** Fever, for example, increases BMR.
4. **Hormones:** Thyroid hormones have a stimulatory effect on the metabolism of the body and, therefore, BMR. Thus, BMR is raised in hyperthyroidism and reduced in hypo-thyroidism.
5. **Age:** Mmetabolic rate declines with age. In infants and children, BMR is higher and in adults, it is less.
6. **Diet:** Starvation or serious abrupt calorie-reduction can dramatically reduce BMR (30%). Restrictive low-calorie weight loss diets may cause BMR to drop as much as 20%.
7. **Pregnancy/breast feeding:** These increase metabolic rate.
8. **Environment:** In cold climates, the BMR is higher compared to warm climates.
9. **Disease states:** BMR is higher in cardiac failure, leukemias, and hypertension. It is marginally lowered in Addison's disease.
10. **Weight:** The heavier our weight, the higher our BMR.
    Example: The metabolic rate of obese women is 25 percent higher than the metabolic rate of thin women.
11. **Exercise:** Physical exercise not only influences body weight by burning calories, it also helps raise our BMR by building extra lean tissue.

Calculation of BMR

The first step in designing a personal nutrition plan for ourselves is to calculate how many calories we burn in a day; our total daily energy expenditure (TDEE). TDEE is the total number of calories that our body expends in 24 hours, including all activities.

Methods of determining caloric needs

Quick method (based on total body weight).

Equations based on BMR: A much more accurate method for calculating TDEE is to determine basal metabolic rate (BMR) using multiple factors, including height, weight, age and sex, then multiply the BMR by an activity factor to determine TDEE. BMR is the total number of calories that our body requires for normal bodily functions. BMR usually accounts for about two-thirds of total daily energy expenditure. BMR may vary dramatically from person to person depending on genetic factors.

The Harris-Benedict formula (BMR based on total body weight): The Harris-Benedict equation is a calorie formula using the factors of height, weight, age, and sex to determine basal metabolic rate (BMR). This makes it more accurate than determining calorie needs based on total body weight alone. The only variable it does not take into consideration is lean body mass. Therefore, this equation will be very accurate in all, but the extremely muscular and the extremely over fat.

Men: BMR = 66 + (13.7 × wt in kg) + (5 × ht in cm) – (6.8 × age in years)

Women: BMR = 655 + (9.6 × wt in kg) + (1.8 × ht in cm) – (4.7 × age in years)

Note: 1 inch = 2.54 cm

1 kilogram = 2.2 lb

Example

Female, 30 years old, 5' 6" tall (167.6 cm), weighing 120 lb (54.5 kg)

BMR = 655 + 523 + 302 – 141 = **1339 calories/day**

To determine TDEE from BMR, you simply multiply BMR by the activity multiplier:

Activity Multiplier

Sedentary = BMR × 1.2 (little or no exercise, desk job)

Lightly active = BMR × 1.375 (light exercise/sports 1–3 days/week)

Moderately active = BMR × 1.55 (moderate exercise/sports 3–5 days/week)

Very active = BMR × 1.725 (hard exercise/sports 6–7 days/week)

Extra active = BMR × 1.9 (hard daily exercise/sports and physical job or 2X day training, i.e. marathon, contest, etc.)

Example

Your BMR is 1339 calories per day

Your activity level is moderately active (work out 3–4 times per week)

Your activity factor is 1.55

Your TDEE = 1.55 × 1339 = **2075 calories/day**

Specific dynamic action

- Ingestion of food is accompanied by an increased rate of heat production. The extra heat production by the body, over and above the calculated caloric value, when a given food is metabolized by the body, is called as specific dynamic action. Various names for this effect have been suggested, including specific dynamic action (SDA), specific dynamic effect, heat increment of a feeding, calorigenic effect of foods, and thermogenic effect.

- Imagine that a man requires 1800 cal/day to maintain his basal metabolic requirement. His heat output may exceed 1800 cal (by about 180 cal) after eating a food. This means that the excess calories would have to come from his own tissues, and maintain his weight, he has to take about 2000 (1800 + extra 10% (180)) cal. If he continues with 1800 cal, he would loose weight.
- The SDA values vary according to the type of food taken. If eats 25 gm of protein, we expect his heat output is 100 cal (25 × 4 cal, a caloric value of protein). But his actual heat output is 130 cal (a rise of 30%). So the SDA for protein is 30%.
- The SDA value for carbohydrate is 5%. (After he consumes 25 gm carbohydrate, the heat output is 105 cal instead of 100 cal).
- The SDA value for fat is 12%. (After he consumes 11 gm fat, the heat output is 111 cal instead of 100 cal). (11 × 9 + 12).
- For a mixed diet, the SDA is 10%. This is because of the presence of carbohydrates and fats which reduce the SDA of protein.
- The significance of SDA of a protein is the maintenance of body temperature in cold climate. The higher SDA for protein indicates that it is not a good source of energy.

1. The energy requirement of a man (age 20 years, BMR = 42 cal/sqm body surface/ hr, body surface area = 1.7 sq m) engaged in light work.

The energy demand depends on three important factors:
a. basal metabolic rate
b. physical activity and
c. specific dynamic action

The food provides energy for:

➢ Basal metabolism (8 hours)
➢ *Simple activities:* Standing, sitting, walking, dressing and writing (8 hours)
➢ *Professional work:* (i) light work, (ii) moderate work, (iii) heavy work, (iv)very heavy work
➢ Other 10 % as SDA

The daily energy requirement is a variable which depends on age, sex, and body size

- Sleep basal level (8 hours) BMR × body surface area × 8 hours

$$= 42 × 1.7 × 8 = 571 \text{ cal}$$

- Simple activities (8 hours)
  At basal level   = 571 cal
  For simple activities at 25 calories/hour over basal level 25 × 8   = 200 cal
- For professional work (light work):
  At basal level   = 571 cal
  For professional work at 55 calories/hour over basal level 55 × 8   = 440 cal

  Sub total   = 2353 cal
- Extra 10 % for SDA   = 235 cal

Total   = 2588 cal/day

2. **The energy requirement of dental student (age 18 years, BMR = 40 cal/sq m body surface/hr, body surface area = 1.7 sq m) engaged in moderate work.**

- Sleep-basal level (8 hours) BMR × body surface area × 8 hours
  $$= 40 \times 1.7 \times 8 = 544 \text{ cal}$$
- Simple activities (8 hours)

  At basal level   = 544 cal

  For simple activities at 25 calories/hour over basal level 25 × 8   = 200 cal
- For professional work (light work)

  At basal level   = 544 cal

  For professional work at 75 calories/hour over basal level 75 × 8   = 600 cal

  Sub total   = 2432 cal
- Extra 10 % for SDA,   = 243 cal

  Total = 2675 cal/day

3. **The energy requirement of men (age 25 years, BMR = 40 cal/sq m body surface/hr, body surface area = 1.7 sq m) engaged in heavy work.**

- Sleep-basal level (8 hours) BMR × body surface area × 8 hours
  $$= 40 \times 1.7 \times 8 = 544 \text{ cal}$$
- Simple activities (8 hours)

  At basal level   = 544 cal

  For simple activities at 25 calories/hour over basal level 25 × 8   = 200 cal
- For professional work (heavy work):

  At basal level   = 544 cal

  For professional work at 150 calories/hour over basal level 75 × 8   = 1200 cal

  Sub total   = 3032 cal
- Extra 10 % for SDA,

  = 303 cal
  Total = 3335 cal/day

From the above calculations, the reference ranges of caloric requirements of various types of work for an adult per day is as follows:

Light work	2100–2600
Moderate work	2500–3000
Heavy work	3000–3500
Very heavy work	3500–4000

Biological value of a protein (BVP)

It is a measurement of protein quality expressing the rate of efficiency with which protein is used for growth. A protein with high BV has all the essential amino acids in the right proportion.

The BVP can be calculated by using a formula.

$$BVP = \frac{N \text{ intake} - (N \text{ excretion in urine and feces}) \times 100}{N \text{ intake} - N \text{ excretion in feces}} = \frac{N \text{ retained} \times 100}{N \text{ absorbed}}$$

Egg contains the highest quality food protein is known. It is so nearly perfect, in fact, that egg protein is often the standard by which all other proteins are judged. Based on the essential amino acids, it provides egg protein is second only to mother's milk for human nutrition. On a scale with 100 representing top efficiency, these are the biological values of proteins in several foods.

Whole egg	93.7	Rice, polished	64.0
Milk	84.5	Wheat, whole	64.0
Fish	76.0	Corn	60.0
Beef	74.3	Beans, dry	58.0
Soyabeans	72.8		

Protein from animal sources (meat, fish, dairy products, egg white) is considered high biological value protein or a "complete" protein because all nine essential amino acids are present in these proteins. An exception to this rule is collagen-derived gelatin which is lacking in tryptophan.

Nitrogen balance

➤ This is when a person's daily intake of nitrogen from proteins equals to the daily excretion of nitrogen.

➤ If a person excretes more nitrogen than he consumes, his body will breakdown muscle tissue to get the nitrogen it needs (**Negative nitrogen state**). Muscle loss occurs.

➤ If a person consumes more nitrogen than he excretes, he will be in an anabolic-muscle building-state (**positive nitrogen state**).

Balanced diet

A balanced diet includes a variety of foods from all 5 food groups (carbohydrates, proteins, fats, vitamins and minerals). It should provide enough calories to ensure a desirable weight and should include all the necessary daily nutrients (Table 17.1).

The healthiest combination for a balanced diet is **low fat, low refined carbohydrates + healthy carbohydrates + moderate protein**. For example, as a general rule:

Table 17.1: *Sample menu*

Breakfast	Lunch	Dinner

• grapefruit 1/2
• oatmeal 3/4 cup
• raisins 2 Tbsp
• whole wheat toast
  2 slices
• margarine 2 tsp
• jelly/jam 2 Tbsp
• skim milk 1 cup
• coffee 3/4 cup
	• vegetable soup 1 cup
	• lean hamburger patty 3 oz
	• bun 1
	• tomato 1 small
	• lettuce
	• baked beans 1/2 cup
	• medium apple 1
	• oatmeal cookie 1
	• skim milk 1 cup
	• rice ½ cup
	• yogurt 1/2 cup
		• garden salad:
		  lettuce 1 cup
		  cucumber 1/8 cup
		  tomato 1/2 med
		  bean sprouts 1/8 cup
		  salad dressing 2 Tbsp
		• broiled chicken 3 oz
		• brown rice 1/2 cup
		• broccoli with
		  cheese sauce 1/2 cup
		• pumpernickel bread 1 slice
		• margarine 1 tsp
		• strawberries 1/2 cup
		  with plain low-fat
		• skim milk 1 cup

Snacks		
• bran muffin or one slice bread • orange juice 1/2 cup		
This sample diet provides		
Calories	2491	Fat 89 gm
Protein	121 gm	Sodium 3585 mg
Carbohydrates	318 gm	Fiber 38 gm

- About 50 percent of your calories should come from complex carbohydrates.
- About 20 percent should come from protein.
- About 30 percent should come from all fats. (Of this, a maximum of one third may be saturated fat).

Protein energy malnutrition (PEM) or protein calorie malnutrition (PCM)

Protein calorie malnutrition (PCM) is present when sufficient energy and/or protein is not available to meet metabolic demands, leading to impairment in normal physiologic processes.

- Kwashiorkor is a condition which develops when there is gross protein deficiency though nonprotein calorie intake may be adequate.
- Marasmus occurs with deficiency of both protein and calories.

Causes

- Inadequate dietary intake
- Poor quality dietary proteins
- Increased metabolic demands
- Increased nutrient losses

KWASHIORKOR

Its a high mortality deficiency disease known as kwashiorkor meaning red boy. The name comes from the odd reddish orange color of the hair, as well as from the skin rash, characteristics of the disease. Moderate to severe growth failure is present kwashiorkor.

For the 1st a few months of life, the breast fed infant in the developing countries grows at a rate that is comparable to that of well-fed infants, but thereafter symptoms starts occurring of a kwashiorkor child, if the nutrition is not adequate.

Symptoms

- The increase in stature and retarded tissue development.
- Poorly developed in muscle and lack of tone
- Severe edema
- Potbelly (protruding of the stomach)
- Swollen legs and face
- Anorexia and diarrhea are common. Poor sanitation is cause of diarrhea
- Whimpering, but does not cry or scream
- The child is not interested in or curious about his surrounding, but remains seated whenever he is put down

Pathologic and biochemical changes

- Fatty infiltration of the liver.
- Decreased serum levels of triglycerides, phospholipids, and cholesterol.
- Reduced amylase, lipase and trypsin.
- Serum proteins and albumin fractions are markedly reduced.
- Low Hb levels, especially, if parasite infestation is also present.
- Vitamin A levels are usually reduced. This could be a serious complication leading to blindness and death in some children.

MARASMUS

It is a protein caloric malnutrition caused by a diet deficient in both protein and carbohydrates. Severe growth failure and emaciation are the most striking characteristics of the marasmic infant. Marasmus differs from kwashiorkor in several important aspects as shown in Table 17.2.

Table 17.2

Marasmus	Kwashiorkor
1. The onset is earlier, usually in the first year of life.	Onset is later, after the breastfeeding is stopped.
2. Growth failure is more pronounced.	Not very pronounced.
3. There is no edema.	Edema is present.
4. Blood protein concentration is reduced less markedly.	Blood protein concentration is reduced very much.
5. Skin changes are seen less frequently.	Red boils and patches are classic symptoms.
6. Liver is not infiltrated with fat.	Fatty liver is seen.
7. Recovery is much longer.	Recovery period is short.

Self Test

1. Mention the caloric values for proteins, carbohydrates and fats.
2. What is respiratory quotient and mention its significance?
3. What are complete and incomplete proteins?
4. How do you explain protein and weight gain?
5. Add a note on protein and weight loss.
6. Write the importance of carbohydrates.
7. Briefly discuss the dietary fiber and its importance.
8. What is protein calorie malnutrition?
9. How do you differentiate kwashiorkor from marasmus?
10. Give the signs and symptoms of kwashiorkor.
11. What is biological value of protein and write the formula to calculate it?
12. Discuss the components of balanced diet.
13. What is specific dynamic action and mention its importance?
14. Define BMR and mention the factors affecting BMR.
15. Briefly discuss the negative and positive nitrogen balance.
16. Calculate the energy requirement of allied health student (age 18 years, BMR = 40 cal/sq m body surface/hour, body surface area = 1.7 sq m) engaged in moderate work.
17. What is resting metabolic rate?
18. How do you differentiate soluble fiber from insoluble fiber?

18

Nucleic Acids

Nucleic acids are complex structures used to maintain **genetic information**.

Nucleotides are found primarily as the monomeric units comprising the major nucleic acids of the cell, RNA and DNA.

They are required for other important functions within the cell. They are:

➤ Serving as **energy stores** for future use in phosphate transfer reactions. These reactions are predominantly carried out by ATP.

➤ Forming a part of several important coenzymes such as **NAD$^+$, NADP$^+$, FAD and coenzyme A.**

➤ Serving as **mediators** of numerous important cellular processes such as second messengers in signal transduction events. The predominant second messenger is cyclic-AMP (cAMP), a cyclic derivative of AMP formed from ATP.

➤ **Controlling numerous enzymatic reactions** through allosteric effects on enzyme activity.

➤ Serving as **activated intermediates** in numerous biosynthetic reactions. These activated intermediates include S-adenosylmethionine (S-AdoMet) involved in methyl transfer reactions as well as the many sugar coupled nucleotides involved in glycogen and glycoprotein syntheses.

Deoxyribonucleic acid (DNA) serves as the master copy for most information in the cell.

Ribonucleic acid (RNA) are different types, they act to transform information from DNA to the rest of the cell.

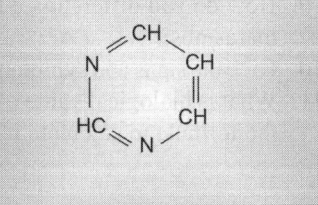

The primary structures of both DNA and RNA are similar.

Each consists of **sugar/phosphate** backbone to which a **nitrogenous base** is attached.

The nucleotides found in cells are derivatives of the heterocyclic highly basic compounds, **purine** and **pyrimidine**.

There are five major bases found in cells.

The **purine** bases are **adenine** and **guanine**.

Pyrimidine bases are **thymine, cytosine** and **uracil**. The common abbreviations used for these five bases are **A, G, T, C** and **U**.

Table 18.1: *Nitrogenous bases*

Base formula	Base	Nucleoside	Nucleotide
	Cytosine, C	Cytidine	Cytidine monophosphate CMP
	Uracil, U	Uridine, U	Uridine monophosphate UMP
	Thymine, T	Thymidine, T	Thymidine monophosphate TMP
	Adenine, A	Adenosine, A	Adenosine monophosphate AMP
	Guanine, G	Guanosine, G	Guanosine monophosphate GMP

- The purine and pyrimidine bases in cells are linked to carbohydrate and they are termed as **nucleosides**.
- When **nucleosides** are coupled to **D-ribose** or **2′-deoxy-D-ribose** through a β-N-glycosidic bond between the anomeric carbon of the ribose and the N^9 of a purine or N^1 of a pyrimidine.
- Nucleosides are found in the cell primarily in their phosphorylated forms. These are termed **nucleotides**.
- The most common site of phosphorylation of nucleotides found in cells is the hydroxyl group attached to the 5′-carbon of the ribose. The carbon atoms of the ribose present in nucleotides are designated with a prime (′) mark to distinguish them from the backbone numbering in the bases.
- Nucleotides can exist in the mono-, di-, or tri-phosphorylated forms.

Structure of DNA

➤ The structure of DNA is illustrated by a right handed double helix.

➤ Contains 10 nucleotide pairs per helical turn.

➤ Each spiral strand, composed of a sugar phosphate backbone and attached bases, is connected to a complementary strand by hydrogen bonding (non-covalent) between paired bases, adenine (A) with thymine (T) and guanine (G) with cytosine (C).

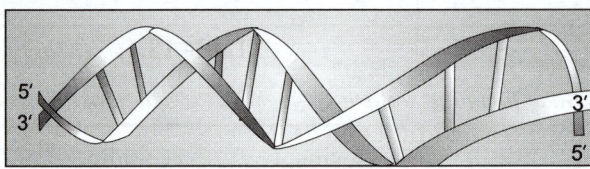

Figure 18.1

➤ There are 4 different bases in a DNA molecule:

Adenine (a purine)

Cytosine (a pyrimidine)

Guanine (a purine)

Thymine (a pyrimidine)

➤ The number of purine bases equals the number of pyrimidine bases.

➤ The number of adenine bases equals the number of thymine bases.

➤ The number of guanine bases equals the number of cytosine bases.

➤ Two DNA strands form a helical spiral, winding around a helix axis in a right-handed spiral.

➤ The two polynucleotide chains run in opposite directions.

   Within the double helix, adenine and thymine are connected by two hydrogen bonds (non-covalent) on the opposite strands while guanine and cytosine are connected by three hydrogen bonds.

Why base pairing takes place?

• Replication of DNA requires non-covalent strand separation.

• Stability of DNA delicate because of phosphates on outside are very acidic and repulsion between phosphates tends to de-stabilizes the DNA.

• Uniform structure, identical shape and size of base pairs formed.

The transfer of genetic information takes place with three processes.

1. **Replication** is the process by which an identical copy of DNA is made. Replication occurs every time when a cell divides so that information can be preserved and transferred to offspring.

2. **Transcription** is the process by which the genetic messages contained in DNA are "read" or "transcribed". The product of transcription, known as messenger RNA (mRNA), leaves the cell nucleus and carries the message to the sites of protein synthesis.

3. **Translation** is the process by which the genetic messages carried by mRNA are decoded and used to build proteins.

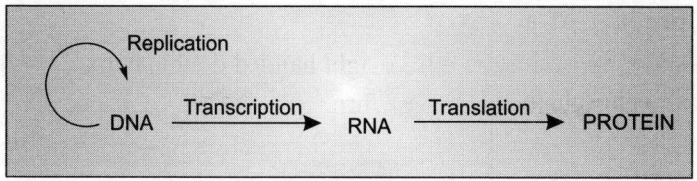

Figure 18.2

Structure and function of RNA

Both RNA and DNA are sugar-phosphate polymers and both have nitrogen bases attached to the sugars of the backbone but:

- They differ in composition.
  1. The sugar in RNA is ribose and deoxyribose in DNA.
  2. The base present in RNA is uracil instead of thymine.
- They also differ in size and structure.
  1. RNA molecules are smaller (shorter) than DNA molecules.
  2. RNA is single-stranded, not double-stranded like DNA.
- DNA storing only the genetic information in its sequence of nucleotide bases.
- But there are three types of ribonucleic acid, each with their own function.

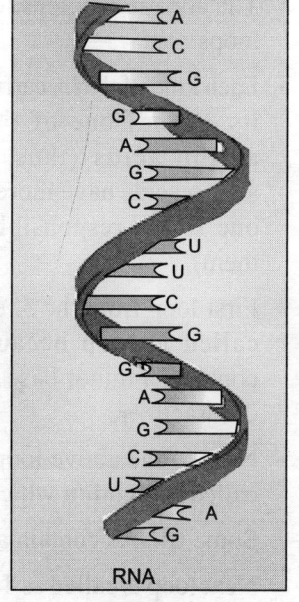

RNA

Figure 18.3

1. **Ribosomal RNAs (rRNAs)** exist outside the nucleus in the cytoplasm of a cell in structures called **ribosome**. Each ribosome is a complex consisting of about 60% ribosomal RNA **(rRNA)** and 40% protein.

These are 4 kinds. In eukaryotes, these are:

- **18S rRNA**. One of these molecules, along with some 30 different protein molecules, is used to make the **small subunit** of the ribosome.
- **28S, 5.8S, and 5S rRNA**. One each of these molecules, along with some 45 different proteins, is used to make the **large subunit** of the ribosome.

The S number given in each type of rRNA reflects the rate at which the molecules sediment in the ultracentrifuge.

The larger the number, the larger the molecule.

The 28S, 18S, and 5.8S molecules are produced by the processing of a single primary transcript from a cluster of identical copies of a single gene. The 5S molecules are produced from a different cluster of identical genes.

2. **Messenger RNAs** are the nucleic acids that "record" information from DNA in the cell nucleus and carry it to the ribosomes and are known as messenger RNAs **(mRNA)**.

3. **Transfer RNAs:** The function of transfer RNAs **(tRNA)** is to transfer amino acids one by one, to protein chains, growing at ribosomes.

There are some 3' different kinds of tRNA in a typical eukaryotic cell.

- Each is the product of a separate gene.
- 5′ end starts with a phosphate and guanine.
- They are small (~ 4S), containing 73–93 nucleotides.
- Many of the bases in the chain pair with each other forming sections of double helix.
- The unpaired regions form 3 loops.
- Each kind of tRNA carries (at its 3′ end) one of the 20 **amino acids** (thus most amino acids have more than one tRNA responsible for them).
- First loop from the 5′ end is called D loop because it contains a minor base dihydrouracil.

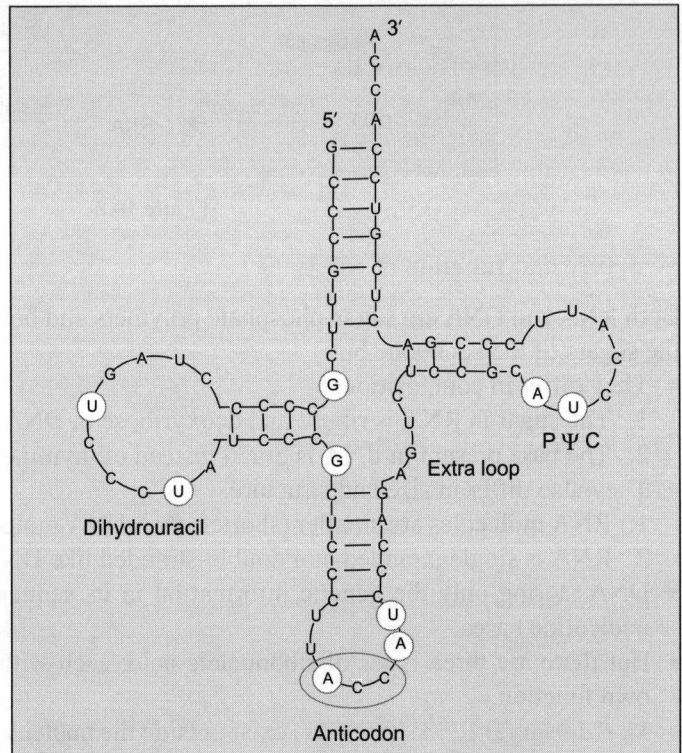

Figure 18.4

- Next to the above loop is an anticodon loop. It contains a sequence of 3 unpaired bases called **anticodon** which is complementary to the 3 bases (codon) of mRNA.
- Some tRNAs contain an extra arm next to the anticodon small loop.
- Next loop is called as T ψ C loop. This contains minor bases like thymine and pseudouracil.
- Base pairing between the anticodon and the complementary codon on an mRNA molecule brings the correct amino acid into the growing polypeptide chain.
- 3′ end—ends with a sequence C-C-A.

4. **Small nuclear RNA (snRNA):** DNA transcription of the genes for mRNA, rRNA, and tRNA produces large precursor molecules (**primary transcripts**) that must be processed within the nucleus to produce the functional molecules for export to the cytosol. Some of these processing steps are mediated by snRNAs.

5. **Small nucleolar RNA (snoRNA):** These RNAs within the nucleolus have several functions.

6. **MicroRNA (miRNA):** These are tiny (~22 nts) RNA molecules that appear to regulate the expression of messenger RNA (mRNA) molecules.

Genetic Code

The code consists of at least three bases, according to astronomer George Gamow. To code for the 20 essential amino acids, a genetic code must consist of at least a 3-base set (triplet) of the 4 bases. If one considers the possibilities of arranging four things 3 at a time ($4 \times 4 \times 4$), we get 64 possible code words, or codons (a 3-base sequence on the mRNA that codes for either a specific amino acid or a control word).

Table 18.2: *Inhibitors of replication, transcription and translation*

Inhibitors of replication	
Mitomycin C and novobiocin	Inhibitors of inhibit cell division and they also inhibit DNA polymerase.
Inhibitors of transcription	
Rifampicin and actinomycin D Adriamycin HCl	Inhibit RNA polymerase Inhibits DNA and RNA syntheses by forming complexes with DNA.
Inhibitors of translation	
Chloramphenicol	Inhibits prokaryotic peptidyl transferase.
Streptomycin	Inhibits prokaryotic peptide chain initiation, also induces mRNA misreading.
Tetracycline	Inhibits prokaryotic aminoacyl-tRNA binding to the ribosome small subunit.
Neomycin	Inhibits prokaryotic peptide chain initiation, also induces mRNA misreading.
Erythromycin	Similar in activity to streptomycin and inhibits prokaryotic translocation through the ribosome large subunit.
Puromycin	Resembles an aminoacyl-tRNA, interferes with peptide transfer, resulting in premature termination in both prokaryotes and eukaryotes.

Self Test

1. Briefly discuss the structure of DNA.
2. Differentiate nucleosides from nucleotides.
3. Name the purine and pyrimidine bases.
4. Add a note on the structure of tRNA.
5. Briefly explain the genetic code.
6. Mention the functions of mRNA and tRNA.
7. Name the inhibitors of transcription and replication.
8. Mention the action of chloramphenical.
9. Name some nucleotides which are used or generated in the metabolism of carbohydrates.

19

Organ Function Tests

LIVER FUNCTION TEST (LFT)

- Liver plays a major role in storing blood (acts as a reservoir of blood)
- The parenchymal cells of the liver are related to the breakdown of hemoglobin to bilirubin and the removal of pigments
- It plays a central role in the metabolism of:
  - Carbohydrates (Glycogenesis, glycogenolysis, gluconeogenesis and alcohol metabolism)
  - Proteins (Transamination, oxidative deamination of amino acids, urea synthesis and protein synthesis)
  - Lipids
  - Hormones
  - Vitamins
  - Bilirubin
  - Bile acids.
- The hepatobiliary tree represents hepatic cells and biliary tract cells.
- Inflammation of the hepatic cells results in the elevation of alanine aminotransferase (ALT), aspartate aminotransferase (AST) and possibly the bilirubin.
- Inflammation of the biliary tract cells results predominantly in an elevation of the alkaline phosphatase (ALP).
- In liver disease, there are crossover between purely biliary disease and hepatocellular disease.
- To interpret these, the physician will look at the entire picture of the hepatocellular and biliary tract diseases to determine which is the primary abnormality.

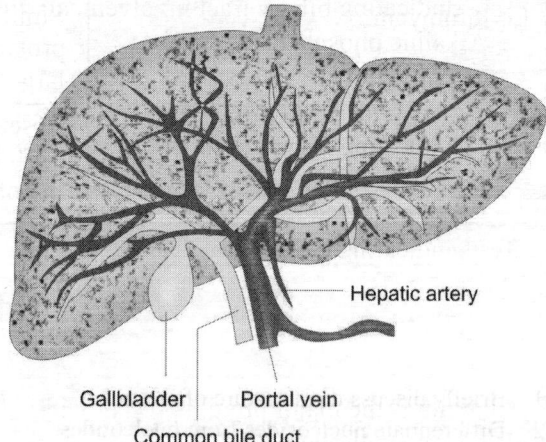

Figure 19.1: *Hepatobiliary tree representing hepatic cells and biliary tract cells*

230

Indications of LFT

- LFTs are useful in the differential diagnosis of jaundice.
- Detection of liver diseases
- Assessment of severity and progress of liver disease.

Basic Processes in Liver Diseases

Liver cell damage: This may vary from areas of local damage to destruction of most of the liver cells leading to liver failure.

Causes

Acute hepatitis: May be viral.

Chronic hepatitis: Due to the continuing action of infective or toxic agents or that associated with autoimmune response.

Cirrhosis: Destruction of hepatic cells.

Biliary tract involvement: The involvement of biliary tract is associated with obstruction to bile flow (cholestasis) and may present as obstructive jaundice.

There are 2 types of obstruction:

Intrahepatic cholestasis: Mainly arises with liver cell destruction.

Causes: Viral hepatitis, use of steroids (during pregnancy or in the case of woman taking oral contraceptives).

Extrahepatic cholestasis:

Causes: Gallstone in the common bile duct, carcinoma of the pancreas

Cirrhosis of the bile duct: The liver function tests are considered under the following categories:

- Tests which indicate the liver cell damage:
  - Aspartate transaminase (AST)
  - Alanine transaminase (ALT)
- Tests indicating biliary tract involvement:
  - Alkaline phosphatase (ALP)
  - Gamma glutamyl transferase (GGT)
  - 5-nucleotidase
- Tests indicating impaired function:
  - Serum proteins
  - Bilirubin
- Tests indicating etiology.

Total Protein, Albumin and Globulin

Albumin

- Albumin is the major protein present within the blood.
- The liver synthesizes albumin.
- It represents a major synthetic protein and is a marker for the ability of the liver to synthesize proteins.

- It is one of the proteins synthesized by the liver. However, since it is easy to measure, it represents a reliable and inexpensive laboratory test for physicians to assess the degree of liver damage present in the particular patient. When the liver has been chronically damaged, the albumin may be low. This would indicate that the synthetic function of the liver has been markedly diminished.
- Such findings suggest a diagnosis of cirrhosis. Malnutrition can also cause low albumin with no associated liver disease.
  The important tests related to protein metabolism.

Serum Total Protein Estimation

- Albumin estimation
- Globulins estimation
  Methods: The serum proteins are estimated by differential precipitation of albumin and globulin fractions.
- Biuret method
- Albumin by Dye binding method

Serum Protein Electrophoresis

- This is an evaluation of the types of protein present in serum.
- With an electrophoresis, major proteins can be separated and this results in four major types of proteins.
  – Albumin
  – Alpha globulins
  – Beta globulins
  – Gamma globulins.

Normal range:
- Total protein : 5.0 – 7.5 g/dL
- Albumin   : 3.5 – 4.5 g/dL
- Globulin   : 2 – 3 g/dL
- g-globulin   : 0.5 – 1.5 g/dL

Prothrombin Time
- Liver synthesizes clotting factors like prothrombin, fibrinogen, factors V, VII and X.
- The PT is prolonged in the cases of hepatocellular damage. The ability of the parenchymal cells to synthesize clotting factors is impaired.

Jaundice

- Jaundice comes from French word jaune, which means yellow.
- Normal serum bilirubin concentration is around 1.2 mg/100 ml.
- Whenever the level exceeds more than the normal range, it diffuses into the tissues.
- The skin and sclera of the eye turns yellow.

- The condition is called jaundice (icterus).
- The yellowish coloration is caused by an excess amount of bilirubin in the skin.
- Bilirubin is a yellowish-red pigment.
- Normally, small amounts of bilirubin are found in everyone's blood.
- When too much bilirubin is made, the excess is dumped into the bloodstream and is deposited in tissues for temporary storage.
- Jaundice in the infant appears first in the face and upper body and progresses downward towards the toes.

Formation and Metabolism of Bilirubin

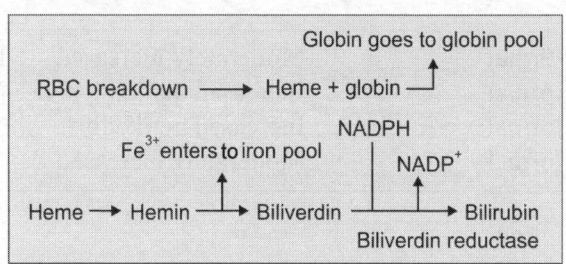

Figure 19.2: *Flowchart showing the formation of blirubin*

- Bilirubin formed, binds to albumin and is transported to liver.
- In the liver, it is separated from the albumin.
- The liver cells take up the bilirubin.
- In the liver, the UDP glucuronyl transferase enzyme conjugates the bilirubin with two molecules of UDP glucuronic acid to form a conjugated bilirubin called bilirubin diglucuronide.
- Normally, the bilirubin is secreted into the bile through the bile duct.
- The conjugated bilirubin reaches to the intestine through the bile.
- The intestinal bacteria act on it and deconjugate the conjugated bilirubin.
- The free bilirubin then gets reduced to colorless tetrapyrrole urobilinogen. Twenty percent of this urobilinogen is reabsorbed from the intestine and returned to the liver by portal blood. The urobilinogen is again re-excreted.
- The urobilinogen is excreted through the blood is negligible.
- The urobilinogen is further reduced to stercobilinogen and excreted through feces (around 200–300 mg/day).
- The urobilinogen and stercobilinogen are colorless compounds but when they are exposed to atmospheric oxidation, they are converted to a colored urobilin and stercobilin respectively.

There are three different types of jaundice:

1. Hemolytic jaundice
2. Hepatic jaundice
3. Obstructive or pos-thepatic jaundice

Table 19.1: *Causes and biochemical findings of different types of jaundice*			
Causes	Abnormal red cells; antibodies; abnormal hemoglobin	Viral hepatitis; toxic hepatitis; intrahepatic cholestasis of bile duct; drugs, and toxins	Extrahepatic cholestasis; gallstones; tumor Carcinoma of pancreas
Blood			
Unconjugated bilirubin	Present (++)	Present (++)	Normal
Conjugated bilirubin	Normal	Increases in early phase and later decreases	Present (++)
Serum enzymes			
ALP	Normal	Moderately increased	Increased markedly
ALT	Normal	Increased markedly	Moderately increased
AST	Normal	Increased markedly	Moderately increased
GGT	Normal	Moderately increased	Increased markedly

van den Bergh's Reaction

Direct van den Bergh's Test

- The conjugated water-soluble bilirubin when treated with diazoreagent ($NaNO_3$ + Sulfanilic acid), gives red color immediately. This is called direct van den Bergh Test.
- The conjugated bilirubin reacts directly without adding methanol then it is also called as direct bilirubin.

Indirect van den Bergh's Test

- The water-insoluble unconjugated bilirubin gives a positive van den Bergh's Test only if methanol is added to the serum. This is called indirect van den Bergh's test.
- This is also called as indirect bilirubin.

Fouchet's Test for Urine Bilirubin

Two ml of barium chloride solution (100 g/L) to about 10 ml of urine in a test tube. Filter, dry the filtrate on a filter paper and add a drop of Fouchet's reagent (25 g TCA + 10 ml ferric chloride (100 g/L) + 100 ml water) on the filtrate. A greenish color due, an oxidation product of bilirubin is obtained, if bilirubin is present in the sample.

Hay's Test for Bile Salts

Sprinkle the sulfur powder on the urine sample in a test tube. The sulfur powder sinks to the bottom of the tube, if bile salts are present in the urine because bile salts have the property of lowering the surface tension.

In jaundice, with unconjugated hyperbilirubinemia, there is no excretion of bilirubin and bile salts in the urine and the urine is of a normal color. The jaundice with conjugated hyperbilirubinemia, there is an excretion of bilirubin and bile salts in urine which results in deep yellow or dark color of urine. This will be seen usually in regurgitation jaundice, infective or toxic hepatitis.

Urobilinogen in Urine and Feces

- The presence of urobilinogen in a test sample can be shown by a test based on the production of red color when urobilinogen reacts with Ehrlich's aldehyde reagent.
- In hemolytic jaundice, there is increased formation of bilirubin, excretion into the intestine through the bile, therefore, there will be increased formation of urobilinogen in the intestine and increased level in the urine and feces.

Normal Values

- Total bilirubin: 0.2–1.0 mg%
- Direct bilirubin: 0–0.2 mg%
- Indirect bilirubin: 0–0.8 mg%

Serum Enzymes in Liver Disease

The assay of serum enzymes is very useful in the differential diagnosis and monitoring of various hepatobiliary disorders.

There are 3 types of enzyme:

1. Enzymes, which are normally, present inside the hepatocytes released into the blood when there is hepatocellular damage—markers for hepatocellular damage (Viral hepatitis, cirrhosis of the liver).
2. Enzymes which are primarily membrane bound (plasma membrane or side of hepatocytes)—marker for cholestasis.
3. Enzymes, which are synthesized in the hepatocyte—indicates disturbances in the hepatocellular synthesis.

Serum Transaminases: AST and ALT

- ALT is specific for liver.
- Its level increases more than the normal in liver diseases (viral hepatitis, cirrhosis of the liver).
- But AST is not specific to liver and its level varies in other forms of tissue damage such as myocardial infarction, muscle necrosis and renal disorders.

Alkaline Phosphatase

- The serum ALP estimation is the most widely used biochemical test to put in evidence for cholestasis of intrahepatic or extrahepatic origin.
- Normal level = 4–13 kA units or 40–140 IU/l
- Increase in serum level of alkaline phosphatase from liver is a very sensitive indicator of cholestasis.

- Increased ALP level in cholestasis may be due to 2 features:
  - Regurgitation of ALP from bile to blood
  - Increased synthesis from the cells lining the biliary canaliculi.

Gamma-glutamyl Transferase (GGT) Estimation

- This enzyme catalyzes the transfer of g-glutamyl group from glutamyl peptides to another peptide or an amino acid.
- It is a marker of cholestasis.
- The GGT level increases both in liver disease and in cholestasis, but it is very high in cholestasis.
- It is also considered as a marker enzyme in the patients of cirrhosis in chronic alcoholics. *Normal value*: 10 to 30 U/l.

RENAL FUNCTION TESTS

Introduction

- Kidneys are the very important and vital organ.
- They perform many important functions to regulate the internal environment of the human body.
- It is the main regulator of all the substances of body fluids and responsible for maintaining homeostasis.

Functions of Kidney

The functional unit of a kidney is nephron.

Kidney has five important functions:

1. Urine formation
2. Regulation of fluid and electrolyte balance
3. Regulation of acid-base balance
4. Hormonal function
5. Excretion of non-protein nitrogenous (NPN) substances.

Kidney function tests are grouped under two categories:

1. The tests measuring GFR: Clearance tests.
   - Inulin clearance test
   - Urea clearance test
   - Creatinine clearance test.
2. Study of elimination of NPN substances: Tests measuring the retention of NPN substances in serum are: Determination of urea, uric acid, creatinine, amino acids and ammonia.

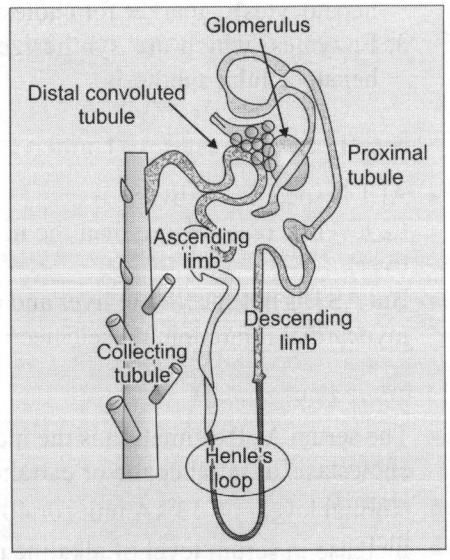

Figure 19.3: *Structure of nephron*

Clearance Test

Creatinine Clearance Test

It is the volume of plasma that completely cleared off the creatinine which is excreted in the urine.

Formula: $\dfrac{UV}{P}$ or $\dfrac{U \times V \times 1.73/A}{P}$

where
- U = Urine creatinine
- P = Plasma
- 1.73 = Generally accepted body surface urea
- A = Body surface area of the patient, under investigation

- The creatinine clearance is very convenient to measure GFR.
- It is fulfilling all the requirement of the substance which is ideal for measuring GFR
- The amount of creatinine produced is relatively constant and also it is not affected by the dietary intake.

Normal values:

- Males 105 + 20 ml/min
- Female 95 + 20 ml/min.

Abnormal results are lower than normal GFR measurements, and they indicate:
- Acute tubular necrosis
- Congestive heart failure
- Dehydration
- Glomerulonephritis
- Shock
- Acute nephrotic syndrome
- Acute and chronic renal failures.

Study of Elimination of NPN Substances (Non-protein Nitrogenous Substances)

The intermediate or the end products of protein metabolism includes urea, creatinine, uric acid, amino acid and NH_3.

Urea

- Urea constitutes about 45% of NPN substances.
- Study of their elimination can be done with blood and urine.
- One of the methods available for the determination of urea is diacetyl monoxime (DAM) method.

Normal values:

Serum/plasma urea: 15 to 45 mg/dL
2.49 to 7.47 mmol/dL
BUN: 7 to 21 mg/dL

Clinical Significance

Causes for urea increase are:

- Prerenal causes:
  - Cardiac decompensation
  - Water depletion due to decreased intake or excessive loss
  - Increased protein breakdown
- Renal causes:
  - Acute glomerulonephritis
  - Chronic nephritis
  - Polycystic kidney
  - Nephrosclerosis
  - Tubular necrosis
- Postrenal causes:
  - Any obstruction to urine flow (Stone, tumor, enlarged prostate)

Normal value: 15–35 mg%.

Creatinine

- Creatinine is a breakdown product of creatine, which is an important part of muscle.
- The most important source of energy inside cells is the ATP molecule, with its high-energy phosphate bonds.
- When one of these bonds is broken, energy is released, and ATP becomes ADP.
- Creatine phosphate represents a backup energy source for ATP because it can quickly reconvert ADP back to ATP.
- Overtime, the creatine molecule gradually degrades to creatinine.
- Creatinine is a waste product, that is, it cannot be used by cells for any constructive purpose.
- The daily production of creatine, and subsequently creatinine, depends on muscle mass, which fluctuates little in most normal people over long periods of time.
- Creatinine is excreted from the body entirely by the kidneys.
- With normal kidney function, the serum creatinine level should remain constant and normal.

Interpretation

- Normal value: 0.8 to 1.4 mg/dL
- Normal value ranges may vary slightly among different laboratories
- Higher than normal levels may indicate:
  - Nephrotic syndrome
  - Chronic glomerulonephritis
  - Acute tubular necrosis
  - Dehydration
  - Diabetic nephropathy
  - Reduced renal blood flow
  - Pyelonephritis
  - Renal failure
  - Urinary tract obstruction

- Lower than normal levels may indicate:
  - Muscular dystrophy (late stage)
  - Myasthenia gravis.

Uric Acid

Normal Value: 2.5–7 mg%
Value increases in:
- Renal failure
- Acute gout
- Pneumonia
- Sepsis
- Leukemia
- Polycythemia vera
- Anemia

Value decreases in: Acromegaly.

Tests measuring tubular function:
- Excretory function test
- Phenolsulfonphthalein test (PSP test)
- Tests to measure the concentrating and diluting ability:
  - Specific gravity determination
  - Osmolality determination

Calcium and Phosphorus

In chronic renal failure, there is impaired excretion of phosphate and progressive hyper-phosphatemia occur. This results in the decreased plasma calcium concentration giving rise to secondary hyperparathyroidism.

Determination of Amino Acids

- Amino acids are the part of NPN.
- Their determination is helpful only in some congenital renal disorders.
- If there is defect in reabsorption, more amino acid will appear in the urine, this condition is called aminoaciduria.
  Example: Cystinuria, homocystinuria

Aminoaciduria

Aminoaciduria may be primary or secondary.
- Primary aminoaciduria is due to an inherited enzyme deficiency, this is also called as an inborn error of metabolism. The defect is located in the pathway by which amino acid is metabolized or in the renal tubular system by which the amino acid is absorbed.

- Secondary aminoaciduria may be due to disease of the liver or renal tubular dysfunction or protein energy malnutrition. In both the conditions, metabolites of amino acids accumulated in the blood are excreted in the urine. There are several tests to detect these amino acids and their metabolites in the urine.

Pathological Conditions of the Kidney

Acute Glomerulonephritis (AGN)

It is an acute inflammation of the glomeruli which results in:
- Oliguria
- Hematuria
- Proteinuria
- Anemia
- Increased blood urea and creatinine
- Decreased GFR

The presence of RBCs in the urine is an insufficient evidence for AGN. Because of the appearance of blood may be from urinary tract.

Nephrotic Syndrome

- It is a clinical entity characterized by massive proteinuria, edema, hypoalbuminemia, hyperlipidemia and lipiduria.
- The syndrome is having multiple causes.
- Increased membrane permeability leads to massive proteinuria (mainly albumin loss). There will be reduction in plasma osmotic pressure and the fluid movement from vascular to interstitial space that leads to edema.

Tubular Disease

- Proximal renal tubular acidosis (Reduced proximal tubular HCO_3 reabsorption)
- Distal renal tubular acidosis (DRTA): There is an inability of tubular cells to create and maintain the usual pH difference between tubular and blood.

Urinary Tract Infection (UTI)

- Infection may occur in the bladder (cystitis) or it may involve in the kidneys.
- Diagnosis is made by the presence of bacterial concentration of more than 1 lakh colonies/ml of urine.

THYROID FUNCTION TESTS

The function of the thyroid gland is to take iodine, found in many foods, and convert it into thyroid hormones: Thyroxine (T4) and triiodothyronine (T3).

Thyroid cells are the only cells in the body which can absorb iodine. These cells combine iodine and the amino acid tyrosine to make T3 and T4. T3 and T4 are then released into the blood stream and are transported throughout the body where they control metabolism. Most of the cells in the body depend upon thyroid hormones for regulation of their metabolism.

- The hypothalamus, pituitary gland and the thyroid, all play a part in the feedback and regulatory mechanisms involved in the production of thyroxine (T4) and triiodothyronine (T3) from the thyroid gland.
- Thyroid releasing hormone (TRH) is secreted by the hypothalamus and stimulates the production of the polypeptide thyroid stimulating hormone (TSH) from the anterior pituitary.
- TSH then stimulates the production and release of T4 and T3 from the thyroid.
- Once released, T4 and T3 then exert a negative feedback mechanism on TSH production.
- T4 is the main hormone produced by the thyroid.
- T3 is mainly produced by peripheral conversion of T4.
- T3 and T4 both act via nuclear receptors to increase cell metabolism.
- The normal thyroid gland produces about 80% T4 and about 20% T3, however, T3 possesses about four times the hormone "strength" as T4.
- The 70–80% of T3 and T4 are transported in plasma by a thyroid binding globulin (TBG), a plasma protein.
- The remaining 20–30 % of T3 and T4 is transported by thyroxine binding prealbumin (TBPA) and albumin.
- Only the unbound or 'free' portion (FT3, FT4) is active.
- It is the free portion of the thyroid hormones and is the true determinant of the thyroid status of the patient.
- The evaluation of the thyroid status is not a simple procedure because it does not depend mainly on the measurement of circulating thyroid hormones.
- The one or more factors may be abnormal and they are:
  - The TBG concentration and its degree of saturation with T3 and T4.
  - Concentration of free T3 and T4.
  - The state of the hypothalamus and anterior pituitary with their respective outputs of TRH and TSH.
  - The response of pituitary to TRH and response of the thyroid gland.

Thyroid disease is common, presents with many non-specific symptoms so needs to be considered in many differentials and, once diagnosed, needs to be regularly monitored for therapy. As a consequence, TFTs are the most commonly used endocrine test. Therefore, laboratory investigations of thyroid functions are useful in distinguishing patients with euthyroidism from those with hyperthyroidism and hypothyroidism.

Common Thyroid Problems

- *Goiters*: A thyroid goiter is an enlargement of the thyroid gland. Goiters are often removed because of cosmetic reasons or, more commonly, because they compress other vital structures of the neck including the trachea and the esophagus making breathing and swallowing difficult. Sometimes goiters will actually grow into the chest where they can cause trouble as well.
- *Thyroid cancer*: It is a fairly common malignancy; however, the vast majorities have excellent long-term survival.
- *Solitary thyroid nodules*: There are several characteristics of solitary nodules of the thyroid which make them suspicious for malignancy. Although as many as 50% of the population

will have a nodule somewhere in their thyroid, the overwhelming majority of these are benign. Occasionally, thyroid nodules can take on characteristics of malignancy and require either a needle biopsy or surgical excision.

- *Hyperthyroidism*: It means too much thyroid hormone. Current methods used for treating a hyperthyroid patient are radioactive iodine, anti-thyroid drugs, or surgery. Each method has advantages and disadvantages and is selected for individual patients.

- *Hypothyroidism*: It means too little thyroid hormone and is a common problem. In fact, hypothyroidism is often present for a number of years, before it is recognized and treated. Hypothyroidism can even be associated with pregnancy.

- *Thyroiditis*: It is an inflammatory process ongoing within the thyroid gland. Thyroiditis can present with a number of symptoms such as fever and pain, but it can also present as subtle findings of hypo- or hyperthyroidism.

The thyroid function tests ate grouped into *in vitro* and *in vivo*.

The *in vitro* tests are:
- Total serum T3 and T4
- Free serum T3 and T4
- Blood TBG
- Resin-uptake test
- Serum TSH
- Thyroid autoantibodies

In vivo tests are:
- Thyroid iodine uptake
- TRH stimulation test
- TSH stimulation test

Total serum T3 and T4 determination by immunoassay (RIA or ELISA) and Chemiluminescence method:

- It is a direct measurement of the total T3 and T4 in the blood. The serum T4 assays are more reliable than T3, because it is the major secretory product of thyroid gland. The majority of the T3 comes from peripheral deiodination of T4. This test mainly helps to rule out hyperthyroidism and hypothyroidism.

- Normal range: T4 = 5–12.5 μg/dl

  T3 = 80–180 ng/dl

- Value increased in hyperthyroidism and decreased in hypothyroidism.

- The values also decreased in when TBG concentration goes down due to loss in urine and liver diseases.

Free T3 and T4 Determination

This is a measure of circulatory T4 and T3 that exists in the free form in the blood. The free thyroid hormone concentration is independent of changes in the concentration and affinity of thyroid binding proteins and provides more reliable means of diagnosing thyroid dysfunction than measurement of total T3 and T4 hormones.

Normal values: Free T4 = 10–27 pmol/l
                    Free T3 = 3–9 pmol/l
Value increased in hyperthyroidism and thyrotoxicosis and decreased in hypothyroidism.

Hyperthyroidism

Hyperthyroidism occurs as a consequence of excessive thyroid hormone activity. Common causes include: thyroiditis, Graves' disease and toxic nodular goiter.

Diagnosis

- The initial lab investigation with a possible diagnosis of hyperthyroidism should be a sensitive serum TSH assay which will show reduced circulating levels of TSH.
- Low serum TSH is not specific for hyperthyroidism—it may also occur with "non-thyroidal illness" or with the use of some commonly prescribed drugs.
- Patients who have a low TSH may then go on to have further investigations.
  - Free T4 and T3 assays—a subnormal TSH, should trigger the measurement of FT4. If this is not elevated, FT3 should be measured to identify cases of T3-thyrotoxicosis.
  - Thyroid autoantibodies, e.g. thyroid peroxidase antibodies (TPOAb), TSH receptor antibodies (TRAb).
  - Radioactive iodine uptake—thyroid scanning with either 131I (most frequent) or ^{99m}Tc helps to determine cause of hypothyroidism, e.g. diffuse pattern of uptake in Graves' disease compared to one or more 'hot' nodules in toxic nodular hyperthyroidism.

Hypothyroidism

- Primary hypothyroidism occurs as a result of undersecretion of thyroid hormone from the thyroid gland.
- Causes include as Hashimoto's thyroiditis, irradiation and drugs such as lithium. Secondary hypothyroidism may occur as a result of damage or disease of the pituitary or hypothalamus.

Diagnosis

- To diagnose primary hypothyroidism, needs to measure both TSH and FT4 where TSH is >10 mU/l and FT4 below reference range, the diagnosis is overt primary hypothyroidism and the patient needs treatment with thyroid replacement therapy.
- Secondary hypothyroidism is suggested by low, within or mildly elevated TSH combined with a low FT4. Differentiating this from non-thyroidal illness can be difficult and clinical history, FT3 and sometimes anterior pituitary hormone tests are necessary.
  Additional diagnostic tests may include:
  - Thyroid autoantibodies—antithyroid peroxidase and antithyroglobulin antibodies
  - Thyroid scan

Subclinical Disease

Subclinical thyroid disease is common in American population. Diagnosis is based solely on test results. When to treat subclinical disease is contentious.

Subclinical Hyperthyroidism

- Is diagnosed by low serum TSH, normal FT4 and FT3, in the absence of non-thyroidal illness or relevant drug therapy.
- May increases risk of developing AF and CVD.
- TFTs should be repeated at 3–6 months or earlier, if elderly or, if patient has pre-existing CVD, to determine whether full blown hyperthyroidism has developed or, if the subclinical picture has persisted.

Self Test

1. List the tests under LFT panel.
2. What are the indications of LFT?
3. What are the functions performed by the liver?
4. Name the tests related to protein metabolism.
5. Give the normal values for:
   a. Total protein
   b. Albumin
   c. Alanine transaminase
   d. Aspartate transaminase
   e. Total bilirubin
   f. Direct bilirubin
6. Write the flowchart to show the formation of bilirubin from the RBC.
7. What are the steps involved during the bilirubin excretion?
8. Mention the conditions in which bilirubin metabolism and excretion is disturbed.
9. Define jaundice.
10. What are the different types of jaundice?
11. Write the biochemical findings of any two types of jaundice.
12. What is direct and indirect van den Bergh's tests?
13. Which test is used to find the bilirubin in the urine and write its procedure?
14. Why bile salts sinks to the bottom of the solution, if it is present in the urine?
15. Which enzymes are considered as marker enzymes for hepatocellular damage?
16. Mention the enzymes, which are used as marker enzymes to detect the cholestasis.
17. How many isoenzyme forms of ALP are there?
18. Give the normal value of alkaline phosphatase.
19. Name the functions performed by the kidney.
20. List the tests under RFT.
21. Define creatinine clearance.
22. Give the formula to calculate creatinine clearance.
23. Give the procedure for performing creatinine clearance.
24. Why creatinine is selected for measuring GFR?
25. Mention the conditions in which creatinine clearance decreases.
26. Write the normal values for the following:
    a. Urea
    b. Creatinine
    c. Uric acid
27. Mention the causes in which urea level decreases.
28. Write short notes on:
    a. Nephrotic syndrome
    b. Glomerulonephritis
29. Which tests are used to identify the amino acids?
30. Give the normal creatinine clearance value.

Lab Manual

REACTIONS OF CARBOHYDRATES

Carbohydrates are polyhydroxy aldehydes and ketones or substances that hydrolyze to yield polyhydroxy aldehydes and ketones. The monosaccharides are glucose, fructose, galactose, ribose, etc. The two monosaccharides combine together to form disaccharides which include sucrose, lactose and maltose. Starch and cellulose are polysaccharides which consist of many monosaccharide residues.

Molisch's Test

This is a common test for all carbohydrates. The test is on the basis that pentoses and hexoses are dehydrated by conc. sulfuric acid to form furfural or hydroxymethylfurfural, respectively. These products condense with α-naphthol to form purple condensation product.

Benedict's Test

The free aldehyde or keto group in the reducing sugars reduces cupric hydroxide in alkaline medium to red colored cuprous oxide. Depending on the concentration of sugars, yellow to green color is developed. All monosaccharides are reducing sugars as they all have a free reactive carbonyl group. Some disaccharides like maltose have exposed carbonyl groups and are also reducing sugars but less reactive than monosaccharides.

Barfoed's Test

Barfoed's test is used to detect the presence of monosaccharide (reducing) sugars in solution. Barfoed's reagent, a mixture of ethanoic (acetic) acid and copper (II) acetate, is combined with the test solution and boiled. A red copper (II) oxide precipitate is formed, will indicates the presence of reducing sugar. The reaction will be negative in the presence of disaccharide sugars because they are weaker reducing agents. This test is specific for monosaccharides. Due to the weakly acidic nature of Barfoed's reagent, it is reduced only by monosaccharides.

245

Seliwanoff's Test

It is a color reaction specific for ketoses. When concentrated HCl is added, ketoses undergo dehydration to yield furfural derivatives more rapidly than aldoses. These derivatives form complexes with resorcinol to yield deep red color. The test reagent causes the dehydration of ketohexoses to form 5-hydroxymethylfurfural. 5-hydroxymethylfurfural reacts with resorcinol, present in the test reagent, to produce a red product within two minutes (reaction not shown). Aldohexoses reacts so slowly to form the same product.

Iodine Test

This test is used for the detection of starch in the solution. The blue-black color is due to the formation of starch-iodine complex. Starch contains polymer of α-amylose and amylopectin which forms a complex with iodine to give the blue-black color.

Osazone Test

The ketoses and aldoses react with phenylhydrazine to produce a phenylhydrazone which further reacts with another two molecules of phenylhydrazine to yield the osazone. Needle-shaped yellow osazone crystals are produced by Glucose, fructose and mannose whereas lactosazone produces mushroom-shaped crystals. Crystals of different shapes will be shown by different osazones. Flower-shaped crystals are produced by maltose.

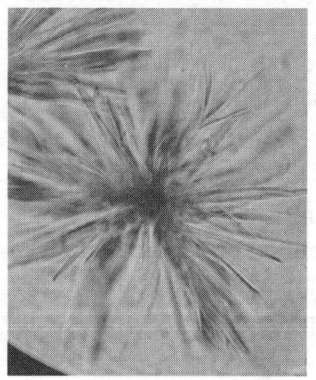

Maltosazone
Sunflower-shaped

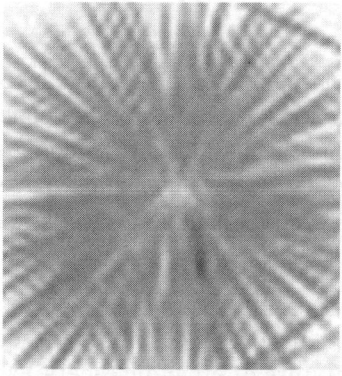

Lactosazone Powder puff

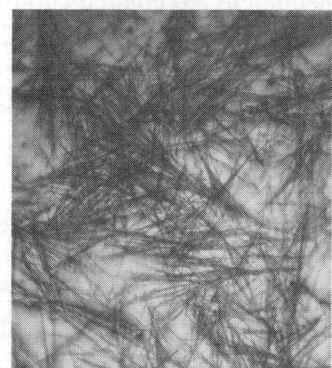

Glucosazone/Fructosazone
Needle or Broom stick-shaped

Reactions of Monosaccharide—Glucose

Sr. No.	Test	Observation	Inference	Reaction
1.	**Molisch's test** 2–3 drops of α-naphthol + 2 ml of the test solution. Very gently add 1 ml of Conc. H_2SO_4 along the side of the test tube.	A deep violet coloration is produced at the junction of two layers. Presence of carbohydrates.	Presence of carbohydrates.	This is due to the formation of an unstable condensation product of α-naphthol with furfural (produced by the dehydration of the carbohydrate).
2.	**Benedict's test** 5.0 ml of Benedict's solution + 1 ml of the test solution and shake the test tube. Place the tube in a boiling water bath and heat for 3 minutes. Remove the tube from the heat and allow it to cool.	Formation of a green, red, or yellow precipitate.	Presence of reducing sugars.	If the saccharide is a reducing sugar, it will reduce Copper [Cu] (11) ions to Cu (1) oxide, a red precipitate.
3.	**Barfoed's test** 2.0 ml of the solution to be tested is added with 2 ml of freshly prepared Barfoed's reagent. Place the test tube into a boiling water bath and heat for 3 minutes. Allow it to cool.	A deep blue color is formed with a red ppt. settling down at the bottom or sides of the test tube.	Presence of reducing sugars [appearance of a red precipitate as a thin film] at the bottom of the test tube within 3–5 min is indicative of reducing monosaccharide. If the ppt. formation takes more time then it is a reducing disaccharide.	If the saccharide is a reducing sugar, it will reduce Cu (11) ions to Cu (1) oxide.
4.	**Seliwanoff's test** 3 ml of Seliwanoff's reagent + 1 ml of the test solution, boil in a water-bath for 2 minutes.	A cherry red colored precipitate within 5 minutes is obtained. A faint red color produced.	Presence of ketoses. [Sucrose gives a positive ketohexose test] Presence of aldoses.	When reacted with Seliwanoff reagent, ketoses react within 2 minutes forming a cherry red condensation product. Aldopentoses react slowly forming the colored condensation product.
5.	**Osazone Test** 2 ml of the test solution + 3 ml of phenyl hydrazine hydrochloride solution and mix them. Keep it in a boiling water bath for 30 minutes. Cool the solution and observe the crystals under microscope.	Formation of beautiful yellow crystals of osazone. Needle shaped crystals.	Presence of glucose/fructose.	Reducing sugars form osazone on treating with phenylhydrazine.

Reactions of Monosaccharide—Fructose

Sr. No.	Test	Observation	Inference	Reaction
1.	**Molisch's test** 2–3 drops of α-naphthol solution + 2 ml of the test solution. Very gently add 1 ml of conc. H_2SO_4 along the side of the test tube.	A deep violet coloration is produced at the junction of two layers.	Presence of carbohydrates.	Fructose is a carbohydrate. This is due to the formation of an unstable condensation product of α-naphthol with furfural (produced by the dehydration of the carbohydrate).
2.	**Benedict's test** 5.0 ml of Benedict's solution + 1 ml of the test solution and shake the test tube. Place the tube in a boiling water bath and heat for 3 minutes. Remove the tube from the heat and allow it to cool.	Formation of a green, red, or yellow precipitate.	Presence of reducing sugars.	Fructose is a reducing sugar. If the saccharide is a reducing sugar, it will reduce Copper [Cu] (11) ions to Cu (1) oxide, a red precipitate.
3.	**Barfoed's test** 2.0 ml of the solution to be tested is added with 2 ml of freshly prepared Barfoed's reagent. Place the test tube into a boiling water bath and heat for 3 minutes. Allow to cool.	A deep blue color is formed with a red ppt. settling down at the bottom or sides of the test tube.	Presence of reducing sugars [appearance of a red ppt as a thin film] at the bottom of the test tube within 3–5 min is indicative of reducing monosaccharide. If the ppt. formation takes more time then it is a reducing disaccharide.	Fructose is a monosaccharide. If the saccharide is a reducing sugar, it will reduce Cu (11) ions to Cu (1) oxide.
4.	**Seliwanoff's test** 3 ml of Seliwanoff's reagent +1 ml of the test solution, boil in water bath for 2 minutes.	A cherry red colored precipitate within 5 minutes is obtained A faint red color produced.	Presence of ketoses [Sucrose gives a positive ketohexose test] Presence of aldoses.	Fructose is a ketohexose. When reacted with Seliwanoff reagent, ketoses react within 2 minutes forming a cherry red condensation product. Aldopentoses react slowly forming the colored condensation product.
5.	**Osazone test** Take 2 ml of the test solution + 3 ml of phenyl hydrazine hydrochloride solution and mix them. Keep in a boiling water bath for 30 min. Cool the solution and observe the crystals under microscope.	Formation of beautiful yellow crystals of osazone. Needle shaped/broom stick shaped crystals.	Presence of fructose.	Fructose forms fructosazone. Reducing sugars forms osazone on treating with phenylhydrazine.

Reactions of Disaccharides—Lactose and Maltose

Sr. No.	Test	Observation	Inference	Reaction
1.	**Molisch's test** 2–3 drops of α-naphthol solution + 2.0 ml of the test solution. Very gently add 1ml of Conc. H_2SO_4 along the side of the test tube.	A deep violet coloration is produced at the junction of two layers.	Presence of carbohydrates.	Lactose/maltose is a carbohydrate. This is due to the formation of an unstable condensation product of α-naphthol with furfural (produced by the dehydration of the carbohydrate).
2.	**Benedict's test** 5.0 ml of Benedict's solution + 1 ml of the test solution and shake tube. Place the tube in a boiling water bath and heat for 3 minutes. Remove the tube from the heat and allow it to cool.	Formation of a green, red, or yellow precipitate.	Presence of reducing sugars.	Lactose/maltose is a reducing sugar. If the saccharide is a reducing sugar, it will reduce Copper [Cu] (11) ions to Cu (1) oxide, a red precipitate.
3.	**Barfoed's test** 2 ml of the solution to be tested is added with 2 ml of freshly prepared Barfoed's reagent. Place the test tube into a boiling water bath and heat for 3 minutes. Allow to them cool.	No deep blue color is formed with a red ppt. settling down at the bottom or sides of the test tube.	Presence of reducing sugars [appearance of a red ppt as a thin film] at the bottom of the test tube within 3–5 min. is indicative of reducing monosaccharide. If the ppt. formation takes more time then it is a reducing disaccharide.	Lactose/maltose is a reducing disaccaride sugar. If the saccharide is a reducing sugar, it will reduce Cu (11) ions to Cu (1) oxide.
4.	**Osazone test for maltose** Take 2.0 ml of the test solution + 3 ml of phenyl hydrazine hydrochloride solution and mix. Keep it in a boiling water bath for 30 min. Cool the solution and observe the crystals under microscope.	Formation of beautiful yellow crystals of osazone. Sunflower shaped crystals.	Presence of maltose.	Maltose forms maltosazone. Reducing sugar forms osazone on treating with phenylhydrazine.
5.	**Osazone test for lactose** 2.0 ml of the test solution + 3 ml of phenyl hydrazine hydrochloride solution and mix them. Keep it in a boiling water bath for 30 min. Cool the solution and observe the crystals under microscope.	Formation of beautiful yellow crystals of osazone. Power puff shape crystals	Presence of lactose.	Lactose forms lactosazone. Reducing sugar forms osazone on treating with phenylhydrazine.

Reactions of non-reducing Disaccharide—Sucrose

Sr. No.	Test	Observation	Inference	Reaction
1.	**Molisch's test** 2–3 drops of α-naphthol solution +2 ml of the test solution. Very gently add 1 ml of conc. H_2SO_4 along the side of the test tube.	A deep violet coloration is produced at the junction of two layers.	Presence of carbohydrates.	Sucrose is a carbohydrate. This is due to the formation of an unstable condensation product of α-naphthol with furfural (produced by the dehydration of the carbohydrate).
2.	**Benedict's test** 5 ml of Benedict's solution + 1 ml of the test solution and shake the test tube. Place the tube in a boiling water bath and heat for 3 minutes. Remove the tube from the heat and allow it to cool.	No formation of a green, red, or yellow precipitate	Absence of reducing sugars.	Sucrose is a non-reducing sugar. So the saccharide does not reduce copper [Cu](11) ions to Cu (1) oxide, a red precipitate.
3.	**Acid hydrolysis** 5 ml of test solution in a clean dry test tube + 4 drops of conc. hydrocloric acid and keep this solution in a boiling water bath for 10 minutes. Cool under running water and then neutralize by adding 5 drops of 10% sodium carbonate.	Red litmus paper turns blue.	Presence of non-reducing sugars.	Sucrose is a non-reducing sugar. The sucrose is hydrolyzed.
4.	**Benedict's test after hydrolysis** 5 ml of Benedict's solution + 1 ml of the hydrolysate test solution and shake the test tube. Place the tube in a boiling water bath and heat for 3 minutes. Remove the tube from the heat and allow it to cool.	Formation of a green, red, or yellow precipitate.	Presence of reducing sugars.	Hydrolysate is a reducing sugar. If the saccharide is a reducing sugar, it will reduce Copper [Cu] (11) ions to Cu (1) oxide, a red precipitate.
5.	**Seliwanoff's test** 3.0 ml of Seliwanoff's reagent + 1 ml of the hydrolysate test solution, boil in a water bath for 2 minutes.	A cherry red colored precipitate within 5 minutes is obtained. A faint red color produced.	Hydrolysate consists of keto sugar. Presence of ketoses. [Sucrose gives a positive ketohexose test] Presence of aldoses.	Fructose is a ketohexose. When reacted with Seliwanoff reagent, ketoses react within 2 minutes forming a cherry red condensation product. Aldopentoses react slowly forming the colored condensation product.

Reactions of Polysaccharide—Starch

Sr. No.	Test	Observation	Inference	Reaction
1.	**Molisch's test** — 2-3 drops of α-naphthol solution + 2 ml of the test solution. Very gently add 1 ml of conc. H_2SO_4 along the side of the test tube.	A deep violet coloration is produced at the junction of two layers.	Presence of carbohydrates.	Starch is a carbohydrate. This is due to the formation of an unstable condensation product of α-naphthol with furfural (produced by the dehydration of the carbohydrate).
2.	**Iodine test** 4–5 drops of iodine solution + 1 ml of the test solution and mix the contents gently.	Blue color is observed.	Presence of polysaccharide.	Starch is a polysaccharide. Iodine forms colorred adsorption complexes with polysaccharides.
3.	**Benedict's test** 5 ml of Benedict's solution + 1 ml of the test solution and shake the test tube. Place the tube in a boiling water bath and heat for 3 minutes. Remove the tube from the heat and allow it to cool.	No formation of a green, red, or yellow precipitate	Absence of reducing sugars.	Starch is not a reducing sugar. So the saccharide does not reduce Copper [Cu] (11) ions to Cu (1) oxide, a red precipitate.
4.	**Acid hydrolysis** 5 ml of test solution in a clean dry test tube + 4 drops of conc. hydrochloric acid and keep this solution in a boiling water bath for 10 minutes. Cool under running water and then neutralize by adding 5 drops of 10% sodium carbonate.	Red litmus paper turns blue.	The solution is hydrolyzed.	Starch is a polysaccharide and a non-reducing sugar.
5.	**Benedict's test after hydrolysis** 5 ml of Benedict's solution + 1 ml of the hydrolysate test solution and shake the test tube. Place the tube in a boiling water bath and heat for 3 minutes. Remove the tube from the heat and allow it to cool.	Formation of a green, red, or yellow precipitate.	Presence of reducing sugars.	Hydrolysate is a reducing sugar. It will reduce copper [Cu](11) ions to Cu (1) oxide, a red precipitate.

Scheme for identification of unknown carbohydrate

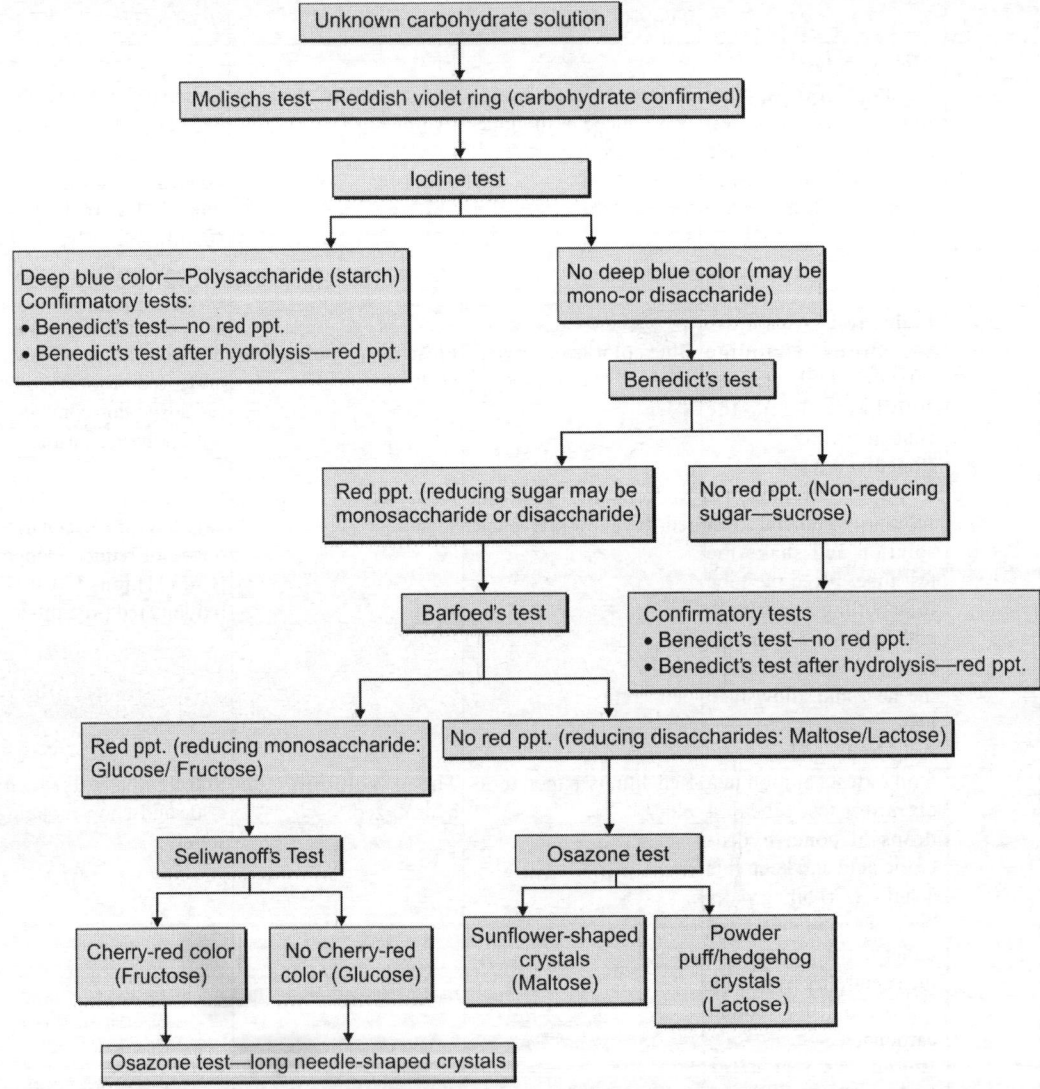

IDENTIFICATION OF PHYSIOLOGICAL IMPORTANT CONSTITUENTS

Physical characteristics:

a. Volume

b. Color

c. Odour

d. Reaction to litmus

IDENTIFICATION OF UNKNOWN PROTEIN

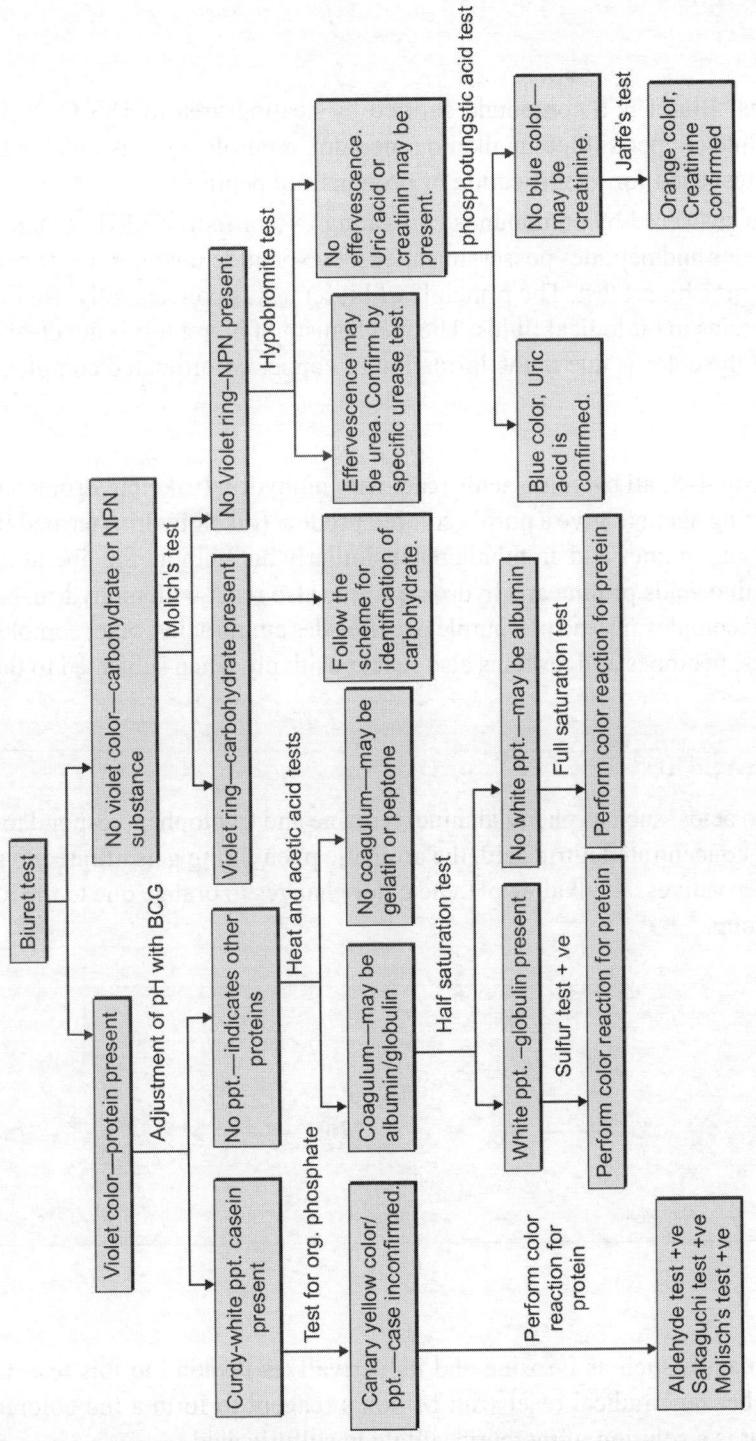

COLOR REACTIONS OF PROTEINS

Principle

Biuret reactions: Biuret is a compound formed by heating urea to 180°C. When biuret is treated with dilute copper sulfate in alkaline medium, a purple color is obtained. This is the basis of biuret test used for identification of proteins and peptides.

Biuret test is answered by compounds containing two or more CONH group, i.e. peptide bonds. All proteins and peptides possessing atleast two peptide linkages, i.e. tripeptides (with 3 amino acids) give biuret test. The principle of biuret test is conveniently used to detect the presence of proteins in biological fluids. The mechanism of biuret test is not clearly known. It is believed that the color is due to the formation of copper co-ordinated complex.

Ninhydrin Test

In the pH range of 4–8, all α-amino acids react with ninhydrin (triketohydrindene hydrate), a powerful oxidizing agent to give a purple colored product (diketohydrin) termed Ruhemann's purple. All primary amines and ammonia react similarly but without the liberation of carbon dioxide. The imino acids proline and hydroxyproline also react with ninhydrin, but they give a yellow colored complex instead of a purple one. Besides amino acids, other complex structures such as peptides, peptones and proteins also react positively when subjected to the ninhydrin reaction.

Xanthoproteic Acid Test

Aromatic amino acids, such as phenylalanine, tyrosine and tryptophan, respond to this test. In the presence of concentrated nitric acid, the aromatic phenyl ring gets nitrated to give yellow colored nitro-derivatives. At alkaline pH, the color changes to orange due to the ionization of the phenolic group.

Millon's Test

Phenolic amino acids such as tyrosine and its derivatives respond to this test. Compounds with a hydroxybenzene radical react with Millon's reagent to form a red colored complex. Millon's reagent is a solution of mercuric sulfate in sulfuric acid.

Pauly's diazo Test

This test is specific for the detection of tryptophan or histidine. The reagent used for this test contains sulfanilic acid dissolved in hydrochloric acid. Sulfanilic acid upon diazotization in the presence of sodium nitrite and hydrochloric acid results in the formation a diazonium salt. The diazonium salt formed, couples with either tyrosine or histidine in alkaline medium to give a red colored chromogen (azo dye).

Hopkins-Cole Test

This test is a specific test for detecting tryptophan. The indole moiety of tryptophan reacts with glyoxylic acid in the presence of concentrated sulfuric acid to give a purple colored product. Glyoxylic acid is prepared from glacial acetic acid by exposed to sunlight.

Sakaguchi reactions: Arginine, containing guanidine group, reacts with α-naphthol and alkaline hypobromite to form a red colored complex.

Sulfur Test

This is a test specific for sulfur containing amino acids namely cysteine and cystine, but not methionine.When cysteine and cystine are boiled with sodium hydroxide, organic sulfur is converted to inorganic sodium sulfide.This reacts with lead acetate to form a black precipitate of lead sulfide. Methionine is not split by alkali.

Pauly's Test

This reaction is specific for histidine (imidazole ring). Diazotised sulfanilic acid reacts with imidazole ring in alkaline medium to form a red colored complex.

Histidine Test

This test was discovered by Knoop. This reaction involves bromination of histidine in acid solution, followed by neutralization of the acid with excess of ammonia, and heating of alkaline solution, develops a blue or violet coloration.

Sakaguchi Test

Under alkaline condition, α-naphthol (1-hydroxy naphthalene) reacts with a mono-substituted guanidine compound like arginine, which upon treatment with hypobromite or hypochlorite, produces a characteristic red color.

Lead Sulfide Test

Sulfur containing amino acids, such as cysteine and cystine upon boiling with sodium hydroxide (hot alkali) yield sodium sulfide. This reaction is due to partial conversion of the organic sulfur to inorganic sulfide, which can be detected by precipitating it to lead sulfide, using lead acetate solution.

$$S \text{ (Proteins)} + 2NaOH \longrightarrow Na_2S$$
$$Na_2S + (CH_3COO)_2Pb \longrightarrow PbS + 2CH_3COONa$$

Folin's McCarthy Sullivan Test

Imino acids such as proline and hydroxyproline condense with isatin reagent under alkaline condition to yield blue colored adduct. Addition to sodium nitroprusside [$Na_2Fe(CN)_5NO$] to an alkaline solution of methionine followed by the acidification of the reaction yields a red color. This reaction also forms the basis for the quantitative determination of methionine.

Neumann's Test

The organic phosphate in phosphoproteins is converted to inorganic phosphate on boiling with strong sodium hydroxide solution. Inorganic phosphate reacts with ammonium molybdate in presence of nitric acid to form ammonium phosphomolybdate precipitate, which is canary yellow in color.

Color Reactions of Albumin/Casein/Gelatin/Peptone

Experiment	Observation	Inference
Biuret test: 1 ml of albumin/casein/gelatin/peptone solution + 1 ml of 5% NaOH and 2 drops of copper sulfate. Mix them.	Violet color	Albumin/casein/gelatin/peptone is a protein.
Ninhydrin test: 2 ml of albumin/casein/gelatin/peptone Solution + 2 drops of 0.2% ninhydrin solution. Mix and boil for 2–3 minutes.	Purple color (Ruhemann's purple)	Albumin/casein/gelatin/peptone contains free amino groups.
Xanthoproteic test: 3 ml of albumin/casein/peptone solution + 1 ml of conc. nitric acid. Mix boil solution for 3 min. Cool under tap water. Divide contents into 2 parts. To one part, add few drops of 40% NaOH.	Yellow color Orange color	Albumin/casein/peptone contains aromatic amino acids.
3 ml of gelatin solution + 1 ml conc. nitric acid. Mix boil solution for 3 min. Cool under tap water. Divide contents into 2 parts. To one part, add few drops of 40% NaOH.	Light yellow color Light orange color	Gelatin contains traces of aromatic amino acids: Tyrosine and tryptophan.
Millon's test: 1 ml of albumin/casein/gelatin/peptone solution + 1 ml of Millon's reagent. Boil for 2 min. Cool + 2 drops of freshly prepared 1% sodium nitrate. Mix them.	Red color ppt.	Albumin/casein/gelatin/peptone contains tyrosine.

(contd.)

Hopkin-Cole test: 1.0 ml of albumin/casein/gelatin/peptone solution + 1 drop of 0.2% formalin. Add a drop of 10% mercuric sulfate. Mix and add 1 ml of conc. H_2SO_4 along the sides of the test tube.	Violet colored ring is seen at the junction between the two liquids.	Albumin/casein/peptone contains tryptophan.
	No Violet colored ring is seen at the junction between the two liquids.	Gelatin does not contain tryptophan.
Sakaguchi test: 1 ml of albumin/casein/gelatin/peptone solution + 2 drops of 40% NaOH and 4 drops of 1% α-naphthol. Add few drops of bromine water. Mix well.	Cherry red color	Albumin/casein/gelatin/peptone contains arginine.
Sulfur test with albumin/peptone solution: 2 ml of albumin/peptone solution + equal volume of 40% NaOH and boil for a minute. Cool and add 2–3 drops of lead acetate. Mix well.	Brown/black color	Albumin/peptone contains sulfur containing amino acids (cystine and cysteine).
Sulfur test with casein/gelatin solution: 2 ml of casein/gelatin solution + equal volume of 40% NaOH and boil for a minute. Cool and add 2–3 drops of lead acetate. Mix well.	No Brown/black color	Casein/gelatin does not contain sulfur containing amino acids
Pauly's diazo test: 0.5 ml of sulfanilic acid + equal volume of 0.5 % sodium nitrite. After standing for 1 min + 1 ml albumin/casein/gelatin/peptone solution. Mix well. Add 1 ml of 10% sodium carbonate to make the solution alkaline.	Cherry-red color	Albumin/casein/gelatin/peptone contains histidine.
Neumann's test for casein: 5 ml of casein solution + 0.5 ml of 40% NaOH. Heat strongly. Cool under tap water. Add 0.5 ml conc. Nitric acid. Filter the precipitate. To the filtrate add a pinch of ammonium molybdate and warm gently.	Canary yellow precipitate.	Casein is a phosphoprotein.
Molish's test for albumin: 1 ml of albumin solution + 2 drops of Molish's reagent. Mix and add 1–2 ml of conc. H_2SO_4 carefully along the sides of the test tube.	Reddish violet ring at the junction of 2 layers.	Albumin is a glycoprotein.

PRECIPITATION AND COAGULATION REACTIONS OF PROTEINS

Proteins are made up of L-α-amino acids having large molecular weight and form colloidal solutions. Proteins can be precipitated either by removal of water layer (dehydration), denaturation, adjusting the isoelectric pH or by neutralization of charge present on protein molecule.

Principle: Precipitation by ammonium sulfate: Concentrated salt solutions cause precipitation of proteins by removing the water shell around the protein molecule. This process is known as salting out. Albumin has large number of molecules of water, and therefore, needs a full saturated ammonium sulfate than globulins to get precipitated.

Isoelectric precipitation: The pH at which the molecules of a protein bear no net charge, is called its isoelectric point. The isoelectric pH varies with different proteins. Proteins have minimum solubility at their isoelectric point. Many proteins are precipitated from their solution on adjusting the pH close to their isoelectric point by addition of an acid or alkali. The best example is casein, which forms a flocculent precipitate at its isoelectic pH 4.6 and redissolves in highly acidic or alkaline solutions.

Coagulation of proteins: The disruption of secondary, tertiary and quaternary structures of protein molecules is called denaturation. The aggregate of denatured proteins is called a coagulum, and the process is called coagulation. Albumin and globulins are easily coagulated by heat at their isoelectric points. On addition of acetic acid, there is a derease in pH, when pH approaches to the isoelectric pH of albumin/globulin, coagulation occurs spontaneously since the solution is pre-heated. This is called heat and acetic acid test.

Precipitation by strong mineral acids: Concentrated mineral acids like HNO_3, H_2SO_4 and HCl cause denaturation of proteins. This is the basis for the formation of white ring at the junction of two layers.

Precipitation by heavy metal salts: In an alkaline medium, the proteins acquire a negative charge. This is neutralized by the positive charge of heavy metals of these reagents, have negative charges which neutralize positive charges of proteins. Proteins acquire positive charge in acidic medium.

Precipitation by alcohol: Organic solvents like ethanol precipitate proteins from aqueous solution. They remove shell of hydration and reduce dielectric constant of the medium. This favors coalescence and precipitation of proteins.

Experiment	Observation	Inference

1. Precipitation by ammonium sulfate:
  a. **Half saturation test:**
    2 ml of protein solution. Add 2 ml of saturated ammonium sulfate solution and mix well. Keep it for some time.
	White ppt. is formed	Globulin gets precipitated on half saturation.

(contd.)

b. Full saturation test: 3 ml of protein solution + excess amount of ammonium sulfate crystals (some crystals should be left undissolved after thorough mixing)	White ppt is formed.	Albumin gets precipitated on full saturation.
2. Isoelectric precipitation: **Adjustment of pH 4.6 with BCG:** a. 3 ml of 1% casein solution + 2 drops of BCG	Blue color	pH >5.4
b. Add 1% of acetic acid drop by drop until the solution turns green in color.	Curdy white ppt.	At pH 4.6, casein is precipitated, the indicator color changes to green at this point.
3. Coagulation of proteins: **Heat and acetic acid test:** 10 ml of proteins solution, heat the upper layer of solution and add 1% of acetic acid drop by drop.	Coagulum seen	Albumin and globulin are coagulated by heat at their isoelectric pH.
4. Precipitation by strong mineral acids: Heller's nitric acid ring test: 3 ml of conc. HNO_3 in a clean dry test tube. To that, add 3 ml of protein solution along the sides of the test tube.	White ring at the junction of two layers	Proteins get precipitated.
5. Precipitation of heavy metal salts: 3 ml of protein in a clean dry test tube + 2 drops of 2% Na_2CO_3 solution and 1 drop of lead acetate solution	White ppt.	Proteins get precipitated.
6. Precipitation by alkaloid reagents: a. 3 ml of protein solution in a clean dry test tube + 5 drops of 10% trichloroacetic acid and mix them.	White ppt.	Proteins get precipitated.
b. 3 ml of protein solution + 3–4 drops of 20% sulfosalicylic acid and mix them.	White ppt.	Proteins get precipitated.
7. Precipitation by alcohol: 1 ml of protein solution in a clean dry test tube + 2 ml of absolute alcohol. Mix them.	Scanty-white ppt.	Proteins get precipitated.

REACTIONS OF UREA, URIC ACID AND CREATININE

Procedure	Observation	Inference
Tests for urea:		
1. **Sodium hypobromite test:** 3 ml of sample in a test tube. Add 1 ml of sodium hypobromite solution.	Effervescence is seen.	Indicates the presence of urea.
2. **Specific urease test:** 3 ml of sample in a test tube. Add 4–6 drops of phenolphthalein indicator and 1 ml of urease solution. Mix the contents well and keep it for a few minutes.	Pink color develops	Confirms the presence of urea.
Tests for uric acid: **Benedict's uric acid reagent test:** 3 ml of sample in a test tube. Add 1 spoonful of sodium carbonate crystals and mix well. Then add 1 ml of Benedict's blue color uric acid reagent and mix.	Formation of deep blue color	Shows the presence of uric acid.
Confirmatory test: **Schiff's test:** Wet piece of filter paper with few drops of ammonical silver nitrate solution. Add 1 or 2 drops of sample on the same paper.	Black color formed after sometime.	Confirms presence of uric acid.
Tests for creatinine: 1. **Jaffe's test:** Mix 5 ml of picric acid and 5 ml of 5% NaOH and divide this solution into two parts:		
i. To one part add 5 ml of sample	Orange red color	Creatinine is present.
ii. To another part add 5 ml of water.	No color	This is control test.
2. **Sodium nitroprusside test:** 5 ml of sample in a test tube + 5 drops of sodium nitroprusside solution. Then add 2 ml of 10% NaOH solution.	Red color changes to yellow.	Shows the presence of creatinine.

QUALITATIVE ANALYSIS OF GASTRIC JUICE—NORMAL AND ABNORMAL CONTENTS

Introduction

Gastric jucie is a composite secretion from stomach of three different types of cell
  i. Parietal cells—secrete HCl and intrinsic factor.
 ii. Chief cells—secrete Pepsinogen
iii. Mucous secreting cells—secrete mucous.

Characteristics of Normal Gastric Juice

* **Color:** Light colored fluid
* **Volume:** 2–4l
* **pH:** Highly acidic (1–2)
* **Specific gravity:** 1.007
* **Important constituents:** HCl, pepsin, mucin, and intrinsic factor
* **Abnormal constituents:** Lactic acid, blood, bile salt and bile pigment

Tests for Normal Constituents

Procedure	Observation	Inference
1. Test for hydrochloric acid (HCl): a. **Topfer's indicator test:** 2 ml of gastric juice + 2 drops of Topfer's indicator	Red color is formed.	Presence of HCl in gastric juice. Gastric juice has low pH. Topfer's indicator gives red color at this pH.
Note: Topfer's indicator may give false positive test when concentration of organic acids is high. A sensitive and confirmatory test for HCl is Gunzberg's test, which is done as follows.		
b. **Gunzberg's test:** Mix a few drops of gastric juice with an equal volume of Gunzberg's reagent in a china dish. Evaporate carefully over a low flame.	A red deposit is formed.	Geunzberg's reagent contains phloroglucinol and vanillin. On evapouration gastric juice, conc. HCl increases. Under this acid conc, phloroglucinol condenses with vanillin to form a red colored complex.
2. Test for pepsin: Label two test tubes as 'test' and 'control'. *Test*: 2 ml of gastric juice + 5 ml of casein solution *Control*: 2 ml of gastric juice and boil for one minute to inactivate pepsin enzyme. Add 5 ml casein solution.	A very little precipitate is formed. A maximum precipitate is formed.	Presence of pepsin in gastric juice. Pepsin converts casein to peptone and smaller peptides, which are soluble at pH 4.6. So the test shows less precipitate indicating the digestion of casein by pepsin.

(contd.)

Mix and incubate both tubes for 30 min. Then add 10% of sodium acetate solution drop by drop (counting) to 'C' tube with mixing till maximum precipitate occurs. Add same number of drops of sodium acetate solution to 'T' tube. Compare the amount to precipitate in the tubes.		Maximum precipitate indicates that, casein is not digested by heat-inactivated pepsin enzyme

Note: If the amount of precipitates are same in 'C' and 'T', this suggests that the gastric juice given has no pepsin. When both HCl and pepsin are absent in gastric jice, the condition is known as 'achyla gastrica'.

A. Test for bile salts		
1. **Hay's sulfur powder test:** 3 ml of gastric juice in a test tube and sprinkle small quantity of sulfur powder without shaking.	Sulfur powder sinks to the bottom.	Bile salts present.
2. **Fouchet's test:** 10 ml of gastric juice in a test tube and 3–4 ml of barium chloride solution + 1–2 drops of ammonium sulfate. Filter and dry the ppt. between the folds of the filter paper. Then add 1–2 drops of Fouchet's reagent on the ppt.	Formation of green color.	Bile pigments present.

Note: The gastric juice can be contaminated with bile mainly due to regurgitation of intestinal contents. The color of gastric juice will be yellow or green under this condition.

3. **Test for blood:** **Benzidine test:** Prepare a mixture with 2–3 drops of benzidine solution + 2 drops of hydrogen peroxide. 2 ml of gastric juice + 2 drops of the mixture	Blue or green color is formed immediately and disappears in few seconds (it turns brown).	Presence of blood in gastric juice.

Note: Fresh red blood may be present in gastric juice as a result of injury caused by introduction of stomach tube (Ryle's tube). Occult or hidden blood may be present in a gastric ulcer or cancer in stomach. Under the latter conditions, gastric juice may have dark brown color.

4. **Test for starch:** **Iodine test:** 2 ml of gastric juice + few drops of iodine solution and mix.	Blue color is formed.	Presence of starch in gastric juice.

Note: Dietary starch leaves the stomach within 2 to 3 hours after food intake. Detection of starch in the post absorptive period indicates a delay in emptying of the stomach contents.

URINE ANALYSIS: NORMAL CONSTITUENTS OF URINE

Principles:

1. **Test for chlorides:** Chlorides present in urine react with silver nitrate to form a white ppt. of silver chloride (AgCl).

2. **Test for calcium:** Calcium present in the urine reacts with potassium oxalate to form a white ppt. of calcium oxalate.

3. **Test for phosphates:** Phosphates present in the urine react with ammonium molybdate to form a canary yellow colored ppt. of ammonium phosphomolybdate.

4. **Test for sulfates:** Sulfates present in the urine reacts with barium chloride to form white precipitate of barium sulfate.

5. **Sodium hypobromite test:** The effervescence is due to liberation of nitrogen gas from the decomposition of urea into N_2 and CO_2 by the action of sodium hypobromite and CO_2 evolved reacts to form sodium carbonate.

6. **Specific urease test:** The enzyme urease splits urea present in urine to form ammonium carbonate. The ammonium carbonate makes the urine alkaline. The change in the pH is indicated by development of pink color by phenolphthalein indicator.

7. **Test for ammonia:** In an alkaline medium, the ammonium salt present in the urine decomposes to ammonia on boiling. The ammonia present in the vapours turns red litmus to blue color.

8. **Benedict's uric acid reagent test:** Uric acid is a reducing agent. In an alkaline medium, it reduces phosphotungstic acid to deep, blue colored tungsten blue.

9. **Schiff's test:** Uric acid reduces ammoniacal silver nitrate to metallic silver which is black in color.

10. **Jaffe's test:** Creatinine present in urine reacts with picric acid in an alkaline medium to give orange red colored compound, creatinine picrate.

11. **Sodium nitroprusside test:** The red colored complex is oxidized to give yellow color.

Physical characteristics:

a. Volume

b. Color

c. Odour

d. Reaction to litmus

e. Specific gravity

f. Deposits or turbidity

Tests for inorganic constituents:

Procedure	Observation	Inference
Tests for chlorides: 3 ml of urine in a test tube. Add 1 ml of conc. HNO_3 + 1 ml of silver nitrate and mix.	Formation of white ppt.	Shows the presence of chlorides.
Tests for calcium: 3 ml of urine in a test tube. Make it alkaline by adding few drops of liquor ammonia. Then Add 1 ml of potassium oxalate turbidity solution and mix.	Formation of white turbity	Shows the presence of calcium.
Tests for phosphates: 3 ml of urine in a test tube. Add 1 ml of conc. HNO_3 and 5 ml of ammonium molybdate solution. Then boil and cool under tap water.	Formation of canary yellow ppt.	Shows the presence of phosphates.
Tests for sulfates: 3 ml of urine in a test tube. Add 4 drops of conc. HCl and 2 ml of barium chloride solution and mix.	Formation of white ppt.	Shows the presence of sulfates.

Tests for organic constituents:

Procedure	Observation	Inference
Tests for urea: 1. **Sodium hypobromite test** 3 ml of urine in a test tube. Add 1 ml of sodium hypobromite solution.	Effervescence is seen.	Indicates the presence of urea.
2. **Specific urease test** 3 ml of urine in a test tube. Add 4–6 drops of phenolphthalein indicator and 1 ml of urease solution. Mix the contents well and keep it for a few minutes.	Pink color develops.	Confirms the presence of urea.
Tests for uric acid: **Benedict's uric acid reagent test:** 3 ml of urine in a test tube. Add 1 spoonful of sodium carbonate crystals and mix well. Then add 1 ml of Benedict's blue color uric acid reagent and mix.	Formation of deep blue color.	Shows the presence of uric acid.

(contd.)

Confirmatory test: Schiff's test: Wet piece of filter paper with few drops of ammonical silver nitrate solution. Add 1 or 2 drops of urine sample on the same paper.	Black color formed after some-time.	Confirms presence of uric acid.
Test for ammonia: 3 ml of urine in a test tube. Add 2 ml of 10% NaOH solution. Boil and hold a red litmus paper to vapours at the mouth of the test tube.	Red litmus turns blue.	Shows the presence of ammonia.
Tests for creatinine: 1. Jaffe's test: Mix 5 ml of picric acid and 5 ml of 5% NaOH and divide it into two parts: (i) to one part add 5ml urine, (ii) to another part add 5ml of water.	Orange red color No color	Creatinine is present. This is control test.
2. Sodium nitroprusside test: 5 ml of urine in a test tube + 5 drops of sodium nitroprusside solution. Then add 2 ml of 10% NaOH solution.	Red color changes to yellow.	Shows the presence of creatinine.

URINE ANALYSIS: ABNORMAL CONSTITUENTS OF URINE

Physical Characteristics
a. Volume
b. Color
c. Odour
d. Reaction to litmus
e. Specific gravity
f. Deposits or turbidity

Tests for Abnormal Constituents

Principle:
1. **Sulfosalicylic acid test:** The protein present in the urine is precipitated by sulfosalicylic acid by neutralizing the charges on the protein.
2. **Heat and acetic acid test:** Albumin is the major protein excreted in proteinuria. It is a heat coagulable protein and, hence, easily coagulated by heating the urine sample containg it. Formation of turbidity is due to protein or phosphate present in the urine. Presence of turbity upon addition of dil. Acetic acid indicates the presence of protein.
3. **Benedict's test:** Ref. carbohydrate
4. **Rothera's test:** Sodium nitroprusside in alkaline medium reacts with ketone groups of acetone and acetic acid to form permanganate ring at the junction of the two liquids.

5. **Gerhardt's test:** Acetoacetic acid gives red color with ferric chloride.
6. **Benzidine glacial acetic acid test:** Heme part of hemoglobin has peroxidase like activity which acts on hydrogen peroxide to release nascent oxygen. This nascent oxygen oxidizes benzidine to give green color.
7. **Hay's sulfur powder test:** Bile salts lower the surface tension of urine and, hence, the sulfur powder sinks to the bottom of the test tube.
8. **Fouchet's test:** The bile pigment present in the urine gets adsorbed onto the precipitate of barium sulfate which is separated by filtration. The dried precipitate is then treated with fouchet's reagent which contains ferric chloride. Ferric chloride is an oxidizing agent and it oxidizes bilirubin to biliverdin to give green color.

Procedure	Observation	Inference
(B) Tests for proteins:		
5. **Sulfosalicylic acid test:** 3 ml of urine in a test tube. Add 1 ml of sulfosalicylic acid and mix.	Formation of white ppt.	Proteins present.
6. **Heller's nitric acid test:** 3 ml of conc. HNO_3 in a test tube. Add 3 ml of urine by touching inside wall of test tube.	Formation of a white ring at the junction of two liquids.	Proteins or phosphates present.
7. **Heat and acetic acid tests:** 10 ml of urine in a test tube and heat the upper column. Acidify the urine by adding few drops of dil. acetic acid.	Coagulum or ppt. appears	Confirms the presence of proteins.
(C) Test for reducing sugars:		
8. **Benedict's test:** 5 ml of Benedict's reagent in a test tube and boil. Then add 8 drops of given urine. Boil again and cool under tap water.	Formation of colored ppt. (green 0.5%, yellow 1%, orange 1.5%, red 2%)	Reducing sugar present.
(D) Test for ketone bodies:		
9. **Rothera's test:** (for acetone and acetoacetic acid) 5 ml of urine in a test tube and saturate with ammonium sulfate. Then add 2–3 drops of sodium nitroprusside solution and 1 ml of liquor ammonia dropwise by the inside wall of test tube.	Appearance of permanganate ring at the junction of the two liquids.	Ketone bodies present.
10. **Gerhardt's test:** 3 ml of urine in a test tube + few drops of 10% ferric chloride solution	Red color is formed.	Acetoacetic acid present.

(E) Test for blood: **11. Benzidine glacial acetic acid test:** 2 ml of benzidine glacial acetic acid and 2 ml of hydrogen peroxide solution and divide this solution into two parts: • one part add equal amount of urine • another part add equal amount of water	Formation of blue or green color. Stable only for few minutes then changes to brown.	Blood present.
(F) Test for bile salts: **12. Hay's sulfur powder test:** 3 ml of urine in a test tube and sprinkle small quantity of sulfur powder without shaking	Sulfur powder sinks to the bottom.	Bile salts present.
(G) Tests for bile pigments: **13. Gmellin's test:** 3 ml conc. HNO_3 in a test tube. Add 2 ml of urine and just shake the test tube.	Play of colors are seen.	Bile pigments present.
14. Fouchet's test: 10 ml of urine in a test tube and 3–4 ml of barium chloride solution + 1–2 drops of ammonium sulfate. Filter and dry the ppt. between the folds of the filter paper. Then add 1–2 drops of Fouchet's reagent on the ppt.	Formation of green color.	Bile pigments present.

DETERMINATION OF CREATININE CONTENT IN URINE, CALCULATION OF CREATININE CLEARANCE

Principle: Creatinine in urine is determined by its reaction with picric acid in alkaline medium to form orange colored tautomer of creatinine picrate. Sicne creatinine content of urine is high, it is suitable to diluted. Equal volume of diluted urine, standard and blank is treated with picric acid and NaOH. The intensity of orange color is read using green filter (540 nm). The concentration of creatinine is calculated for 100 ml.

Procedure: Dilute 5 ml of urine in 50 ml volumetric flask. Label three test tubes as B, S, T. Add 5 ml of distilled water into B and 5 ml standard into S. Pipette 5ml of diluted urine into T. To each, add 2 ml of picric acid solution and 2 ml of 0.75M NaOH. Mix and read OD after 15 min.

$$\text{Serum creatinine in mg/dL} = \frac{\text{OD of T} - \text{OD of B}}{\text{OD of S} - \text{OD of B}} \times 100$$

If the urine output per day is 1500 ml then creatinine is

$$\text{Serum creatinine in mg/dl} = \frac{\text{OD of T} - \text{OD of B}}{\text{OD of S} - \text{OD of B}} \times 100 \times \frac{15}{10000} \text{ gm}$$

CLEARANCE TEST

Creatinine Clearance Test

It is the volume of plasma completely cleared off creatinine which is excreted in the urine.
Formula: UV/ P or U V / P × 1.73.

$$U = \text{Urine creatinine}$$
$$P = \text{Plasma}$$
$$1.73 = \text{Generally accepted body surface area}$$
$$A = \text{Body surface area of the patient, under investigation.}$$

The creatinine clearance is very convenient to measure GFR.

It fulfills all the requirements of the substance which is ideal for measuring GFR.

The amount of creatinine produced is relatively constant and also it is not affected by the dietary intake.

Normal values:

Males: 105 ± 20 ml/min.

Female: 95 ± 20 ml/min.

Abnormal results are lower than normal GFR measurements, and they indicate:

• Acute tubular necrosis
• Congestive heart failure
• Dehydration
• Glomerulonephritis
• Shock
• Acute nephrotic syndrome
• Acute and chronic renal failure

ESTIMATION OF BLOOD SUGAR

Folin-Wu Method

Principle: Glucose in the protein-free filtrate at higher temperature and alkaline medium reduces Cu^{2+} to Cu^+. The cuprous oxide formed is in turn treated with phosphomolybdic acid, which is reduced proportionally by the cuprous ions to phosphomolybdous acid (molybdenum blue), glue solution. The intesntiy of this blue solution is a measure of the amount of glucose present.

$$\text{Glucose} + Cu^{2+} \xrightarrow{\text{Na}_2\text{SO}_4 \text{ heat}} Cu^+$$

Tartarate in the reagent helps to chelate Cu^{2+} and releases it slowly for reduction to Cu^+, thus, preventing its ppt. as CuO.

$$Cu^+ + \text{phosphomolybdic} \longrightarrow \text{acid phosphomolybdous acid (blue)}$$

Reagents:
a. 10% sodium tungstate
b. 2/3 N H_2SO_4
c. Alkaline copper reagent
d. Standard glucose (0.1 mg/ml)
   Sample: Blood collected in a fluoride and oxalate containing tube.

Part I

Preparation of protein-free filtrate from blood.
   In a test tube, take 7 ml distilled water, 1 ml blood sample, 1 ml of 10% sodium tungstate solution and 1 ml of 2/3N H_2SO_4 solution (dropwise and with shaking). Thus, the dilution of blood sample is 1 in 10. Let it stand for 10 minutes, filter and collect the filtrate in a dry beaker.
   Note:
   I. Oxalate precipitates Ca^{2+} of the blood, hence, prevent coagulation. Fluoride inhibits glycolytic enzymes of RBC to prevent breakdown of glucose before estimation.
   II. The escaped polypeptide bind to Cu^{2+} and forms colored complexes which give high values.

Part II

Procedure

Reagents	Blank	Standard	Test
Water	2 ml	—	—
Standard	—	2 ml	—
Test	—	—	2 ml
Alkaline copper reagent	2ml	2 ml	2 ml
Mix. Keep in a boiling water bath for 8 minutes and cool.			
Phosphomolybdic acid	2 ml	2 ml	2 ml
Add distilled water up to the 25 ml mark and mix the tubes by inverting them.			
Read the absorbance at 420 nm or blue filter.			

   Keeping the tubes in boiling waterbath for more than 8 min will increase the reading due to excess reduction of Cu^{2+}.

Calculation
   Concentration of glucose in mg/100 ml blood:

$$\frac{\text{OD of T} - \text{OD of B}}{\text{OD of S} - \text{OD of B}}$$

$$\frac{\dfrac{\text{OD of T} - \text{OD of B}}{\text{OD of S} - \text{OD of B}}}{\text{-----------------} \quad \text{mg/dl.}} \times 100 \text{ mg\%}$$

ESTIMATION OF GLUCOSE BY O-TOLUIDINE METHOD

Principle: Glucose reacts with o-toluidine in glacial acetic acid on heating to yield a blue-green N-glycosylamine derivative. The intensity of this color is proportional to the concentration of glucose present. The proteins are precipitated in this method with the help of alkaloidal reagent, TCA acid. Glacial acetic acid, heat

$$\text{Glucose} + \text{O-toluidine} \longrightarrow \text{N-glycosylamine derivative (blue-green)}$$

Reagents:

1. 1% o-toluidine reagent in ethanol
2. 10% trichloroacetic acid
3. Saturated glucose solution (0.1 mg/ml)

Part II: Preparation of protein free filtrate (PFF) from blood. 3 ml distilled water, 0.5 ml of blood and 1.5 ml of 10% TCA. Mix, keep for 10 min and filter in a dry TT to obtain a clear solution of PFF.

Part II: Use this PFF for glucose estimation.

Reagents	Blank	Standard	Test
TCA	1 ml	—	—
Standard	—	1 ml	—
PFF	—	—	1 ml
O-toluidine	5 ml	5 ml	5 ml
Mix. Keep in a boiling water bath for 10 minutes and cool.			
Read the absorbance at 630 nm.			

Calculation:

Concentration of glucose in mg/100 ml blood:

$$\frac{\text{OD of T} - \text{OD of B}}{\text{OD of S} - \text{OD of B}} \times \text{conc. of std}$$

$$\frac{\text{OD of T} - \text{OD of B}}{\text{OD of S} - \text{OD of B}} \times 100 \text{ mg\%}$$

$$------------ \text{ mg/dl.}$$

COLORIMETRY

Principles of Spectrophotometry/ Colorimetry

Both these techniques are based on the estimation of light absorbing nature of the substances in solution. In colorimetry, only the colored compounds or the compounds capable of forming color complexes by reacting with reagents can be analyzed. In this, the intensity of the color reflects the concentration of the substance. Whereas, in spectrophotometry not only colored but also colorless solution can be studied by means of ultraviolet spectral analysis. These techniques are based on 2 laws:

1. **Beer's law:** "Absorbance of a solution is directly proportional to the concentration of the solution" (i.e. $A \propto C$) or "transmittance of a solution decreases exponentially with the increase in the concentration of the solution" (i.e. $T = e-kc$).

2. **Lambert's law:** "Absorbance of a solution is directly proportional to the thickness of the optical path" (i.e. $A \propto t$) or "Transmittance of a solution decreases exponentially with the increase in the thickness of the optical light path" (i.e. $T = e-kt$) (Figure 19.4).

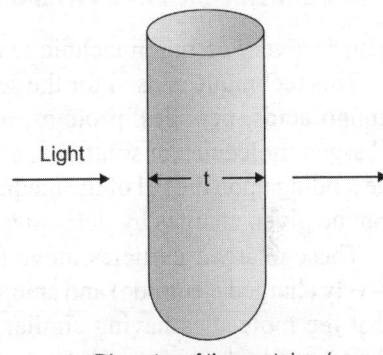

Light

t—Diameter of the container/
Width of the solution layer/
Thickness of the optical path

Lambert's law C

Instrumentation

Components of colorimeter/spectrophotometer:

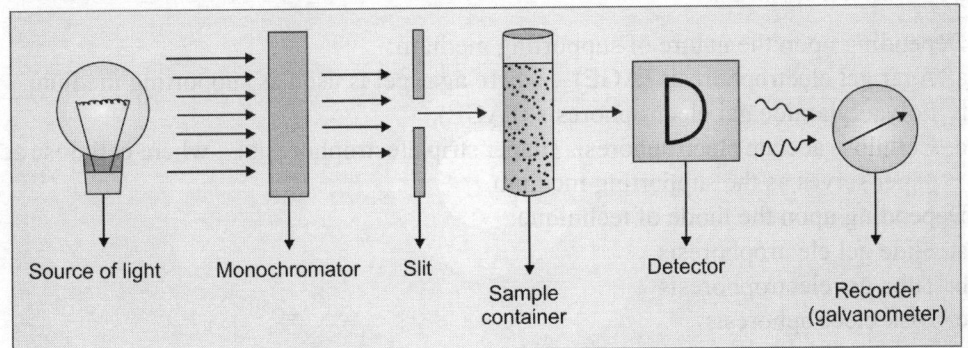

Source of light   Monochromator   Slit   Detector

Sample
container

Recorder
(galvanometer)

Figure: Components of colorimeter or spectrophotometer

ELECTROPHORESIS AND CHROMATOGRAPHY

ELECTROPHORESIS

Introduction

Electrophoresis and chromatography are the popular methods for the separation of closely related compounds like mixture of proteins, amino acid, carbohydrates, steroid hormones and drugs.

General Principle of Electrophoresis

This is a very common technique used in clinical and research laboratories.

This technique is used for the separation of charged particles. Biological materials such as amino acids, peptides, proteins, nucleic acids possess ionisable groups and hence exist as charged molecules in solutions, either as cations (+vely charged) or anions (–vely charged), depending upon the pH of the medium. Even typical nonpolar substances such as carbohydrates can be given charges by derivatization, for example as borate or phosphates.

These charged particles move (migrate) in an electric field, i.e. cations towards cathode (–vely charged electrode) and anions towards anode (+vely charged electrode). So, it is obvious that the molecules having similar charges move in the same direction. But because of the difference in their molecular mass the extent to which they move differs.

Hence, the difference in charge: Mass ratio (C/M) forms the basis for the differential migration of particles in an applied electric field. And this forms the general principle of electrophoresis.

The following example of an amino acid shows how the extent of ionization and direction of migration is dependent on pH.

Types of Electrophoresis

i. Depending upon the nature of supporting medium:
    a. Agar gel electrophoresis (AGE)—where agar gel is used as supporting medium.
    b. Polyacrylamide gel electrophoresis (PAGE).
    c. Cellulose acetate electrophoresis (Paper strip electrophoresis)—where cellulose acetate paper serves as the supporting medium.
ii. Depending upon the mode of technique:
    a. Slide gel electrophoresis
    b. Tube gel electrophoresis
    c. Disk electrophoresis
    d. Low and high voltage electrophoresis.

Applications

1. In separating serum proteins for diagnostic purposes
2. Hemoglobin electrophoresis
3. Lipoprotein electrophoresis
4. Isozyme analysis
5. Nucleic acid studies

CHROMATOGRAPHY

Chromatography is one of the most popular tools of biochemistry. This technique is used for the separation of a number of similar components in a mixture from each other so that these could be determined with a minimum of interference. These closely related compounds include proteins, peptides, amino acids, lipids, carbohydrates, vitamins and drugs. This technique is working on the principle of adsorption, partition, ion-exchange and exclusion properties.

General Principle

Chromatography usually consists of a mobile phase and a stationary phase. The mobile phase refers to the mixture of substance to be separated in a liquid or a gas. The stationary phase is a porous solid matrix through which the sample contained in the mobile phase percolates. The interaction between the stationary phase and the mobile phase causes the separation of compounds from the mixture. These interactions include adsorption, partition, ion-exchange and exclusion type of physiochemical properties.

Classification of Chromatography

The type of interaction medium used for stationary phase and mobile phase is the basis of classification of chromatography.

Principle of Partition Chromatography

The molecules which are to be separated undergo continuous redistribution between a stationary phase and a mobile phase. The separation depends on the relative tendencies of the molecule in a mixture to associate more strongly with one or other phases. Since partitioning process is repeated hundreds or thousand times, small difference in partition ratio permits excellent separation.

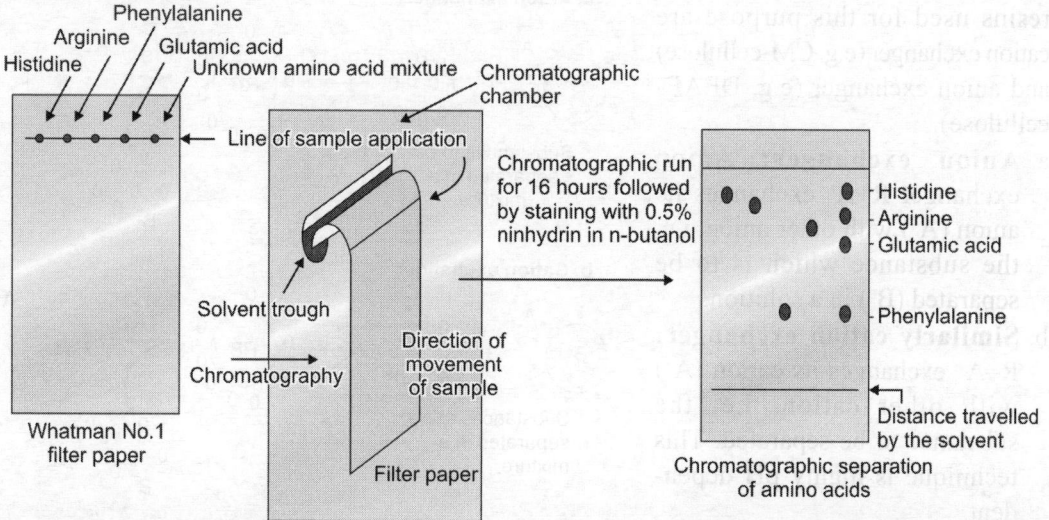

Chromatographic separation of amino acids

In paper chromatography, paper serves as a solid support to hold the stationary phase. The solvent system provides both stationary phase and mobile phase. For amino acid chromatography, butanol, acetic acid and water in the proportion of 4:1:5 v/v is used as solvent system. Butanol with a little acetic acid acts as the mobile phase and water-acetic acid forms the stationary phase which will be held to the paper.

Adsorption Chromatography

In this technique, separation of substances is based on the difference in adsorption on the surface of a solid stationary medium such as silica gel or alumina. During the elution, weekly held substances move fast. Strongly held substances are eluted by changing pH and salt conditions.

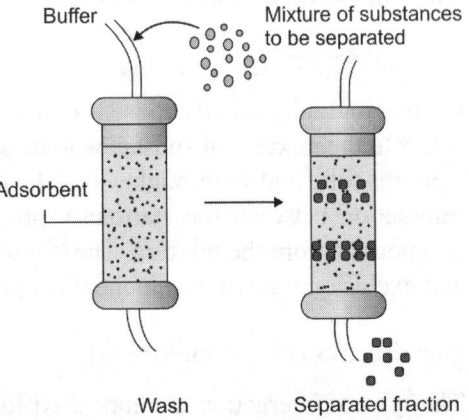

Gas-liquid Chromatography

This is a method of choice for the separation of volatile substances like lipids and drugs. Stationary phase is inert solid material which is impregnated with a nonvolatile liquid like polyethylene glycol. This is packed in a narrow column. Under proper condition volatile material, which is to be separated, is passed through column with the help of an inert gas (Argon). Separation of individual substance is based on partition of components.

Ion-exchange Chromatography

Here separation of molecules is based on their charges. Ion-exchange resins used for this purpose are cation exchanger (e.g. CM-cellulose) and anion exchanger (e.g. DEAE-cellulose).

a. **Anion exchanger:** Anion exchanger R+A$^-$ exchanges its anion (A$^-$) with other anion, i.e. the substance which is to be separated (B$^-$) in a solution.

b. **Similarly cation exchanger:** R–A$^+$ exchanges its cation (A$^+$) with other cation, i.e. the substance to be separated. This technique is highly pH dependent.

Gel Filtration Chromatography

Here the separation is based on size, shape and molecular weight of the substance to be separated. The gel serves as a molecular sieve for these substances. The larger particles cannot pass through the pores of the gel and, therefore, move faster. On the other hand smaller particles enter to the gel beads and are left behind, which come out of the column very slowly, e.g. for gel filtration materials are Sephadex G-100, Bio gel P-10.

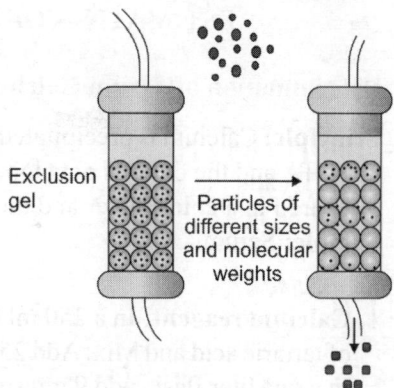

Affinity Chromatography

The principle is based on the specific and noncovalent binding of substances (like proteins and enzymes) to a specific ligand (cofactor or substrates) attached to the gel matrix. For example, separation of lactate dehydrogenase from RBC using NAD^+ ligand linked to an affinity gel.

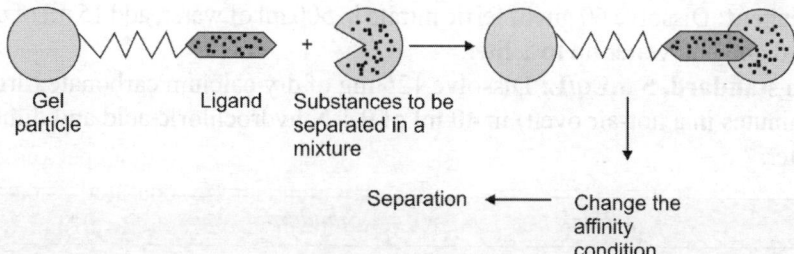

ESTIMATION OF SERUM CALCIUM AND PHOSPHOROS

Determination of Serum Calcium by Trinder Method

Principle: Calcium is precipitated with naphthylhydroxamic acid. The precipitate is dissolved in EDTA and the color is developed with ferric nitrate. The absorbance of color compound is measured in a colorimeter and the calcium level is determined.

Sample: Serum.

Reagents:

1. **Calcium reagent:** In a 250 ml beaker, add 100 ml water and 5 ml ethanolamine. Add 2 gm of tartaric acid and Mix. Add 250 mg of naphthylhydroxamic acid and dissolve by warming. In a one liter flask, add 9 gm sodium chloride and 500 ml of water. Pour the contents of the beaker into the 1 L flask containing sodium chloride solution. Add water up to 1 L mark. mix. Filter through Whatman No. 40 filter paper. The reagent is stable for months.

2. **EDTA solution:** Dissolve 2 gm of disodium ethylene diamine tetraacetate in 1 L of 0.1 N NaOH.

3. **Color reagent:** Dissolve 60 gm of ferric nitrate in 500 ml of water, add 15 ml of concentrated nitric acid and add water up to 1 liter.

4. **Calcium standard, 5 mEq/L:** Dissolve 125 mg of dry calcium carbonate (dried at 120°C for 30 minutes in a hot-air oven) in 40 ml of 0.1 N hydrochloric acid and dilute to 500 ml with water.

Reagents	Blank	Standard	Test
Serum	—	—	0.2 mL
Standard calcium	—	0.2 mL	—
Calcium reagent	5.0 mL	5.0 mL	5.0 mL
Mix. Stand for 30 minutes at room temperature. Centrifuge and Pour off supernatant			
EDTA solution	1.0 mL	1.0 mL	1.0 mL
Keep in boiling water bath for 10 minutes and cool.			
Color reagent	3.0 mL	3.0 mL	3.0 mL
Read the absorbance at 450 nm or Blue filter.			

Calculation

$$\text{Serum calcium in mEq/L} = \frac{\text{OD of T} - \text{OD of B}}{\text{OD of S} - \text{OD of B}} \times 10$$

To convert the result to mg% multiply mEq/L by 2.

Note

The glasswares must be perfectly clean.

O-Cresolphthalein Complexone Method

Principle: Calcium in the serum forms a violet colored complex with O-Cresolphthalein complexone. 8-Hydroxyquinoline included in the reagent prevents interference by magnesium.

Reagents:

Reagent A: Transfer 210 gm of diethanolamine to about 900 ml of double distilled water into a one liter beaker. Dissolve the crystals. Adjust the pH to 11.7 with acetic acid. Transfer to a 1 liter flask and make up to 1 liter with double distilled water. The reagent is stable at least for one month.

Reagent B: Dissolve 64 mg of O-Cresolphthaleincomplexone, 1.16 gm of 8-Hydroxyquinoline and 2.5 ml glacial acetic acid in 250 ml of ethanol. Make up the volume to 1 liter with double distilled water. The reagent is stable for at least one month.

Working reagent: Mix equal volumes of reagent A and reagent B just before use (calculate the approximate volume of reagent required and prepare the required volume of reagent for the day).

Calcium standard: 10 mg/100 ml or 5 mEq/L. Dissolve 125 mg of dry calcium carbonate in 40 ml of 0.1 N HCl and dilute to 500 ml with water.

Procedure

Pipette 0.2 ml serum and 1.8 ml water to a test tube and mix. Transfer 0.5 ml from this to a test tube marked test (T). Add 5 ml of working reagent.

To a second test tube add 0.2 ml of calcium standard solution and 1.8 ml of water. Transfer 0.5 ml from this to Standard (S). Add 5 ml of working reagent and mix.

Label a 3rd test tube as Blank (B) and add 0.5 ml water and 5 ml of working reagent and mix.

Read absorbance of B, S and T at 578 nm or using green filter.

Calculation

$$\text{mg of calcium/100 ml serum} = \frac{\text{OD of T} - \text{OD of B}}{\text{OD of S} - \text{OD of B}} \times 10$$

When mg% is divided by 2, mEq/L is obtained.

Clinical Significance

Normal value ranges from 9–10.6 mg per 100 ml serum or 4.5–5.4 mEq/L.

Hypocalcemia

- Hypoparathyroidism
- Vitamin D deficiency: Decreased dietary intake, decreased sun exposure, defective vitamin D metabolism, ineffective active vitamin D, Intestinal malabsorption
- Magnesium deficiency (hypomagnesemia)

- Eating disorders
- Chronic renal failure: The kidney loses its capacity synthesise 1.25-dihydroxycholecalciferol. Increased PTH secretion in response to hypocalcemia may lead to bone disease, if untreated.
- Pseudohypoparathyroidism is a condition primarily associated with resistance to the parathyroid hormone. Patients have a low serum calcium and high phosphate, but the parathyroid hormone level (PTH) is actually appropriately high (due to the hypocalcemia).

Hypercalcemia

Elevated calcium level in the blood

Causes

- Primary hyperparathyroidism
- Solid tumour with metastasis (e.g. squamous cell carcinoma, which can be PTHrP-mediated)
- Solid tumour with humoral mediation of hypercalcemia (e.g. non-small cell lung cancer or kidney cancer, pheochromocytoma)
- Hematologic malignancy (multiple myeloma, lymphoma, leukemia)
- Hypervitaminosis D (vitamin D intoxication)

Phosphorous

- It is a mineral.
- It is also involved in the release of energy from fat, protein, and carbohydrates during metabolism, and in the formation of genetic material, cell membranes, and many enzymes.
- Helps in the formation of bone and teeth. Inorganic phosphorous is a major constituent of hydroxyapatite in bone, thereby playing an important part in structural support of the body.
- Act as a buffer in blood. Mixture of HPO_4^- and $H_2PO_4^-$ constitutes the phosphate buffer which plays a role in maintaining the pH of the body fluid.
- Helps in the formation of compounds like nucleic acids, nucleotides like ATP, GTP, ADP etc., as organic phosphate esters in glycolysis and other metabolic reactions.
- It is also required in energy metabolism, synthesis of phospholipids, cAMP, phosphoproteins, and coenzymes like TPP, etc.
- The phosphorus concentration in serum is inversely proportional to the calcium concentration.
- The normal value for adults is 2.5 to 4.5 mg % and for children 4–6 mg %.

   Determination of Serum Inorganic Phosphorus by Fiske-Subba Row Method

   Specimen: Serum collected from venous blood. Plasma is also suitable.

Principle

Serum proteins are precipitated by trichloroacetic acid. Molybdic acid added to protein-free filtrate converts phosphate to phosphomolybdate. Alpha-naphthol sulfonic acid added, reduces phosphomolybdate to a blue colored compound. The intensity of blue color is measured photometrically using red filter or at 660 nm.

Reagents:

1. **Trichloroacetic acid, 10%:** Dissolve 10 gm TCA in water and make up to 100 liter.
2. **Molybdate reagent:** To 200 ml of water, add 83 ml sulfuric acid, keeping cold under tap or cold water. Dissolve 25 gm of ammonium molybdate in this solution. Dilute to 1 liter with water. Solution is stable.
3. **1, 2, 4-Amino naphthol sulfonic acid reagent (ANSA):** Dissolve 0.125 gm of 1, 2, 4-amino naphthol sulfonic acid, 7.28 gm of sodium meta-bisulfite and 0.25 gm of anhydrous sodium sulfite in 50 ml of water filter. Store in a brown bottle. There agent is stable for one month kept in refrigerator.
4. **Standard phosphorus solution 0.08 mg/ml solution:** Dissolve 0.351 gm of dried potassium dihydrogen phosphate in about 500 ml water in a liter flask. Add 8 ml concentrated HCl and dilute to one liter. Prepare fresh once a month.

Procedure

Reagents	Blank	Standard	Test
Serum	—	—	1 mL
TCA, 10%	—	—	9 mL
Mix, stand for 5 minutes and filter.			
Water	1 mL	0.5 mL	—
Standard phosphorus solution	—	0.5 mL	—
Filtrate	—	—	5 mL
TCA, 10%	4 mL	4 mL	—
Molybdate reagent	1 mL	1 ml	1 mL
ANSA	0.4 mL	0.4 mL	0.4 mL
Mix and stand for 5 minutes.			
Water	3.6 mL	3.6 mL	3.6 mL
Read at 660 nm or red filter.			

Calculation

$$100 \text{ mL serum contains} = \frac{OD \text{ of } T - OD \text{ of } B}{OD \text{ of } S - OD \text{ of } B} \times 0.04 \times \frac{100}{1} = \frac{T - B}{S - B} \times 4$$

Note

1. The inorganic phosphorus increases when blood is allowed to stand so, determine immediately.
2. Use double distilled water throughout the procedure.

3. The method is employed to determine phosphate in urine, urine is adjusted to pH 5 by adding 1 N HCl. It is diluted to 1 in 10 with water. Proceed same as above. Collect 24 hours sample.

Clinical Significance

Hypophosphatemia (decreased level of phosphorous)

Causes

* Rickets
* Hyperparathyroidism
* Condition associated with decrease in the reabsorption of phosphate from the glomerular filtrate (Fanconi syndrome).
* In the treatment of diabetes, the effect of insulin in causing the shift of glucose into cells also enhances the transport of phosphate into cells, which may result into hypophospatemia.

Symptoms

Clinical symptoms are muscle pain and weakness with respiratory failure and decreased myocardial output.

Hyperphosphatemia (Increased phosphorous level)

Causes

* Hypoparathyroidism
* Hypervitaminosis D
* Renal failure
   Elevated phosphate may cause a decrease in serum calcium concentration. Therefore, it may lead to tetany and seizures.

SERUM BILIRUBIN ESTIMATION BY THE MALLOY AND EVELYN METHOD

Principle

Bilirubin of serum reacts with diazo reagent to form a colored complex which is measured at 540 nm photometrically. Conjugated bilirubin (direct bilirubin) undergoes color reaction directly, whereas urconjugated bilirubin (indirect bilirubin) forms color after the addition of alcohol. Total bilirubin is the sum of direct and indirect bilirubins. Indirect reaction gives the concentration of total bilirubin and direct reaction gives that of direct bilirubin. Concentration of indirect bilirubin is obtained by taking the difference between the total and direct bilirubin.

Reagents

1. Absolute methanol
2. **HCl 1.5 percent:** 4.2 ml conc.HCl diluted with 100 ml distilled water.

3. **Diazo reagent:**

　　Solution A: 0.1 gm of sulfanilic acid is dissolved in 1.5 ml concentrated HCl and made up to 100 ml with water.

　　Solution B: 0.5 gm of sodium nitrite is dissolved in 100 ml of water.

　　Diazo reagent is prepared freshly by mixing 10 ml of solution A and 0.3 ml of solution B.

4. **Standard bilirubin, 0.1 mg/ml:** 5 mg of bilirubin is dissolved in 50 ml of chloroform stored in a brown bottle. Keep it in a dark place.

Procedure

Dilute 1 ml of serum to 20 ml with water in a conical flask and mix.

Total Bilirubin

Label two tubes as Test (Tt) and Blank (Tb). Into Tb, pipette 5 ml of methanol, 1 ml of 1.5 percent HCl and 4 ml of diluted serum (1 in 20).

　　Into Tt, pipette 5 ml of methanol, 1 ml of diazo reagent and 4 ml of diluted serum. Mix both the tubes. Stand at room temperature for 30 min. After 30 min read the absorbance using green filter or at 540 nm.

Direct Bilirubin

Mark two test tubes as Test (Dt) and Blank (Db). Into Db, pipette 5 ml of water, 1 ml of 1.5 percent HCl and 4 ml of diluted serum. Into Dt, pipette 5 ml of water, 1 ml of diazo reagent and 4 ml of diluted serum. Mix both the tubes. Let stand at room temperature for 30 min.

Standard

Label two test tubes as Standard (S) and Blank (Sb). Into S, pipette 8.8 ml of methanol, 1 ml of diazo reagent and 0.2 ml of standard. Into Sb, pipette 8.8 ml of methanol, 1 ml of 1.5% HCl and 0.2 ml serum. Mix and keep at room temperature for 30 min. Read absorbance at 540 nm or using green filter.

Reagents	Tt	Tb	Dt	Db	S	Sb
Methanol (mL)	5	5	—	—	8.8	8.8
Water (mL)	—	—	5	5	—	—
Diazo reagent	1 mL	—	1	—	1	—
1.5% HCl (mL)	—	1	—	1	—	—
Diluted serum	4	4	4	4	—	—
Standard bilirubin (mL)	—	—	—	—	0.2	0.2
Mixed and kept for 20–30 minutes.						
Read the OD at 540 nm (Green).						

Calculation

$$\frac{\text{OD of T} - \text{OD of B}}{\text{OD of S} - \text{OD of Sb}} \times 0.02 \times \frac{20}{4} \times 100$$

100 mL serum contains

$$= \frac{\text{OD of Tt} - \text{OD of Tb}}{\text{OD of S} - \text{OD of Sb}} \times 0.02 \times \frac{100}{0.2}$$

$$= \frac{\text{OD of Dt} - \text{OD of Db}}{\text{OD of S} - \text{OD of Sb}} \times 10$$

Note: Bilirubin deteriorates in light. If the assay is delayed, store the serum in the dark and in refrigerator.

BLOOD UREA DETERMINATION BY DIACETYL MONOXIME (DAM) METHOD

- The urea test is somewhat a routine test used primarily to evaluate renal (kidney) function.
- The test is often performed on patients with many different diseases.
- Urea is formed in the liver as the end product of protein metabolism.
- During digestion, protein is broken down into amino acids.
- Amino acids contain nitrogen, which is removed as NH^{4+} (ammonium ion), while the rest of the molecule is used to produce energy or other substances needed by the cell.
- The ammonia is combined with other intermediates to produce urea.
- The urea makes its way into the blood and it is ultimately eliminated in the urine by the kidneys.
- Most renal diseases affect urea excretion so that urea levels increase in the blood.
- Patients with dehydration or bleeding into the stomach and/or intestines may also have abnormal urea levels.
- Numerous drugs also affect urea by competing with it for elimination by the kidneys.

Principle

Urea reacts with diacetyl monoxime under strongly acidic conditions in presence of ferric ions and thiosemicarbazide to give a pink colored complex.

$$\text{Diacetyl monoxime} + H_2O \xrightarrow{\;H^+\;} \text{Diacetyl} + \text{Hydroxylamine}$$

$$\text{Diacetyl} + \text{Urea} \xrightarrow{\;H^+\;} \text{Diazoderivative, read at 540 nm}$$

Specimen: Serum or plasma can be used.

Reagents

1. **Diacetyl monoxime:** Dissolve 1.56 gm diacetyl monoxime in 250 ml water.
2. **Ferric chloride:** Dissolve 324 mg of ferric chloride in 10 ml of 56 percent orthophosphoric acid. Store in a brown bottle.

3. **Thiosemicarbazide:** Dissolve 41 mg of thiosemicarbazide in 50 ml of water.
4. **Sulfuric acid 20%:** Add 200 ml of concentrated sulfuric acid to 800 ml of water in a beaker slowly with stirring and cooling.
5. **Acid reagent:** Mix 1 liter of 20% sulfuric acid (Reagent 4) with 1 ml of ferric chloride reagent (Reagent 2).
6. **Trichloroacetic acid, 10%:** Dissolve 10 g of TCA in water and make up to 100 ml.
7. **Preservative diluent for standard:** Boil 250 ml water and add 40 mg of phenyl mercuric acetate, mix to dissolve. Transfer to 1 liter graduated cylinder. Add 0.3 ml concentrated sulfuric acid and make up the volume to 1 liter and mix. The use of preservative diluent is optional.
8. **Stock standard urea:** 0.5 mg per ml. Dissolve 50 mg of urea (GR Grade) in 100 ml of preservative diluent (Reagent 7) or can be dissolved in deionized water and it is stable for a week, if it is refrigerated.
9. **Standard urea for use:** 0.01 mg per ml. Dilute 1 ml of stock standard (Reagent 8) solution to 50 ml with deionized water.

Procedure

Reagents	Blank	Standard	Test
Water	—	—	3.4 mL
Serum	—	—	0.1 mL
TCA, 10%	—	—	1.5 mL
Mix. Wait for 10 minutes and centrifuge.			
Supernatant	—	—	1.0 mL
Water (mL)	1.0	—	—
Standard urea for use	—	1.0 mL	—
Diacetyl monoxime	1.0 mL	1.0 mL	1.0 mL
Thiosemicarbazide	1.0 mL	1.0 mL	1.0 mL
Acid reagent	3.0 mL	3.0 mL	3.0 mL
Place in a boiling water bath exactly for 15 minutes and cool.			
Read the absorbance at 540 nm or blue filter.			

Calculation

$$\text{mg urea in 100 ml of blood} = \frac{T-B}{S-B} \times \frac{5}{1} \times 0.01 \times \frac{100}{0.1}$$

$$= \frac{\text{OD of T} - \text{OD of B}}{\text{OD of S} - \text{OD of B}} \times 50$$

Clinical Significance

Normal values

Serum/plasma urea: 8.0 – 40 mg/dL, 2.49 – 7.47 mmol/L, BUN: 7 – 21 mg/dL

Greater than normal levels may indicate:

a. *Prerenal causes*:
  - Congestive heart failure
  - Myocardial infarction
  - Hypovolemia due to burns, shock or dehydration
  - Excessive protein catabolism
  - Gastrointestinal bleeding

b. *Renal causes*:
  - Acute glomerulonephritis
  - Chronic nephritis
  - Pyelonephritis
  - Nephrotic syndrome
  - Acute tubular necrosis

c. *Postrenal causes*:
  - Urinary tract obstruction to urine flow (Stone, tumor, enlarged prostate)

ESTIMATION OF PLASMA PROTEINS

Determination of serum protein, albumin, globulin and their ratio by Biuret method:

Principle

Proteins react with the Biuret reagent to form a violet colored complex, which has a maximum absorbance at 540–560 nm. Biuret reagent consists of cupric ions (Cu^{2+}) which react with the N atoms of the peptide bonds of peptides and proteins, in an alkaline medium (presence of peptide bonds is the minimum requirement). The density of the purple color is directly proportional to the concentration of protein.

Biuret reagent consists of copper sulfate, sodium hydroxide, sodium potassium tartrate and potassium iodide.

- The NaOH provides alkalinity to the solution.
- Sodium potassium tartarate keeps the Cu^{2+} ions in solution.
- The conversion of Cu^{2+} to Cu^+ ions is prevented by potassium iodide.

Reagents

1. **Sodium chloride:** 0.9 percent. Dissolve 900 mg of sodium chloride in 80 ml of water and make up to 100 ml.
2. **0.2 N sodium hydroxide:** Dissolve 8 gm of sodium hydroxide in about 400 ml of water in a one liter flask. Make up to one liter.

3. **Biuret reagent:** Dissolve 45 gm of sodium potassium tartarate in 400 ml of 0.2 N sodium hydroxide (Reagent 2). Add 15 gm of copper sulfate by stirring continuously. Add 5 gm of potassium iodide. Dissolve and make up to one litre with 0.2 N sodium hydroxide. This is the stock Biuret reagent. Store in a polythene bottle. It is stable for months.

4. 0.2 N sodium hydroxide containing 5 g of potassium iodide per liter. Add 5 gm of potassium iodide per liter to Reagent 2 and dissolve.

5. **Biuret reagent for use:** Dilute 50 ml of stock Biuret reagent (Reagent 3) to 250 ml with 0.2 N sodium hydroxide containing 5 gm potassium iodide per liter (Reagent 4).

6. Standard protein solution 6 mg/ml:

   Dissolve 714.3 mg of bovine albumin and 100 mg of sodium azide used as preservatives in 100 ml water. Store at 4°C.

7. **Sodium sulfite:** 28 percent. Dissolve 28 gm of anhydrous sodium sulfite in about 70 ml of water. Make up to 100 ml.

8. Ether, AR grade.

Procedure

Reagents	B	S	A	Tp
Sodium sulfite, 28%	—	—	5.8 mL	
Serum	—	—	0.2 mL	
Ether	—	—	2.0 mL	
Mix gently, centrifuge for 5 minutes. Aspirate and discard the ether layer. Pipette the lower layer for albumin estimation.				
Supernatant	—	—	3.0 mL	—
Sodium chloride, 0.9%	3.0 mL	2.0 mL	—	2.9 mL
Serum (mL)	—	—	—	0.1
Standard protein solution	—	1.0 mL	—	—
Biuret reagent for use (mL)	3.0	3.0	3.0	3.0
Mix and stand for 10 minutes. Read OD at 540 nm or green filter.				

Calculation

$$G \text{ of total protein}/100 \text{ mL} = \frac{T-B}{S-B} \times \frac{100}{serum} \times \text{Concentration of standard}$$

$$G \text{ of Tp}/100 \text{ mL taken} = \frac{T-B}{S-B} \times \frac{100}{0.1} \times 6 \times \frac{1}{1000}$$

$$G \text{ of albumin}/100 \text{ mL} = \frac{T-B}{S-B} \times \frac{\text{Total solution}}{\text{Taken solution}} \times \text{Concentration} \times \frac{100}{\text{Serum taken}}$$

$$= \frac{T-B}{S-B} \times \frac{6}{3} \times 6 \times \frac{100}{0.2} \times \frac{1}{1000}$$

Globulins = Total proteins – Albumin

A: G ratio is obtained by dividing albumin by globulin level.

For example, say, Albumin = 4 gm% , Globulin = 2 gm%   Then, A:G Ratio = 4/2 = 2:1

Note: When calculating for A: G ratio, globulin is always considered as one.

Clinical Significance

The change in the plasma protein value takes place either due to change in albumin or globulin fraction. A reduced plasma protein level is mainly due to a decrease in albumin levels. Whereas, increased total protein is usually due to an increase in the globulin levels.

The conditions in which albumin is reduced are:

1. Nephrotic syndrome (more protein is excreted in urine)
2. Burns (dehydration)
3. Severe blood loss
4. Reduced synthesis of proteins in liver diseases like cirrhosis of liver, hepatitis.
5. Impaired digestion and absorption of proteins as in peptic ulcer, carcinoma of stomach, cancer of pancreas and intestinal diseases, etc.
6. Increased breakdown of proteins as seen in fever, acute infections, untreated diabetes mellitus and hyperthyroidism.
7. Due to protein malnutrition (Insufficient dietary protein intake)
8. In liver diseases like cirrhosis, albumin is decreased and globulin is increased.
9. Increased globulin levels are seen in few conditions like multiple myeloma, infections.

PREPARATION OF HEMIN CRYSTALS

Test	Observation	Inference
Spread a drop of blood on a slide in the form of a thin film. Dry it over a low flame. Add 2 drops of Nippe's fluid. Place a cover glass in position. Heat gently over a low flame until gas bubbles formed and the solution boiled. Run one or two drops of Nippe's fluid underneath the cover glass. Cool and examine under the microscope.	brown crystals	On heating with acid, hemoglobin is denatured and heme is oxidized to hematin.

DISCUSSION OF CLINICAL CHARTS—GLUCOSE TOLERANCE TEST (GTT)

Glucose Tolerance Tests (GTT)

- A normal person should be able to reduce a glucose load from his blood within a specified time. This is known as normal tolerance.
- If the person has an elevated blood glucose concentration for longer than the normal time, the condition is called as reduced tolerance.
- If the glucose concentration becomes very low or normal very early than the normal time then the condition is called as increased tolerance.
- The tests that are used to measure these changes in blood glucose after a glucose load are called glucose tolerance tests.

There are 2 types of GTT: (i) oral GTT, (ii) intravenous GTT. They are mainly used in the detection of diabetes. Oral GTT is more commonly used in all the laboratories. It is convenient to give glucose through oral route.

Conditions where GTT performed are:
1. When someone having family history of diabetes mellitus.
2. Signs and symptoms comparable with diabetics without any complications.
3. Glucosuric patients with normal fasting blood sugar.
4. Border line postprandial blood sugar.
5. Reactive hypoglycemia for 3 hours or longer period after food intake.
6. Pregnancy with history of abortions, stillbirths or a large baby.

Method

The test is usually carried out in the early morning after fasting overnight.

Fasting blood sample and urine is then collected. 75 gm (or 100 gm) of glucose dissolved in about 150–200 ml of water is given to drink.

Venous blood for the estimation of blood glucose is collected at ½ hour intervals for 2 – 2½ hours or hourly intervals for 3 hours after the ingestion of glucose. Urine specimens are also collected at the same time.

Blood glucose is estimated in each sample and the urine is tested for the presence of the sugar.

Interpretation

Normal Glucose Tolerance Curve

The normal curve has the following features.
1. The fasting blood glucose in this category is usually within the range of 60–100 mg/dl.
2. The blood glucose does not rise above 160 mg/dl.
3. The blood glucose at 2 hours after the load is 110 mg/dl.
4. The urine remains free of glucose throughout the test.
5. The timing of the peak value is not defined as a part of the normal pattern of response, but it is usually seen either in 30 minutes or 60 minutes blood sample.

Sample no.	mg glucose/100 ml blood	Urine glucose
Fasting	90	Negative
30 minutes	120	Negative
60 minutes	150	Negative
90 minutes	140	Negative
120 minutes	90	Negative

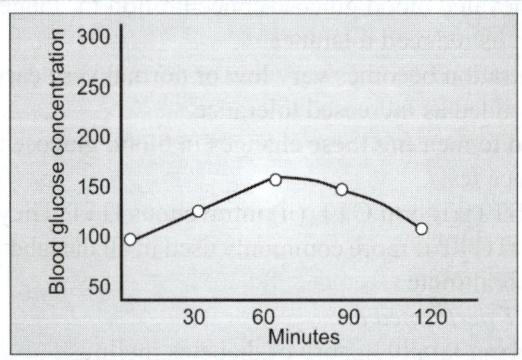

Abnormal Glucose Tolerance Response

Reduced glucose tolerance:

The main features are:

1. The fasting level is above 120 mg.
2. The glucose level crosses 200 mg/100 ml in 30 to 60 minutes.
3. The blood glucose level is more than 110 mg/dl even after 2 hours.
4. There may be glucose in at least two of the urine specimens.

Sample no.	mg glucose/100 ml blood	Urine glucose
Fasting	120	Negative
30 minutes	160	Positive
60 minutes	200	Positive
90 minutes	180	Positive
120 minutes	150	Negative

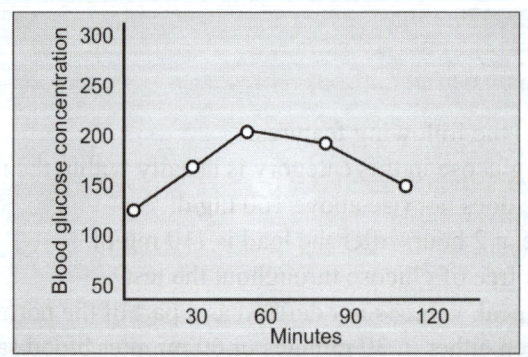

SPOTTERS

Instruments

1. Colorimeter
   - It is an optical device used to measure the optical density of the colored solution.
   - This is used to estimate the concentration of biochemical substances like glucose and urea in biological fluids.
   - Based on the principle of Beer-Lambert law.
2. pH meter
   - To determine the pH of the solution.
   - For potential measurement of electrodes.
3. Centrifuge
   - It is an instrument used to separate the plasma or serum from blood before estimating certain parameters in blood.
   - It is used to separate proteins from a solution, a process called deproteinization.
4. Ryle's tube
   - It is a thin, long rubber tube used to aspirate the gastric contents.
   - Tube has lead beads at the end, which is used to detect the position of tube in gastric antrum by X-ray.
5. Spectroscope
   - This is a simple device that resolves white light into seven component colors.
   - This is used to find out various derivatives of hemoglobin, which have specific absorption spectra in the visible range.
6. Urinometer
   - This is a device used to measure the specific gravity of urine.
   - This is calibrated at 15°C to read the specific gravity in the range of 1.000–1.060.
   - Consists of a heavy bulb with a calibrated tube.
   - The specific gravity of urine, thus measured, is an indication of the solute content of the urine.
7. Esbach's albuminometer
   - This apparatus is used to estimate the concentration of proteins in 24 hours urine sample.
8. Folin-Wu tube
   - This is used in the estimation of blood glucose by Folin-Wu method.
   - Reaction happens in the bulb of the tube and function of the neck of the Folin-Wu tube to reduce the re-oxidation of cuprous oxide by atmospheric oxygen.
9. Flame photometer
   - This instrument is used in quantitative estimation of sodium, potassium, calcium, lithium and magnesium in biological fluids.
   - It consitsts of nebulizer, burner, monochrometer, detector and read out device.
10. Electrophoresis unit
    - This device is used to carry out electrophoresis of proteins, lipoproteins, hemoglobin, isoenzymes, and DNA in biological fluids.
    - It consists of electrophoresis chamber and power pack.

Indicators

Phenolphthalein—used to estimate the total acidity of gastric juice specific urease test to detect urea in urine.

Chlorophenol red—used to adjust the isoelectric pH 5.4 for albumin.

Powders

Ammonium sulfate—used in Rothera's test for acetone and acetoacetic acid. Fractional precipitation of proteins (Half and full saturation tests)

Sodium carbonate—used Benedict's uric acid reagent for uric acid detection. Benedict's qualitative reagent for detection of reducing sugars.

Sulfur powder—used in Hay's sulfur powder test for detection of bile salts.

Reagents and their uses:

Ninhydrin—used in color reactions of proteins as a general test for amino acids and as a dye for amino acid chromatography.

40% NaOH—used in biuret test and xanthoproteic tests.

10% NaOH—used in biuret test and Jaffe's test.

Sulfosalicylic acid—used to identify proteins in urine.

Nitric acid—used in Heller's nitric acid ring test for proteins in urine and in xanthoprotic test.

Sulfuric acid—used in Molisch's test for carbohydrates and Hopkins Cole Aldehyde test for detection of tryptophan in color reactions of proteins.

Copper sulfate—solution used in estimation of blood sugar by Folin-Wu method, Biuret and Benedict's qualitative tests.

Picric acid—used in Jaffe's test for creatinine estimation and in Esbach's reagent for estimation of albumin in 24 hours urine.

Slides

Glucosazone/Fructosazone—broom stick shaped yellow colored crystals.

Lactosazone—ball badminton or powder puff or hedgehog shaped yellow colored crystals

Maltosazone—sunflower-shaped yellow colored crystals.

Reagents, composition and uses:

Benedict's qualitative reagent—sodium carbonate, sodium citrate and copper sulfate—used to identify reducing sugars in urine.

Barfoed's reagent—copper acetate and glacial acetic acid—used to differentiate between monosaccharides and reducing disaccharides.

Seliwanoff's reagent—resorcinol in HCl—used to identify keto sugars.

Fouchet's reagent—10% ferric chloride and TCA.

Biuret reagent—copper sulfate, sodium potassium tartarate and NaOH.

CASE REPORTS

Case 1. *Oral Glucose tolerance test was performed with a 48-year-old person and the results are given below. What is your interpretation?*

Time	Blood glucose (mg%)	Urine sugar
0 (Fasting sample)	60	Blue
0.5	90	Blue
1.0	130	Blue
1.5	90	Blue
2.0	60	Blue

Case 2. *Following are the values of oral glucose tolerance test performed on an individual. Indicate the probable diagnosis.*

Time (Hours)	Blood glucose (mg%)	Urine sugar
0 (Fasting)	60	Blue
0.5	110	Blue
1.0	150	Blue
1.5	120	Blue
2.0	110	Blue

Case 3. *The Oral glucose tolerance test of a pregnant lady showed the following values. What is your interpretation?*

Time (Hours)	Blood glucose (mg%)	Urine sugar
0 (Fasting)	120	Blue
0.5	190	Green
1.0	230	Yellow
1.5	210	Yellow
2.0	180	Green

Case 4. *The following are the biochemical results of a 45-year-old person visited to nephrology clinic. What is your probable diagnosis?*

Blood fasting Glucose	180 mg%
Urine sugar	Positive
Serum creatinine	3.0 mg%
Blood urea	80 mg %

Case 5. *Depending on the following laboratory findings of gastric juice analysis, give your interpretation.*

Free acidity	10 mEq/l
Total acidity	50 mEq/l
Benzidine test	positive
Lactic acid test	positive

Case 6. *The 40-year-old person voluntarily came to the laboratory and was requested the laboratory technician to do his LFT. Give your probable diagnosis depending on the following laboratory findings.*

Serum bilirubin	1.0 mg%
Direct bilirubin	0.2 mg%
Indirect bilirubin	0.8 mg%
AST	18 units/L
ALT	10 units/L
Alkaline phosphatase	25 KA units
Urine bile pigments	Negative
Urine bile salts	Negative
Urobilinogen	Trace
Faeces	Normal color

Case 7. *The sample received from a nephrology ward showed the following biochemical findings. What is your interpretation?*

Blood urea	30 mg%
Serum creatinine	2.0 mg%
Serum cholesterol	560 mg%
Total serum protein	4.0 mg%
Albumin	1.0 gm%
Globulin	3.0 gm%
Urinary protein	10 gm/l

Case 8. *The 50-year-old person was brought to the hospital with a complaint of swelling in the face and abdominal pain. Depending on the following biochemical findings, give your probable diagnosis.*

Blood urea	120 mg%
Serum creatinine	6.0 mg%
Serum uric acid	9.0 mg%
Serum inorganic phosphorous	6.0 mg%

Case 9. *The 30-year-old patient was brought to a hospital with a complaint of weekness, swelling in the face and abdominal pain. His blood and urine samples were sent to the laboratory. The following are the laboratory findings. What is your probable diagnosis?*

Blood urea	90 mg%
Serum creatinine	4.2 mg%
Serum cholesterol	560 mg%
Total plasma protein	4.0 mg%
Albumin	1.2 gm%
Globulin	3.0 gm%
Urinary protein	6 gm/l

Case 10. *The 36-year-old man consulted the physician seeking a treatment for his illness. The physician after through checkup ordered a LET. Give your probable diagnosis depending on the following laboratory findings.*

Serum bilirubin	4.0 mg%
Direct bilirubin	2.2 mg%
Indirect bilirubin	1.8 mg/L%
AST	78 units
ALT	99 units
Alkaline phosphatase	25 KA units
GGT	105 units

Case 11. *The patient visited doctor with a complaint of yellowish skin and sclera of the eye. The doctor suggested him to have blood and urine test in the Biochemistry laboratory. The following are the biochemical findings. What is your probable diagnosis?*

Serum bilirubin	12 mg%
Direct bilirubin	0.4 mg%
Indirect bilirubin	11.6 mg%
AST	18 units
ALT	9 units
Alkaline phosphatase	7 KA units
Urine bile pigments	Negative
Urine bile salts	Negative
Urobilinogen	+++
Feces—Stercobilinogen	+++

Case 12. *The following are the biochemical findings of a patient. What is your interpretation?*

Serum bilirubin	12 mg%
Direct bilirubin	7.0 mg%
Indirect bilirubin	5.0 mg%
AST	280 units/L
ALT	300 units/L
Alkaline phosphatase	25 KA units
Urine bile pigments	++
Bile salts	+
Urobilinogen	+

Case 13. *The following are the biochemical findings of a 20-year-old boy admitted to the hospital. What is your interpretation?*

Serum bilirubin	12 mg%
Direct bilirubin	11.6 mg%
Indirect bilirubin	0.4 mg%
AST	60 units/L
ALT	70 units/L

(contd.)

Alkaline phosphatase	30 KA units
Urine bile pigments	++
Urine bile salts	++
Urobilinogen	Negative
Feces-Stercobilinogen	Negative

Case 14. *The patient's blood after acid-base analysis showed the following results. With the following results, name the acid-base status of the person.*

Blood pH	7.4
pCO_2	40 mm Hg
Plasma HCO_3^-	27 mEq/l
H_2CO_3	1.35 mEq/l

Case 15. *Name the acid-base status of the patient with the following data.*

Blood pH	7.1
pCO_2	40 mm Hg
Plasma HCO_3^-	17 mEq/l
H_2CO_3	1.30 mEq/l

Case 16. *From the following data name the acid base status of the patient.*

Blood pH	7.55
pCO_2	40 mm Hg
Plasma HCO_3^-	37 mEq/l
H_2CO_3	1.32 mEq/l

Case 17. *Name the acid-base status of a patient with the following data.*

Blood pH	7.1
pCO_2	70 mm Hg
Plasma HCO_3^-	27 mEq/l
H_2CO_3	2.6 mEq/l

Case 18. *From the following data obtained after the blood gas analysis of the patient sample, name the acid base status of the patient.*

Blood pH	7.55
pCO_2	20 mm Hg
Plasma HCO_3^-	27 mEq/l
H_2CO_3	0.7 mEq/l

Case 19. *A child was brought to a doctor with a complaint of poor growth and milestones of the child were delayed. On examination the child was found to have cataract in the eye and hepatomegaly (enlargement of liver) urine examination showed reduction with Benedict's reagent but not with glucose oxidase method. What is the probable diagnosis and give reasons.*

Case 20. *A child was brought to the hospital with a complaint of swelling in the abdomen and history of reeling sensation. On examination liver was found to be enlarged. The biochemistry results showed the increased serum uric acid and free fatty acid and associated with hypoglycemia. There was no increase in blood glucose even after intravenous administration of glucagon. What is your probable diagnosis?*

Case 21. *Following are the laboratory findings of a person aged 50. What is your interpretation?*

FBS	200 mg%
Glycated hemoglobin	14% glycosylated Hb
Benedict's test with urine	Yellow

Case 22. *Following are the laboratory findings of a patient admitted in the nephrology ward. What is your probable diagnosis?*

Blood urea	150 mg%
Serum creatinine	7.0 mg%
Seum calcium	5.0 mg%
Serum inorganic phosphorous	6.0 mg%
Seum sodium	120 mEq/l
Albumin	2.0 gm%

Case 23. *The sugar factory workers went on hunger strike. One of the employees was brought to the hospital in an unconscious state. Immediately his blood was sent to the laboratory. From the following laboratory findings, what is your probable diagnosis?*

Blood sugar	40 mg%
Blood pH	7.20
Serum bicarbonate	14 mEq/l
Rothera's test with urine for ketone bodies → Positive	

Case 24. *The patient was brought to the hospital in the coma condition. Following are the laboratory findings of the patient. What is your probable interpretation?*

Blood sugar	280 mg%
Benedict's test with urine	Red
Blood pH	7.20
Serum bicarbonate	14 mEq/l
Rothera's test with urine for ketone bodies → Positive	

Case 25. *A fair chubby boy was brought to the hospital with a complaint of mental retardation. The following are laboratory findings of the boy. What is your probable diagnosis?*

Serum phenylalanine	Very high
Dinitrophenylhydrazine test with urine for phenylacetate, phenyllactae and phenylpyruvate	Positive

Case 26. *A mother sought medical help for her child with a complaint that the diapers used for the child stained black. Blackening of urine was observed on exposure. The doctor immediately asked the child's mother to give the urine and blood samples for the laboratory test. Following are the laboratory findings. What is your diagnosis?*

Benedict's test with urine	Positive
Glucose oxidase test	Negative
Ferric chloride test	Positive

Case 27. *The following are the biochemical findings of a 8-year-old child. What is your probable diagnosis?*

Blood urea	16 mg%
Serum creatinine	1.4 mg%
Serum calcium	7.5 mg%
Serum inorganic phosphorous	1.8 mg%
Serum alkaline phosphatase	670 U/L

Case 28. *A 40-year-old patient was brought to the hospital with a complaint of chest pain radiating to left arm. Following are the laboratory findings. What is your probable diagnosis?*

AST	80 U/L
CK	830 U/L
CKMB	900 U/L
LDH	800 U/L
LD_1	700 U/L

Case 29. *The following are the biochemical findings of a patient. What is your probable diagnosis?*

Urinary creatine	Very high
Serum creatine kinase	Elevated

Case 30. *The patient was brought to the hospital with a complaint of acute abdominal pain. His serum amylase, lipase and urinary amylase were increased. What is your probable diagnosis?*

Case 31. *The CSF analysis of a person showed the following laboratory findings. What is your opinion?*

Color	Clear, colorless
Cells	2×106 cells/L
Protein	30 mg%
Sugar	60 mg%

Case 32. *A child was admitted with a high fever and rigidity of neck. On examination of CSF, showed the following results. Give your opinion.*

Color	Turbid
Cells	800×106 cells/L
Protein	30 mg%
Sugar	25 mg%

Case 33. *A 40-year-old lady visits the doctor with a complaint of sleepiness, constipation and sensitivity to cold. The doctor noticed a slow heart rate and advised her to have a blood test. Following are the biochemical findings. What is your probable interpretation?*

TSH	10 mIU/L
T3	0.2 ng/ml
T4	2.0 microgram/ml

Case 34. *A 40-year-old lady visits the doctor with a complaint of sleeplessness, weight loss, weakness and excessive sweating. The doctor noticed a rapid heart rate and nervousness and advised her to have a blood test. Following are the biochemical findings. What is your probable interpretation?*

TSH	0.1 mIU/L
T3	7.0 ng/ml
T4	20 microgram/ml

Case 35. *A 50-year-old woman was admitted to the hospital due to increased heart rate, severe weakness, weight loss and exophthalmos (abnormal protrusion of the eye). She was extremely irritable, could not tolerate heat and was short of breath. Physical examination revealed bilateral eyelid lag. The plasma levels of T3 and T4 showed high value. What is your probable diagnosis?*

Case 36. *A 30-year-old man was brought to the hospital with multiple symptoms of hypoglycemia, sensitivity to insulin, severe weakness, intolerance to stress and weight loss. The serum and urinary cortisol was also found to be very low. What is your diagnosis?*

Case 37. *A 30-year-old man was brought to the hospital with the symptoms of hyperglycemia, muscle wasting, peculiar redistribution fat, obesity and typical buffalo hump. The serum and urinary cortisol were also found to be very high. What is your diagnosis?*

Case 38. *A 50-year-old chronic smoker visits to the cardiologist with a complaint of indigestion after a meal. He was admitted and ECG was done and it showed an abnormal pattern. The laboratory findings are as shown below. What is your probable interpretation?*

ALT	25 U/L
AST	70 U/L
LDH	600 U/L
LD_1	400 U/L

Case 39. *A 25-year-old man was admitted to the hospital with the symptoms of headache, pain in the flanks, anorexia (loss of appetite). He passed red colored urine and had edema around his eyes. Results of laboratory test are as follows:*
What is your probable diagnosis?

Laboratory test	Result
Blood pressure	160/110 mm Hg
Serum electrolytes	
Sodium	160 mmol/l
Potassium	5.5 mmol/l
Calcium	7.0 mg/dl
Phosphate	5.6 mg/dl
Total protein	7.0 gm/dl
Albumin	4.5 gm/dl
Globulins	2.5 gm/dl
BUN	45 mg/dl
Creatinine	3.0 mg/dl
Hb	9 gm/dl
Urine specific gravity	1.010
Creatinine clearance	50 ml/min

Clinically, this is characterized by a generalized edema, mild hypertension with headache, pain in the flanks and oliguria. Edema, noticeable around eyes is because of diminished glomerular filtration. Tubular function is abnormal, resulting in retention of water and electrolytes.

Case 40. *A 30-year-old man was admitted to the hospital. His blood sample was sent to the laboratory. Following are the laboratory findings. What is your probable diagnosis?*

Total serum protein	10 gm%
Albumin	3.5 gm%
Globulin	6.5 gm%
Electrophoresis showed	"M" band
Bence-Jones protein in urine	Positive

Case 41. *A 40-year-old man was admitted to the hospital with a complaint of abdominal pain. His blood investigation showed following results. What is your interpretation?*

Total serum protein	6.5 gm%
Albumin	2.5 gm%
Globulin	4.0 gm%
ALT	60 units/l
Serum electrophoresis	β-γ bridge

Answers

1. It is a normal response
2. Mild diabetes mellitus
3. Diabetes mellitus
4. Diabetic nephropathy
5. Gastric carcinoma
6. Normal liver function
7. Nephrotic syndrome
8. Chronic renal failure
9. Nephrotic syndrome leading to renal failure
10. Liver cirrhosis
11. Hemolytic jaundice
12. Hepatic jaundice
13. Obstructive jaundice
14. Normal acid-base status
15. Metabolic acidosis
16. Metabolic alkalosis
17. Respiratory acidosis
18. Respiratory alkalosis
19. Galactosemia

    Reason: The galactose converted to galactose-1-phosphate that is then converted to uridinediphosphate glucose with the help of an enzyme galactose-1-phosphate uridyltransferase. Because of the deficiency of this galactose accumulates; galactose, which is reduced to galacitol, may accumulate and leads to cataract.

20. von Gierke's disease
21. Uncontrolled diabetes
22. Chronic renal failure
23. Starvation leading to ketoacidosis
24. Diabetic ketoacidosis
25. Phenylketonuria
26. Alkaptonuria

    The homogentisate oxidase deficiency leads to the accumulation of the metabolite homogentisic acid (reducing substance).

27. Rickets
28. Myocardial infarction
29. Muscular disease
30. Acute pancreatitis

31. Normal CSF analysis
32. Meningitis
33. Primary hypothyroidism
34. Hyperthyroidism
35. Hyperthyroidism
36. Addison's disease
37. Cushing's syndrome
38. An episode of ischemia

    Ischemia is the situation, in which an organ has an inadequate blood supply to maintain its essential function. Patients with an inadequate blood supply to heart often complain of a constricting central chest pressure or pain (angina), which comes on with exertion and is relieved by rest.

39. Glomerulonephritis
40. Multiple myeloma
41. Liver cirrhosis

LABORATORY VALUES

Blood

Tests	Normal values	To diagnose
Fasting glucose	60–110 mg/dl	Diabetes
Postprandial glucose	90–140 mg/dl	Diabetes
Random glucose	90–150 mg/dl	Diabetes
Urea (UN)	8–40 mg/dl	Prerenal and Renal disorder
BUN	7–25 mg/dl	Prerenal and Renal disorder
Creatinine	0.6–1.4 mg/dl	Renal disease and Muscle degeneration
Sodium	130–143 mEq/L	Renal and cardiac disorders
Potassium	3.5–5.0 mEq/L	Renal and cardiac disorders
Chloride	93–110 mEq/L	Renal disorders
Total CO_2	22–26 mEq/L	Renal and acid-base disorders
Anion gap	10–20	Acid-base disorders
Osmolality	270–285 mosm/kg	Renal disorders
Uric acid	3–7 mg/dl	Renal disorder and Gout
Calcium	8.5–10.6 mg/dl	Renal and bone disorder
	4.5–5.4 mEq/dl	
Phosphate	2.5–4.5 mg/dl	Renal disorder
Cholesterol	170–220 mg/dl	Atherosclerosis, diabetes, and hypothyroidism
Triglycerides	40–160 mg/dl	Atherosclerosis, hypothyroidism, liver disease, pancreatitis, myocardial infarction and metabolic disorders
HDL-cholesterol	45–70 mg/dl	High value indicates healthy metabolic system. Low in liver disease
LDL-cholesterol	60–140 mg/dl	atherosclerosis
Total bilirubin	0.2–1.2 mg/dl	Jaundice and Liver disease
Direct bilirubin	0–0.2 mg/dl	Jaundice and Liver disease
Total protein	6.0–8.0 gm/dl	Liver disease, malabsorption Lupus, chronic infections, Alcoholism and leukemia
Albumin	3.5–5.0 gm/dl	Liver disorder, shock and multiple myeloma
Globulin	1.8–3.4 gm/dl	Liver disease and chronic infections, multiple myeloma, rheumatoid arthritis
A/G Ratio	0.8–2.0	Liver disease, chronic infections, and multiple myeloma
Zinc turbidity	2–8 units	Liver disorder
SGOT (AST)	5–40 U/L	Liver and cardiac disease

(contd.)

(*contd.*)

Tests	Normal values	To diagnose
SGPT (ALT)	5–40 U/L	Liver disease
Alk-phosphatase (ALP)	35–125 U/L	Obstructive jaundice and bone disorder
GGT	10–50 U/L	Liver disease, alcoholism, Obstructive jaundice
Amylase	80–240 units	Pancreatitis
Acid phosphatase	Upto 11 U/L	Ca prostate
LDH	0–250 U/L	MI and heart disease
LDH1	Up to 175 U/L	MI and heart disease
LDH1/LDH ratio	Less than 0.4	MI and heart disease
CK	10–80 U/L	MI and heart disease
T3	0.8–2.0 ng/ml	Thyroid disorder
T4	4.5–12.0 µg/dl	Thyroid disorder
TSH	0.3–5.0 µIU/ml	Thyroid disorder
Ferritin	27–300 ng/ml	Anemia
Cortisol		
Morning:	8–26, Cushing's and	
Evening:	5–18 µg/dl	Addison's disease
B-HCG	0–5 mU/ml	Choriocarcinoma
AFP	0–15 ng/ml	Ca Liver and neural tube defect
CEA	0–4 ng/ml	Colon cancer
CA-125	0–35 U/ml	Ovarian cancer
PSA	0–4 ng/ml	Ca prostate
FSH		
Men:	1–12 mIU/ml	
Women:		
Follicular :	3–20	
Mid-cycle:	9–26 Fertility workup	
Luteal:	1–12	
Menopausal:	18–153	
LH		
Men:	2.0 mIU/ml	
Women:		
Follicular:	2–15 Fertility workup	
Luteal:	0.6–19.0	
Menopausal:	16–64	

(*contd.*)

(*contd.*)

Tests	Normal values	To diagnose
Prolactin		
Women:		
Mid-cycle:	5.4–22.5 ng/ml	Fertility workup
Menopausal:	4.5–15 ng/ml	
Testosterone		
Men:	2.8–8.2 ng/ml	Fertility workup
Women:	0.1–4.0 ng/ml	
Progesterone	1–20 ng/ml	Fertility workup
Oestradiol		
Men:	2–50 ng/ml	
Women:		
Follicular:	23–145	
Mid-cycle:	112–443	Fertility workup
Luteal:	48–241	
Menopausal:	0–59	
IgG	1200–1480 mg/dl	Immune disorder
IgA	200–280 mg/dl	Immune disorder
IgM	110–136 mg/dl	Immune disorder
C3	90–150 mg/dl	Immune disorder
C4	15–50 mg/dl	Immune disorder
α-1 Antitrypsin	90–150 U/dl	Acute phase reactant
α-1 Antichymotrypsin	45–75 U/dl	Acute phase reactant
C-Reactive protein	Upto 6.0 mg/L	Immune disorder
Haptoglobin	70–240 mg/dl	Immune disorder
Glu-6-PO_4 dehydrogenase	8–18 U/gm	Immune disorder
Antinuclear antibodies (ANA)	< 20 –ve	Autoimmune disorder
	>160 +ve	
	120–160 borderline	
Anti-ds-DNA antibodies	<50 –ve	Autoimmune disorders
	>65 +ve	
	50–65 borderline	
Anticardiolipin antibodies (ACA)-antiphospholipid	< 10 –ve	Autoimmune disorders
	>15 +ve	
	10–15 borderline	

Urine

Calcium	50–300 mg/24 hr
Phosphorous	400–1300 mg/24 hr
Uric acid	200–500 mg/24 hr
Oxalate	17–53 mg/24 hr
Magnesium	60–120 mg/24 hr
Citrate	300–900 mg/24 hr
Cystine	Negative
Xanthine	Negative
Risk index	600–680
pH	4.5–7.8
Volume	600–2000 ml /24 hr
Urea	10–35 g/24 hr
Creatinine	800–1500 mg/24 hr
Creatinine clearance	60–120 ml/min
Protein	24–180 mg/24 hr
Ammonia	140–1500 mEq/24 hr
Sodium	40–220 mEq/24 hr
Potassium	35–90 mEq/24 hr
Chloride	60–125 mEq/24 hr
Osmolality	50–1400 mOsm/kg
Volume	1000–2000 ml/24 hr
Creatinine	800–1500 mg/24 hr
Estriol	4 mg/24 hr
17-Ketosteroids	
Morning:	8–20 mg/24 hr
Evening:	6–15 mg/24 hr
Catecholamines	Up to 150 μg/24 hr
VMA	2–8 mg/24 hr
HVA	3–28 mg/Creatinine
5-HIAA	1–10 mg/24 hr
Cortisol	Up to 150 μg/24 hr
CSF glucose	60 mg% Meningitis
CSF protein	5–40 mg%

Index